DYSLEXIA

A VISUAL APPROACH

NEURODEVELOPMENTAL DISEASES - LABORATORY AND CLINICAL RESEARCH

Additional books in this series can be found on Nova's website under the Series tab.

Additional e-books in this series can be found on Nova's website under the e-book tab.

NEUROLOGY - LABORATORY AND CLINICAL RESEARCH DEVELOPMENTS

Additional books in this series can be found on Nova's website under the Series tab.

Additional e-books in this series can be found on Nova's website under the e-book tab.

NEURODEVELOPMENTAL DISEASES - LABORATORY AND CLINICAL RESEARCH

DYSLEXIA

A VISUAL APPROACH

CARLO ALECI

NOVA BIOMEDICAL

New York

For permission to use material from this book please contact us:
Telephone 631-231-7269; Fax 631-231-8175
Web Site: http://www.novapublishers.com

Library of Congress Cataloging-in-Publication Data

ISBN: 978-1-62618-534-0

LCCN:2013937387

Published by Nova Science Publishers, Inc. † New York

"To my young pirate Mattia and my little princess Sofia"

Contents

Introduction

This book deals with a challenge.

A scientific challenge to a more and more widespread condition, with devastating effects. The enemy is called developmental dyslexia, the victims are children and teenagers who go to school, who would like to learn but have difficulty in reading. These children are far from lazy, stupid or anything but slow: indeed, the word dyslexia is not a euphemism for sloth, contrary to the opinion of a headmaster in the seventies.[1]

Victims are the parents, too, who happen on a carousel made of rebounds, examinations, interviews with teachers and alleged rehabilitative treatments. For them it is a growing frustration that does not seem to dissolve, an endless string of money, a huge loss of time. A dead end labyrinth.

So far, the paradox of seeing well but not being able to recognize the words has prevented the ophthalmologist from investigating on the crime scene, from facing up to a problem that a century ago was born as a visuperceptive condition and was indeed defined *word blindness*.

Yet, the *scenario* is changing and a novel awareness gives new opportunities and fresh air to the research on developmental dyslexia.

The interest towards the visual aspects is growing: in a month, the number of items found on *Google* by typing in the word *dyslexia* has risen by 1.1% while for *visual dyslexia* it has increased by almost double. Within three years (from July 2008 to July 2011) the rise is approximately linear for *dyslexia* while tends to be exponential for *visual dyslexia.*

We have then decided to report the state of the art on research on developmental dyslexia from the perspective of the visual perception. Common sense and experience confirm that dyslexia is also a visual problem. Not *only* a visual problem but *also* a visual problem. Those who have a *good sight* are not only able to make out two gulls that otherwise would simply be two points away, but even to exploit this capability to their own use. Today, more than yesterday, this need concerns even the lexical function: the ability to read. Aged people (not dyslexic) know how much disabling is to forget the reading glasses, since this simple oversight makes them unable to perform all the functions related to close vision: from reading a newspaper to signing a document.

The fact is that a pair of glasses is not enough to solve the problem of the dyslexics and yet, this does not prevent from thinking that subtle visuoperceptive alterations, not revealed

[1] Episode reported in: Critchley M, Critchley E: Dyslexia defined. Springfield. Il: Charles C. Thomas, 1978.

by a routine examination, can contribute in determining the lexical impairment. In the last 50 years the debate on the visual aspects of dyslexia has regained strength, leading to conflicting opinions in the academic world. The resulting *scenario* is one of the most exciting it can be imagined for the researcher: theories, views, feedbacks, personal experiences and counter evidence. A good starting point for a constructive debate, for a speculative turmoil that would have made happy the ancient Greek philosophers of the Academy, the Lyceum and the Stoà, but at the moment ineffective for the more practical visual rehabilitation. Especially in the neurophtalmological field, it is necessary to use these pieces of knowledge and take stock of the situation to assess what it is probably true and what it is definitely false. In a dialectical effort, these pages are addressed to health professionals who have to do with developmental dyslexia and need some clarification, but also teachers and parents determined to understand more despite the apparent complexity of the subject, as well as those who have the curiosity to learn more about the problem. The goal is to provide an overview on the state of the art of developmental dyslexia from the neuro-ophtalmological perspective, and to promote new investigations aimed at devising rehabilitation treatments based on the scientific method and not just on personal experience. If the reader is looking for definite answers, this is not the right book. If on the contrary, questions arise, our wish and our hope is that through these pages the reader can focus the subject and find out what are the actual acquisitions and which could be the next steps. Although the treatise is meant for a heterogeneous audience, we refused to sacrifice the scientific rigor in exchange for a simpler dissertation. Doubtless, due to the complexity and (in many respects) the contradictory of the argument, some of the concepts are difficult to understand. However, since in our intention this treatise can be read at a double level, those readers who are simply interested in the subject can pass over the more technical passages, while those who are dealing with the problem in a more professional manner can find strict arguments documented by a consistent bibliography.

In the second part, our speculative line is reported. It is based on a phenomenological approach rather than aetiological, therefore moving from the dyslexics' visuoperceptive symptomatology instead of the causal hypotheses and the anatomofunctional data. It is an attempt to present our investigations which have led us to develop a personal hypothesis.

The text is deliberately full of notes, in order to explain concepts that may be unclear to an interdisciplinary audience, to clarify some concepts or to add technical details. This way, it is possible to read on two different levels.

Importantly, in brackets are reported not only the bibliographic references relative to the concepts, as usual, but also the references which are the source, the basis of the personal considerations, in name of the scientific rigor. In this case, personal inferences do not necessarily reflect the concepts reported in the cited study they are derived from.

No doubt the references are far from exhaustive. Here are the most representative studies we have decided to mention. We apologize for the possible faults, but since research on dyslexia has taken a frenetic pace (especially in recent decades), it has been impossible to follow and to report every international publication.

It cannot be ruled out the occurrence of imprecisions and misinterpretations when reporting results from other researches, especially those not strictly related to the neuro-ophthalmological field: after all, this work aims at being a tribute to all researchers in a multidisciplinary context who have contributed with great effort to enrich the knowledge on developmental dyslexia. In case, the author apologizes and if signaled, correction will be done in the next edition. It can be noted a certain redundancy of some concepts. Indeed, the repetition of arguments previously discussed is a useful tool to allow a better comprehension.

Some explanation can seem naïve to an expert reader. He should bear in mind, however, that the book is addressed to a multidisciplinary public.

The reader will judge whether the objectives have been reached.

In the meantime, more than ever, the case is to wish good reading.

Author's Note

Developmental dyslexia is defined in many ways but as “pathological condition” or “illness”. Nevertheless, since it is characterized by a definition, classification, epidemiological description, aetiopathogenetic mechanisms (although not yet completely understood), clinical signs and symptoms, diagnostic criteria and therapeutic proposals (including the pharmacological ones), nothing prevents a doctor from considering it as a real disease. Dyslexia is a disability that hinders academic activities (including the most common ones) and can cause a dramatic drop in the quality of life, leading to psychological suffering that may result in social maladjustment and organic diseases.

Part One.
To See Is not Enough for Reading: State of the Art

Chapter I

A Worldwide Problem

Developmental dyslexia is a pathological condition characterized by a reading delay of at least 2.5 years below that expected for the age, in the presence of normal intellectual quotient, ability in other academic tasks equal to that of normal readers and adequate visual acuity, with no auditory impairment and no gross behavioral problems [Stanley & Hall, 1973]. It is a chronic condition and not a temporary delay in reading skills development. [Scarborough, 1984; Felton et al., 1990; Bruck, 1992; Francis et al., 1996; Shaywitz et al., 1999].

Developmental dyslexia must be distinguished from other forms of lexical disability due to mental retardation, lack of schooling or to pathological conditions such as *hemianopia* (the abolition of vision in half the visual field of both eyes for lesions of the visual pathways or of the cerebral cortex), responsible for that particular clinical entity called h*emianopic dyslexia*.

Developmental dyslexia is the most common lexical form of disability, up to 80% of the total [Lerner, 1989]. It is a worldwide problem, present in countries with languages and graphic systems very different from each other.

Hinshelwood at the beginning of the last century estimated a prevalence of dyslexia in primary school of 1 over 1000 [Hinshelwood, 1917], but according to a less restrictive criterion the figure would rise up to 10% [Orton, 1925].

In more recent times, in the United States the incidence of dyslexia in the school age population ranges from 3 to 10% [Rutter & Yule, 1975, Rutter 1978; Yule, 1988] and more generally in countries which adopt alphabetical systems it ranges from 5 to 10%, up to 17.5% [Interagency Committee on Learning Disabilities, 1987; Shaywitz et al. 1994; Shaywitz, 1998] or even 20-25% [Stedman & Kaestle, 1987].

In 1978, a publication of the National Institute of Health estimated that dyslexic children in US came to 1 million two hundred thousand. From 3 to 20% of schoolchildren were supposed to be dyslexic, with a ratio between males and females of 3:2 or 5:4 according to some sources [Brown, 1978, Shaywitz et al., 1990; Ygge & Lennerstrand, 1992; WHO, 1993], of 2:1 up to 5:1 according to others [Finucci & Childs, 1981].

As a matter of fact, the prevalence in the two genders is similar: 8.7% in males against 6.9% of females, as reported in the Shaywitz Connecticut Longitudinal Study [Shaywitz et al., 1990].

This trend was confirmed first by Wadsworth [Wadsworth et al., 1992], then by Flynn and Rahbar [1994]. The greater involvement of males, therefore, is a bias: the males seem more vulnerable because reading problems in young girls are frequently misunderstood[2]. This argument is supported by the fact that the sex chromosomes are not involved in dyslexia. In the UK, the most optimistic estimates quote a prevalence of severe dyslexia around 3%, reaching 6% when including the mild cases [Miles, 2004]. It has been reported, however, an involvement up to 9.4%, in the school population of Oxford [Stein, 2001] and more than 10% in London [Yule, 1973]. Such an epidemiological situation is quite the same in the Antipodes, for example in Australia (4-8%, government sources). Dyslexics are 5-6% of the school age population in Russia [Kornev, 1995], 3-10% in India [Ramaa, 2000]. In Latin America the situation is not better. On the contrary, it seems even worse in Brazil, where the prevalence reaches up to10-25% if mild cases are included [Capovilla, 2002].

The syndrome does not spare the Far East, in confirmation of the fact that dyslexia is not related to the ability to decode alphabetic writings but extends to those based on ideograms: in line with the western countries, the reported prevalence is 4-8% in China, 7.5% in Taiwan [Stevenson et al., 1982],

In the past decades it was common opinion that Japan was immune: a 1968 study estimated the prevalence of developmental dyslexia in this country to be below 1% (0. 98%), that is up to 10 times lower than in western countries [Makita, 1968]. Subsequent investigations, however, have put the Japanese data in their right perspective, unmasking the myth of the Land of the Rising Sun: the proportion of real Japanese dyslexic children is, in fact, 5.4-6% [Stevenson et al., 1982; Yamada & Banks, 1994, Yamada, 2000].

In the Arab world the prevalence appears very low indeed, reaching about 1% in Egypt [Farrag et al., 1988]. According to the authors of the survey, this is due to the characteristics of the Arabic language; nevertheless, it is likely the data to be biased by methodological differences.

In Italy the official estimate is 4.5%: about 1 million and a half of school-age children. It is interesting to consider that in 1969 the proportion did not exceed 1 .3%. [Faglioni et al., 1969]: the increase of nearly three and a half times over forty years is probably due to a greater attention to the problem rather than to the effective spreading of the disease. It is most worrying, however, that only 20% of all dyslexics are recognized and treated in this country (source: Italian Dyslexia Association).

Epidemiological data are summarized in Figure 1.

So far as we know, no direct epidemiological comparisons among countries are available in literature, apart from an Italian-American work dating back 1985 that reported dyslexia to be more common in the U.S.A. (4.5%) than in Italy (3.6%) [Lindgren et al., 1985]. A similar difference has been found in Europe between the North and South part of the subcontinent (higher prevalence in the first case) [Benton, 1975]. This finding could be due to the lower difficulty in decoding transparent orthographies (such as Italian or Spanish) compared to the northern languages, such as English, less regular and with reduced grapheme-to-phoneme correspondence [Downing, 1973].

Waiting for further comparative population surveys, the epidemiological discrepancies are likely to depend mainly on the lack of shared diagnostic criteria of the disease. In addition, the estimate is made difficult by the presence of a large “grey” area among children that are certainly dyslexic and those who are definitely normal. Therefore, our condition

[2] Yet, some years ago a review of four new epidemiological studies brought this aspect into question, reporting a two-fold prevalence in males than females [Rutter et al.,2004].

would be the tail of a frequency distribution referred to the ability to read, starting from normal readers, going through poor readers and ending with the dyslexics [Bilka, 1982; Shaywitz et al., 1992].

Probably, the lack of continuity between poor readers and dyslexics and the missing of common diagnostic criteria are the main drawbacks for the correct epidemiological assessment in the different countries.

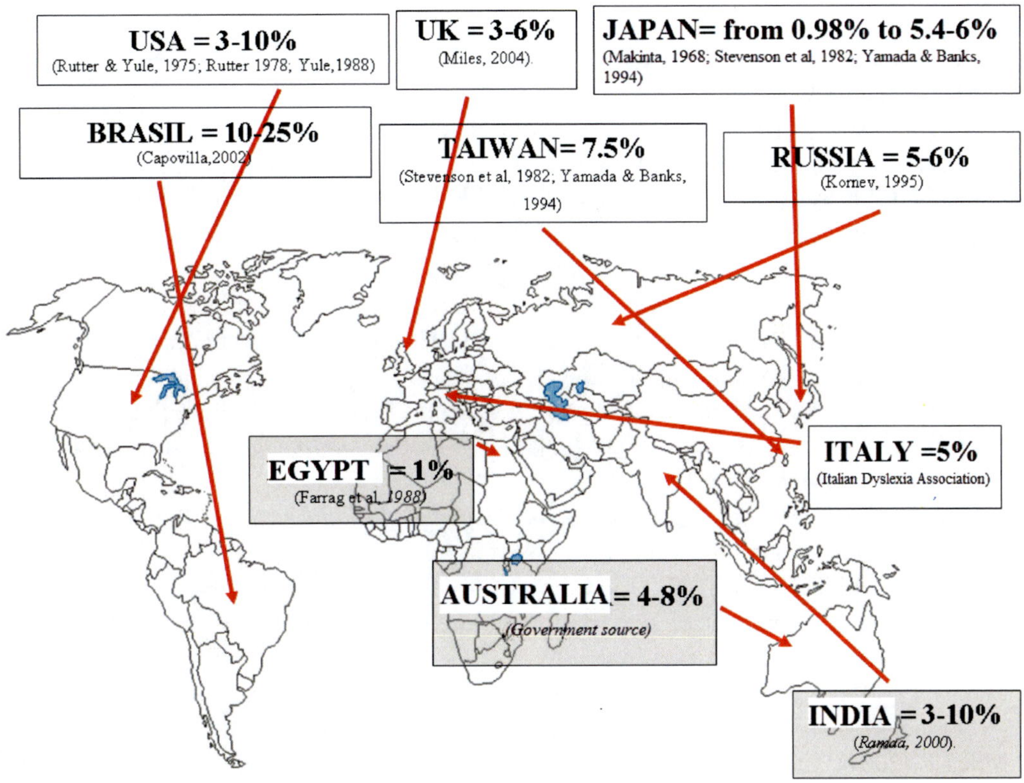

Figure 1. Prevalence of developmental dyslexia in the world.

References

Benton A. (1975) Developmental dyslexia. Neurological aspects. In Friedman W.J. (Ed). *Advances in Neurology: Vol.1, current reviews of higher order nervous system dysfunction.* New York: Raven Press.

Bilka S. (1982). *Ophthalmological findings in pupils of a primary school with particular reference to reading difficulties.* Acta Ophthalmologica, 60: 927-934.

Brown BS. (1978). *Dyslexia: an Appraisal of Current Knowledge.* Benton & Pearl Eds., Oxford University Press, Oxford.

Bruck M. (1992). *Persistence of dyslexics' phonological awareness deficits.* Developmental Psychology, 28: 874-886.

Capovilla AG. (2002). *Compreendo a dislexia: definicão, avaliacão e intervencão.* Cadernos de Psicopedagogia, 2: 36-59.

Downing J. (1973). *Comparative reading,* Downing Ed., MacMillian, New York.

Faglioni P, Gatti B, Paganoni AM, Robutti A. (1969). *A psychometric evaluation of developmental dyslexia in Italian children.* Cortex,5: 15-26.

Farrag AF, el-Behary AA, Kandil MR. (1988). *Prevalence of specific reading difficulty in Egypt.* The Lancet, 2: 837-839.

Felton RH, Naylor CE, Wood FB. (1990). *Neuropsychological profile of adult dyslexics.* Brain and Language, 39: 485-497.

Finucci JM, Childs B. (1981). *Are there really more dyslexic boys than girls?* In: Sex differences in dyslexia. Ansara, Geschwind, Albert & Gartrell Eds., Towson, MD, Orton Dyslexia Society.

Flynn JM, Rahbar MH. (1994). *Prevalence of reading failure in boys compared with girls.* Psychology in the Schools, 31: 66-71.

Francis DJ, Shaywitz SE, Stuebing KK, Shaywitz BA, Fletcher JM. (1996). *Developmental lag versus deficit models of reading disability: a longitudinal, individual growth curves analysis.* Journal of Educational Psychology, 88: 3-17.

Hinshelwood J. (1917). *Congenital word blindness.* HK Lewis & Co. Eds., London.

Interagency Committee on Learning Disabilities. (1987). *Learning disabilities: a report to the U.S. Congress.* Government Printing Office, Washington, D.C.

Kornev AN. (1995). *Dyslexia and dysgraphia in children.* Mim Ed., St.Petersburg.

Lennerstrand G, Ygge J. (1992). *Dyslexia: ophthalmological aspects 1991.* Acta Ophthalmologica, 70: 3-13.

Lerner JW. *Educational interventions in learning disabilities* (1989) Journal of the American Academy of Child & Adolescent Psychiatry, 28: 326-331.

Lindgren SD, De Renzi E, Lichman LC. (1985). *Cross-national comparisons of developmental dyslexia in Italy and the United States.* Child Development, 56: 1404-1417.

Makita K. (1968). *The rarity of reading difficulty in Japanese children.* American Journal of Orthopsychiatry, 38: 599-614.

Miles T. (2004). *Some problems in determining the prevalence of dyslexia.* Electronic Journal of Research in Educational Psychology, 2: 5-12.

Orton ST. (1925). *Word-blindness in school children.* Archives of Neurology and Psychiatry, 14: 581-615.

Ramaa S. (2000). Two decades of research on learning disabilities in India. *Dyslexia,* 6: 268-283.

Rutter M, Yule W. (1975). *The concept of specific reading retardation.* Journal of Child Psychology and Psychiatry, 16: 181-197.

Rutter M. (1978). *Prevalence and types of dyslexia.* In: Dyslexia, an appraisal of current knowledge, Benton & Pearl Eds., Oxford University Press, New York.

Rutter M, Caspi A, Fergusson D, Horwood LJ, Goodman R, Maughan B, Moffitt TE, Meltzer H, Carroll J. (2004). *Sex differences in developmental reading disability-new findings from 4 epidemiological studies.* The Journal of the American Medical Association, 291: 2007-2012.

Scarborough HS. (1984). *Continuity between childhood dyslexia and adult reading.* British Journal of Psychology, 75: 329-348.

Shaywitz SE. (1998). *Dyslexia.* New England Journal of Medicine, 338: 307-312.

Shaywitz SE, Shaywitz BA, Fletcher JM, Escobar MD. (1990). *Prevalence of reading disability in boys and girls: results of the Connecticut Longitudinal Study.* Journal of the American Medical Association, 264: 998-1002.

Shaywitz SE, Escobar MD, Shaywitz BA, Fletcher JM, Makuch R. (1992). *Evidence that dyslexia may represent the lower tail of a normal distribution of reading ability.* New England Journal of Medicine, 326: 145-150.

Shaywitz SE, Fletcher JM, Shaywitz BA. (1994). *Issues in the definition and classification of attention deficit disorder.* Topics in Language Disorders, 14: 1-25.

Shaywitz SE, Fletcher JM, Holahan JM, Shneider AE, Marchione KE, Stuebing KK, Francis DJ, Pugh KR, Shaywitz BA. (1999). *Persistence of dyslexia: the Connecticut Longitudinal Study of adolescence.* Pediatrics, 104: 1351-1359.

Stanley G, Hall R. (1973). *Short term visual processing in dyslexics.* Child Development, 44: 841-844.

Stedman LC, Kaestle CF. (1987). *Literacy and reading performance in the United States, from 1880 to the present.* Reading Research Quarterly, 22: 8-46.

Stein J. (2001). *The magnocellular theory of developmental dyslexia.* Dyslexia,7: 12-36.

Stevenson HT, Stigler JW, Lucker GW, Lee S, Hsu C, Kitamura S. (1982). *Reading disabilities: The case of Chinese, Japanese and English.* Child Development, 53: 1164-1181.

Yamada J. (2000). *The myth of absence of dyslexia in Japan.* Perspectives, 22-23.

Yamada J, Banks A. (1994). *Evidence for and characteristics of dyslexia among Japanese children.* Annals of Dyslexia, 44: 105-119.

Yule W. (1988). *Dyslexia: not one condition but many.* British Medical Journal, 297: 501-502.

Yule M, Rutter M, Berger M, Thompson B. (1973). *Over and under achievement in reading.* British Journal of Educational Psychology, 44: 1-12.

Wadsworth SJ, DeFries JC, Stevenson J, Gilger JW, Pennington BF. (1992). *Gender ratios among reading-disabled children and their siblings as a function of parental impairment.* Journal of Child Psychology and Psychiatry, 33: 1229-1239.

World Health Organization. ICD-10. (1993). *The international classification of diseases: classification of mental and behavioural disorders.* Vol. 10, Geneva.

Chapter II

Historical Background and Morphofunctional Studies

Developmental dyslexia, a word coined in 1887 in Stuttgart, Germany, by the ophthalmologist Rudolf Berlin, was described for the first time as a clinical entity in the late nineteenth century by the Scottish ophthalmologist James Hinshelwood who, in 1895, published in The Lancet (one of the most authoritative international medical journals) *Word blindness and visual memories*. This article was followed one year later by *A case of dyslexia, a peculiar form of word-blindness* and shortly after by *Word and Mind-Blindness* (1900) and *Congenital word blindness* (1917). A few years before (November 7, 1896) GP Pringle Morgan, from Sussex, published in the British Medical Journal the first case report of a fourteen year old patient suffering from dyslexia, "*Percy F,a well-grown lad aged 14, is the eldest son of intelligent parents. He has always been a bright and intelligent boy, quick at games and in no way inferior to others of his age [...]. His greatest difficulty has been -and is now- his inability to learn to read. This inability is so remarkable, and so pronounced, that I have no doubt it is due to some congenital defect [---] he went to school at the age of 7 and the greatest efforts have been made to teach him to read but, in spite of this laborious and persistent training, he can only with difficulty spell out words of one syllable* ". When Percy read aloud, he was unable to read correctly words apart from 'the, of, that'; other words seemed almost unknown to him and he was not even able to pronounce them. In his report, Morgan pointed out the absence of brain lesions and suggested a visual cause, calling the clinical condition "*congenital word blindness*". In line with Morgan, in 1925 the American neuropsychiatrist Samuel Orton was the first to argue the disease can be due to a dysfunction in the visual perception of the text and in 1928 he defined it *strephosimbolìa* (from ancient Greek στρηφος = twisted). According to Orton, reading disability would stem from anomalous brain development, weakening the cerebral dominance of one hemisphere over the other. He believed this impairment to be responsible for inaccurate recognition and positional coding of letters and found a similar anomalous reading pattern in his patients suffering from cerebral ischemia.

More than 30 years before, indeed, autoptic studies in adults had led the French neurologist Jules Dejerine to state that letters and words are processed[3] in a particular region of the cerebral cortex, the left inferoparieotoccipital cortex, more specifically in the left angular gyrus [Dejerine, 1891]. According to Dejerine, therefore, an alteration of this area of the brain would have a key role in the pathogenesis of developmental dyslexia. Twenty-six years later Hinshelwood agreed with this opinion [Hinshelwood, 1917]. The confirmation, however, came in 1968, when the brain of a dyslexic teenager who died for cerebral hemorrhage was examined by the American researcher William Drake. The scientist discovered developmental anomalies, in particular islands of ectopia[4] in the outer layers of the cerebral cortex. The case was considered of paramount importance, so that the abstract of the manuscript, published on the Journal of Learning Disabilities, reads: "*To our knowledge this is the first case history offered to the literature. [...]. The Journal is very proud to publish this manuscript. Dr. Drake and his evaluation team have performed a great service for the field of learning disabilities"*. It was September, 1968.

Nearly 10 years after other investigations focused on the findings of Drake. From 1979 to 1985 Galaburda and his colleagues published histological studies that confirmed the presence of ectopia in the brains of dyslexics, mainly in the left frontal and temporoparietal area, often associated with islands of dysplasia[5] [Galaburda & Kemper, 1979, Galaburda et al., 1985; Hynd & Semrud-Clikeman, 1989]. Interestingly, these clusters localize in corresponding regions of the two hemispheres, connected by fibers crossing the callosal body. Such abnormal islands were found even in the brains of normal subjects, however in these cases they turned out to be less numerous and differently located [Kaufmann & Galaburda, 1989] Furthermore, in three dyslexic patients scars made of glial[6] tissue were detected at the boundary of regions fed by different vascular branches: a sign of a possible development defect of the cortical vascularization [Humphreys et al., 1990]. This observation was confirmed less than a decade later, when positron emission tomography (PET)[7] showed an alteration of blood flow mainly in the left inferior parietal region and in the posterior temporal region (bilaterally) in 17 dyslexics during phonological activities (e.g. reading aloud) [Rumsey et al., 1997a]. Since the change in regional blood flow is indicative of metabolic changes (i.e. activation of abnormal tissue), the results indicate that the dyslexic brains not only have anatomical differences compared with normals, but that these differences lead to a

---

[3] With the term *visual processing* we refer to the perception and processing of a stimulus, that is its retinal transduction, transmission along the visual pathway and its decomposition and recomposition in the visual areas of the cerebral cortex, so as to make it suitable to be experienced. Visual processing is performed by specific anatomofunctional modules, defined *receptive fields*, located on the retina, in the geniculate nucleus as well as in the visual cortical areas. Depending on their hierarchical arrangement, receptive fields are specialized in the analysis of more and more complex characteristics of the stimulus.

[4] Areas of ectopia are clusters of cells localized in the cortex in a position that is not their own as a result of an anomalous migration of embryonic neurons during the intrauterine development [Goldman-Rakic & Rakic, 1984].

[5] A zone of dysplasia is an area where the typical structure of the neurons is subverted.

[6] The glial tissue can be considered the connective tissue of the brain, intermingled with the neurons. Glial cells have a structural function and are responsible for metabolic exchange and elimination of toxic and extraneous substances.

[7] PET is a scintigraphic imaging technique that records the location and intensity of a radioactive track in the human body after a suitable tracer, contained in a biological molecule, is injected intravenously. A radioactive positron-emitting radionuclide supplies the radioactive track. The reaction between electrons and positrons results in the emission of recordable gamma-rays, whose intensity is proportional to the metabolic activity of the tissue. PET is therefore able to describe the intensity of a functional process in an organ, including the brain.

functional activation impairment. The left inferotemporal region seems to be particularly abnormal, especially in its posterior part. The inferotemporal region is an important associative crossroads between areas involved in the visual processing of written words (like the most mesial part of the extrastriate cortex) and the regions aimed to process other kinds of visual stimulation, like MT, responsible for motion perception [Habib, 2000]. Even the posterior parietal cortex, in charge of its importance in the attentive processes, would be compromised in patients, as assessed by blow flow analysis as well as electroencephalographic [Duffy et al., 1980; Wood et al., 1991] and electrophysiological techniques [Schulte-Körne & Bruder, 2010]. Such reports suggest that a visuo-attentional deficit can play a pathogenetical role, as will be discussed hereinafter. In summary, these factors led to believe that the dyslexic brain suffers from a delay of intrauterine maturation occurring around the sixth month of pregnancy, that is to say when the development of the fetus is faster [Stein & Talcott, 1999; Habib, 2000].

Between the twenties and the thirties of the last century, Orton went along a different direction and suggested that reduced hemispheric lateralization in dyslexic causes a delay in the functional specialization of the left hemisphere verbal skills, so that it would ultimately hinder the acquisition of reading [Orton 1925, Orton, 1937].

This theory seems compatible with the hypothesis of the abnormal brain maturation [Habib, 2000] and was verified since the late seventies by subsequent observations, both anatomical [Galaburda et al., 1978; Cohen et al., 1989] and in vivo. By means of magnetic resonance imaging (MRI), the lack of the normal left > right asymmetry of the temporal planum has been described in up to 70% of the patients: in the left hemisphere this structure (rather than being more developed) was observed to be equal or even smaller than the contralateral [Duffy & McAnulty, 1985; Hynd et al., 1990; Larsen et al., 1990; Jernigan et al., 1991] (figure 1).

Although this finding is believed to be linked to a phonological disability [Larsen et al., 1990], on a cellular scale asymmetry failures are reported even in the visual areas: indeed, in normal subjects the cells of the occipital cortex are larger in the left hemisphere, whereas in dyslexics this left/right difference is missing [Jenner et al., 1999][8].

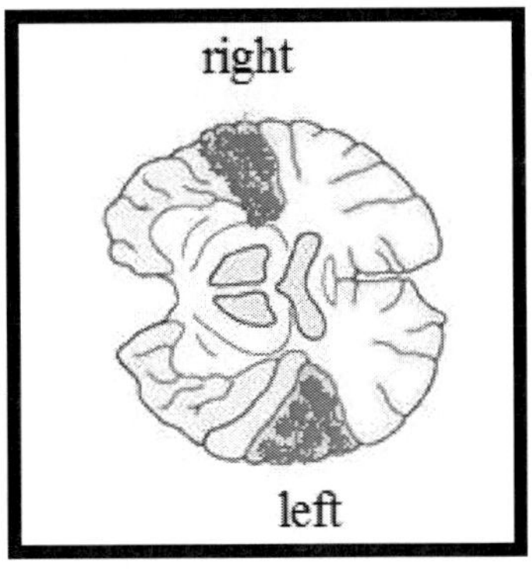

Figure 1. The planum temporale. Note the left> right asymmetry proper of the normal brain and reduced or absent in dyslexic subjects.

[8] The lack of lateralization and the reduced interemisferic asymmetry has been related to the difficulty of many patients in distinguishing left from right and to their ability in using both hands indifferently.

As frequently happens in the academic world, other investigations failed to detect a reduction in the dyslexic's temporal planum asymmetry [Rumsey et al., 1997a,b; Best & Demb, 1999; Heiervang et al., 2000; Robichon et al., 2000; Eckert et al., 2003], while Habib and Robichon [1996] found in subjects with evident phonological problems a reduced asymmetry of a parietal region called the *operculum*[9].

A different investigative line has focused on the corpus callosum, the structure that connects the two cerebral hemispheres[10]. The comparison of the size of the corpus callosum in dyslexic and normal readers supports the theory of the interemispheric asymmetry.

Duara in 1991 and, five years later, Rumsey, measured in their dyslexic samples[11] the size of the corpus callosum [Duara et al., 1991; Rumsey y al, 1996] by means of nuclear magnetic resonance.

The researchers found that the posterior third (in particular the splenium) was wider in patients compared to controls. The increase of the thickness of this structure in its posterior portion was correlated to the reduced asymmetry of the temporal planum and of the posterior parietal cortex [Galaburda et al., 1978]: reduced asymmetry means greater overall amount of tissue, so that corpus callosum has to be thicker to ensure proper interemispheric connection[12] [Habib, 2000].

Therefore, increased size of the caudal portion of the corpus callosum would be related to abnormal interemispheric communication and in particular to defective lateralization of the posterior cortical areas responsible for the linguistic functions [Gross-Glenn & Rothenberg, 1984; Best, 1985; Gladstone et al., 1989; Moore et al., 1995; Markee et al., 1996]. To assess callosal functioning, Markee measured interemispheric transfer time by using visual evoked potentials (VEP)[13] in 21 dyslexics and found them to be delayed [Markee et al., 1996].

Interemispheric communication in dyslexics has been investigated even by means of psychophysical techniques: Gross-Glenn and Rothenberg [1984], measured threshold recognition for letters displayed tachistoscopically in one of the visual hemifields (nasal or temporal). They found in their sample of patients (aged from 11 to 15 years) a marked threshold difference in the two hemifields. The defect in the information transfer between the two hemispheres would involve not only the sensory function but even the motor domain: indeed, when asked to make opposite movements with the hands, the motor coordination of the dyslexic subjects turned out to be defective [Moore et al., 1995].

Once again, counter evidence is reported: making use of magnetic resonance imaging, Larsen first and Pennington later found no substantial differences in the size of the corpus callosum[14] between dyslexics and normal readers [Larsen et al., 1992; Pennington et al.,

[9] Even in the brain of Einstein, who was recognized as adyslexic, the operculum asymmetry was missing [Witelson et al.,1999].

[10] The corpus callosum is a thick layer of white cerebral matter placed in the hemispherical sulcus, curved at its cranial and caudal ends. It is made of fibers stretched between the two hemispheres. In the anteroposterior direction it is made of the following sections: the rostrum, the knee, the truncus and finally the splenium.

[11] 19 and 21 subjects, respectively.

[12] According to Duara's estimates [Duara et al., 1991], the thickness of the corpus callosum is higher in dyslexic females compared to males.

[13] Evoked visual potentials (VEP) are recorded via an electrode placed on the occipital bone and two others applied on the mastoid process on both sides. This way amplitude and latency of the electrical response evoked by a visual stimulation can be measured.

[14] In particolar of the splenium.

1999] whereas Hynd (by using the same technique) has described it as smaller[15][Hynd et al., 1995].

In his review of 1997, Beaton defined as conflictual the findings from the morphometric studies of the corpus callosum and the alleged lack of asymmetry between the cerebral hemispheres and the temporal planum [Beaton, 1997]. Three years later, Habib stated that the reduced asymmetry left> right is necessary but not sufficient as an aetiological factor, since it is found even in one third of the normal population [Habib, 2000].

An additional issue considered relevant, deals with the cerebellum size of dyslexics. By using MRI, Eckhert measured some cerebellar structures in a group of 18 patients[16] and 32 control subjects. They found that the right anterior lobes of the cerebellum of the dyslexics were smaller, and stated that an alteration of cerebellar function is at the basis not only (as already known) of motor alterations but also of the lexical dysfunction [Eckhert et al., 2003].

These results, which add one more factor in the debate on the aetiopathogenesis of dyslexia, are in line with previous neuroimaging [Ito, 1984, 1990, Krupa et al., 1993, Leonard et al., 2001; Finch et al., 2002] and PET studies showing metabolic anomalies in the cerebellum of dyslexics, especially in the right anterior lobe [Nicolson et al., 1999].

Rae compared the metabolic activity of the temporoparietal and cerebellar cortex of 14 dyslexic children with those of 15 normal subjects: in the patients, the activity in the left temporoparietal cortex and in the right cerebellar hemisphere differed from the corresponding contralateral regions, while in normal readers the difference was negligible [Rae et al., 1998]. In addition, in dyslexics the reduced metabolic activation in the anterior cerebellar lobe during sequential fingers movements[17] [Nicolson et al., 1999] and the presence of cerebellar signs as muscular hypotonia, supports the so-called *cerebellar deficit hypothesis* [Nicolson & Fawcett, 1990, Nicolson et al., 2001]. The joined measurement of the size of the cerebellar anterior right lobe and of the *pars triangularis*[18] of the frontal lobe[19] shows a sensitivity of 72% and a specificity of 88% for the diagnosis of developmental dyslexia, with particular reference to its phono-linguistic aspects [Eckert et al., 2003]. A significant correlation was found between such anatomical differences and the lexical function (identification of words and non-words: Eckert et al., 2003[20]]. Furthermore, the size of the cerebellar right anterior lobe in patients is important as it is the only parameter that does not show substantial changes with age [Leonard et al., 2001].

Granted that the probability of a correct diagnosis increases in presence of these morphological findings, it remains to be explained how these elements would have a causal role in determining the reading pattern of dyslexics. Evidently, a single anatomical marker is not enough, given the complexity of the task. The fact remains that these alterations, which have aroused so much interest in the earlier decades, have been studied (and keep on being investigated) more in the perspective of a linguistic- phonological impairment than of the visuoperceptive one [Leonard et al., 2001].

---

[15] Expecially in its most anterior region, the knee.

[16] Mean age: 11 years.

[17] Measured by PET.

[18] The pars triangularis is a portion of Broca's speech area, located in the inferior frontal gyrus and corresponding to Brodmann area 45.

[19] Bilaterally.

[20] While anomalies in the frontal lobe would hamper the grapheme-phoneme conversion [Leonard et al., 2001].

Yet, even excluding in a conjectural way an involvement of the visual system, the results suggest no more than a simple association between brain anomalies and dyslexia, while supporting a cause-effect on the basis of the mere frequency of their distribution in the population is factious. To date, indeed, this relationship is little illuminating about the pathogenesis of the disease.

If we assume that the anatomopathological findings could have in future a decisive role to cast light on the aetiopathogenesis and to devise the best rehabilitative techniques, on the one hand the mechanisms underlying these changes in the brain should be assessed, on the other hand a functional approach to study the way they could be linked should be adopted.

References

Beaton AA. (1997). *The relation of planum temporale asymmetry and morphology of the corpum callosum to handedness, gender, and dyslexia: a review of the evidence.* Brain and Language, 60: 255-322.

Berlin, VP. (1887). *Eine besondere Art der Wortblindheit.* Wiesbaden, Bergmann, Stuttgart.

Best CT. (1985). *Hemispheric function and collaboration in the child.* Best ED., Academic Press, Orlando.

Best M, Demb JB. (1999). *Normal planum temporale asymmetry in dyslexics with a magnocellular pathway deficit.* Neuroreport, 10: 607-612.

Cohen M, Cambell R, Yaghmai F. (1989). *Neuropathological abnormalities in developmental dysphasia.* Annals of Neurology, 25: 567-570.

Dejerine J. (1891). *Sur un cas de cécité verbale avec agraphie, suivi d'autopsie.* Mémoires de la Société de Biologie, 3: 197-201.

Drake WE. (1968). *Clinical and pathological findings in a child with a developmental learning disability.* Journal of Learning Disabilities, 1: 486-502.

Duara R, Kushch A, Gross-Glenn K, Baker W, Jallad B, Pascal S, Loewenstein D, Sheldon J, Rabin L, Levin B, Lubs H. (1991). *Neuroanatomic differences between dyslexic and normal readers on magnetic imaging scans.* Archives of Neurology, 48: 410-416.

Duffy FH, Denckla MB, Bartels PH, Sandini B. (1980) *Dyslexia: regional differences in brain electrical activity by topographical mapping.* Annals of Neurology, 7: 412-420.

Duffy FH, McAnulty GB. (1985). *Brain electrical activity mapping (BEAM): The search for a physiological signature of dyslexia.* In: Dyslexia. A Neuroscientific Approach to Clinical Evaluation, Duffy & Geschwind Eds., Little, Brown and Company, Boston.

Eckert MA, Leonard CM, Richards TL, Aylward EH, Thomson J, Berninger VW. (2003). *Anatomical correlates of dyslexia: frontal and cerebellar findings.* Brain, 126: 482-494.

Finch AJ, Nicolson RI, Fawcett AJ. (2002). *Evidence for a neuroanatomical difference within the olivo-cerebellar pathway of adults with dyslexia.* Cortex, 38: 529-539.

Galaburda AM, Lemay M, Kemper TM, Geschwind N. (1978). *R/L asymmetries in the brain may underlie cerebral dominance.* Science, 199: 852-856.

Galaburda AM, Kemper TL. (1979). *Cytoarchitectonic abnormalities in developmental dyslexia: a case study.* Annals of Neurology, 6: 94-100.

Galaburda AM, Sherman GF, Rosen GD, Aboitiz F, Geschwind N. (1985). *Developmental dyslexia: four consecutive patients with cortical anomalies.* Annals of Neurology, 18: 222-233.

Gladstone M, Best CT, Davidson RJ. (1989). *Anomalous bimanual coordination among dyslexic boys.* Developmental Psychology, 25: 236-246.

Goldman-Rakic P, Rakic P. (1984). *Experimentally modified convolutional patterns in nonhuman primates: Possible relevance of connections to cerebral dominance in humans.* In: Cerebral Dominance: The Biological Foundations, Geschwind & Galaburda Eds., Harvard University Press, Cambridge MA, USA.

Gross-Glenn K, Rothenberg S. (1984). *Evidence for deficit in interhemispheric transfer of information in dyslexic boys.* The International Journal of Neuroscience, 24: 23-35.

Habib M. (2000). *The neurological basis of developmental dyslexia. An overview and working hypothesis.* Brain, 123: 2373-2399.

Habib M & Robichon F. (1996). *Parietal lobe morphology predicts phonological skills in developmental dyslexia.* Brain Cognition, 32: 139-142.

Heiervang E, Hugdahl K, Steinmetz H, Smievoll AI, Stevenson J, Lund A, Ersland L, Lundervold A. (2000). *Planum temporale, planum parietale and dichotic listening in dyslexia.* Neuropsychologia, 38: 1704-1713.

Hinshelwood J. (1895). *Word blindness and visual memories.* The Lancet, 2: 1566-1570.

Hinshelwood J. (1896). *A case of dyslexia; a peculiar form of word-blindness.* The Lancet, 2: 1451.

Hinshelwood J. (1900). *Letter-Word and Mind-Blindness,* HK Lewis & Co. Eds., London.

Hinshelwood J. (1917). *Congenital word blindness.* HK Lewis & Co. Eds., London.

Humphreys P, Kaufmann WE, Galaburda AM. (1990). *Developmental dyslexia in women: neuropathological findings in three patients.* Annals of Neurology, 28: 727-738.

Hynd GW, Semrud-Clikeman M. (1989). *Dyslexia and brain morphology.* Psychological Bulletin, 106: 447-482.

Hynd GW, Semrud-Clikeman M, Lorys AR, Novey ES, Eliopulos D. (1990). *Brain morphology in developmental dyslexia and attention deficit disorder/hyperactivity.* Archives of Neurology, 47: 919- 926.

Hynd GW, Hall J, Novey E, Eliopulos D, Black K, Gonzales JJ, Edomonds JE, Riccio C, Cohen M. (1995). *Dyslexia and corpus callosum morphology.* Archives of Neurology, 52: 32-38.

Ito M. (1984). *The Cerebellum and Neural Control.* Raven Press Ed., New York.

Ito M. (1990). *A new physiological concept on cerebellum.* Journal of Cognitive Neuroscience, 1: 136-152.

Jenner AR, Rosen GD, Galaburda AM. (1999). *Neuronal asymmetries in primary visual cortex of dyslexic and nondsyslexic brains.* Annals of Neurology, 46: 189-196.

Jernigan TL, Hesselink JR, Sowell E, Tallal P. (1991). *Cerebral structure on magnetic resonance imaging in language- and learning-impaired children.* Archives of Neurology, 48: 539-545.

Kaufmann WE, Galaburda AM. (1989). *Cerebrocortical microdysgenesis in neurologically normal subjects: a hystopathologic study.* Neurology, 39: 238-244.

Krupa DJ, Thompson JK, Thompson RF. (1993). *Localization of a memory trace in the mammalian brain.* Science, 260: 989-991.

Larsen JP, Hoien T, Lundberg I, Ødegaard H. (1990). *MRI evaluation of the size and symmetry of the plannum temporale in adolescents with developmental dyslexia.* Brain and Language, 39: 289-301.

Larsen JP, Hølen T, Ødegaard H. (1992). *Magnetic resonance imaging of the corpus callosum in developmental dyslexia.* Cognitive Neuropsychology, 9: 123-134.

Leonard CM, Eckert MA, Lombardino LJ, Oakland T, Kranzler J, Mohr CM, King WM, Freeman A. (2001). *Anatomical risk factors for phonological dyslexia.* Cerebral Cortex, 11: 148-157.

Markee T, Brown WS, Moore LH. (1996). *Callosal function in dyslexia: evoked potential interhemispheric transfer time and bilateral field advantage.* Developmental Neuropsychology, 12: 409-428.

Moore LH, Brown WS, Markee TE, Theberge DC, Zvi JC. (1995). *Bimanual coordination in dyslexic adults.* Neuropsycologia 33: 781-793.

Morgan WP. (1896). *A case of congenital word blindness.* British Medical Journal, 2: 1378.

Nicolson RI, Fawcett AJ. (1990). *Automaticity: a new framework for dyslexia research?* Cognition, 35: 159-182.

Nicolson RI, Fawcett AJ, Berry EL, Jenkins IH, Dean P, Brooks DJ. (1999). *Association of abnormal cerebellar activation with motor learning difficulties in dyslexic adults.* The Lancet, 353: 1662-1667.

Nicolson RI, Fawcett AJ, Dean P. (2001). *Developmental dyslexia: the cerebellar deficit hypothesis.* Trends in Neurosciences, 24: 508-511.

Orton ST. (1925). *Word-blindness in school children.* Archives of Neurology and Psychiatry, 14: 581-615.

Orton ST. (1928). *Specific reading disability-strephosymbolia.* Journal of the American Medical Association, 90; 1095-1099.

Orton ST. (1937). *Reading, writing and speech problems in children.* Chapman & Hall Eds, London.

Pennington BF, Filipek PA, Lefly D, Churchwell J, Kennedy DN, Simon JH, Filley CM, Galaburda A, Alarcon M, DeFries JC. (1999). *Brain morphometry in reading disabled twins.* Neurology, 53: 723-729.

Rae C, Lee MA, Dixon RM, Blamire AM, Thompson CH, Styles P, Talcott J, Richardson A, Stein J. (1998). *Metabolic abnormalities in developmental dyslexia detected by 1H magnetic resonance spectroscopy.* The Lancet, 351: 1849-1852.

Robichon F, Levrier O, Farnarier P, Habib M. (2000). *Developmental dyslexia: atypical cortical asymmetries and functional significance.* European Journal of Neurology, 7: 35-46.

Rumsey JM, Casanova M, Mannheim GB, Patronas N, De Vaughn N, Hamburger SD, Aquino T. (1996). *Corpus callosum morphology, as measured with MRI, in dyslexic men.* Biological Psychiatry, 39: 769-775.

Rumsey JM, Nace K, Donohue B, Wise D, Maisog JM, Andreason P. (1997a). *A positron emission tomographic study of impaired word recognition and phonological processing in dyslexic men.* Archives of Neurology, 54: 562-573.

Rumsey JM, Donohue BC, Brady DR, Nace K, Giedd JN, Paul Andreason P. (1997b). *A magnetic resonance imaging study of planum temporale asymmetry in men with developmental dyslexia.* Archives of Neurology, 54: 1481-1489.

Schulte-Körne G, Bruder J. (2010). *Clinical neurophysiology of visual and auditory processing in dyslexia: A review.* Clinical Neurophysiology, doi:10.1016/j.clinph. 2010.04.028.

Stein JF, Talcott J. (1999). *Impaired neuronal timing in developmental dyslexia-the magnocellular hypothesis.* Dyslexia, 5: 59- 77.

Witelson SF, Kigar DL, Harvey T. (1999). *The exceptional brain of Albert Einstein.* The Lancet, 353: 2149-2153.

Wood F, Felton R, Flowers L, Naylor C. (1991). *Neurobehavioural definition of dyslexia.* In: The reading brain, Dwayne & Grey Eds.. Parkton Press. New York.

Chapter III

Hormonal and Antigenic Factors

Apart from the anatomopathological studies, putative associations between dyslexia and hormonal dysfunction or predisposition to other diseases have been investigated. The presumed greater prevalence of the condition in males[21] led to believe that an anomalous concentration of fetal testosterone, affecting the brain modeling in the later stages of pregnancy, prevents the neuronal depletion responsible for the normal interemispheric asymmetry [Galaburda et al., 1987].

This hypothesis was called the *GBG* theory from the initial letters of its authors: Geschwind, Behan and Galaburda [Geschwind & Behan, 1982; Geschwind, 1984; Geschwind & Galaburda, 1985] or the *hypothesis of testosterone.*

The assumption looks particularly interesting by the light of the documented abnormal size of the corpus callosum in dyslexics, as the development of this structure seems to depend on the concentration of salivary testosterone [Moffat et al., 1997].

Increased concentration of testosterone and/or increased prenatal sensitivity to this hormone would hamper the normal development not only of the cerebral hemispheres and of the corpus callosum but also of the thymus, the fetal gland in charge of the immune T- system maturation (Figure 1).

Indeed, on the short arm of chromosome 6, which is thought to be the carrier of some inherited alterations putatively jointly-responsible for the onset of developmental dyslexia, are located the major histocompatibility complex genes (MHC). The MHC genes modulate the functioning of the antigenic system of histocompatibility HLA[22] [Cardon et al., 1994; Grigorenko et al., 1997; Fisher et al., 1999]: therefore, anomalies at this level would explain on the one hand why dyslexics are more often affected by allergic and autoimmune diseases compared to normal readers, on the other hand why dyslexia tends to be more common in families with autoimmune and atopic diseases such as asthma and eczema[23] [Geschwind & Behan, 1982; Pennington et al., 1987; Hugdahl et al., 1990; Crawford et al., 1994]. It has been suggested, indeed, that a moderate thymus-mediated immune reaction during the

---

[21] See chapter 1.

[22] HLA means Human Leukocyte Antigen and refers to antigens expressed on the leukocyte membranes and codified by the major histocompatibility complex.

[23] Yet, Bryden et al. [1994] provided a counter evidence.

intrauterine life would favor the establishment of these conditions and hinder brain maturation [Geschwind & Behan, 1982; Geschwind & Galaburda, 1987; Hugdahl et al., 1990].

Moreover, it has been advanced that antibodies directed against the magnocellular system (M-system) expressed by the maternal MHC, pass through the placenta during the fetal development and inhibit the maturation of the M-cells of the fetus. The effect MHC would have on the development of the magnocellular system [Corriveau et al., 1998] is revealing since, as we shall write, the M-system is in charge of the visuoperceptive functions required for reading.

In support of this position, in the brains of three dyslexic subjects glial scars due to an immune disorder have been described [Humphreys et al., 1990].

An in vivo experiment supports the relationship between immune over-activity and magnocellular impairment: Vincent injected into pregnant mice the serum obtained from human mothers of at least two dyslexic children: it was observed that serum antibodies, after crossing the placenta, bound to the M-cells of the fetal cerebellum. At birth, mice showed motor coordination problems and changes in their cerebellar metabolism [Vincent et al., 2002].

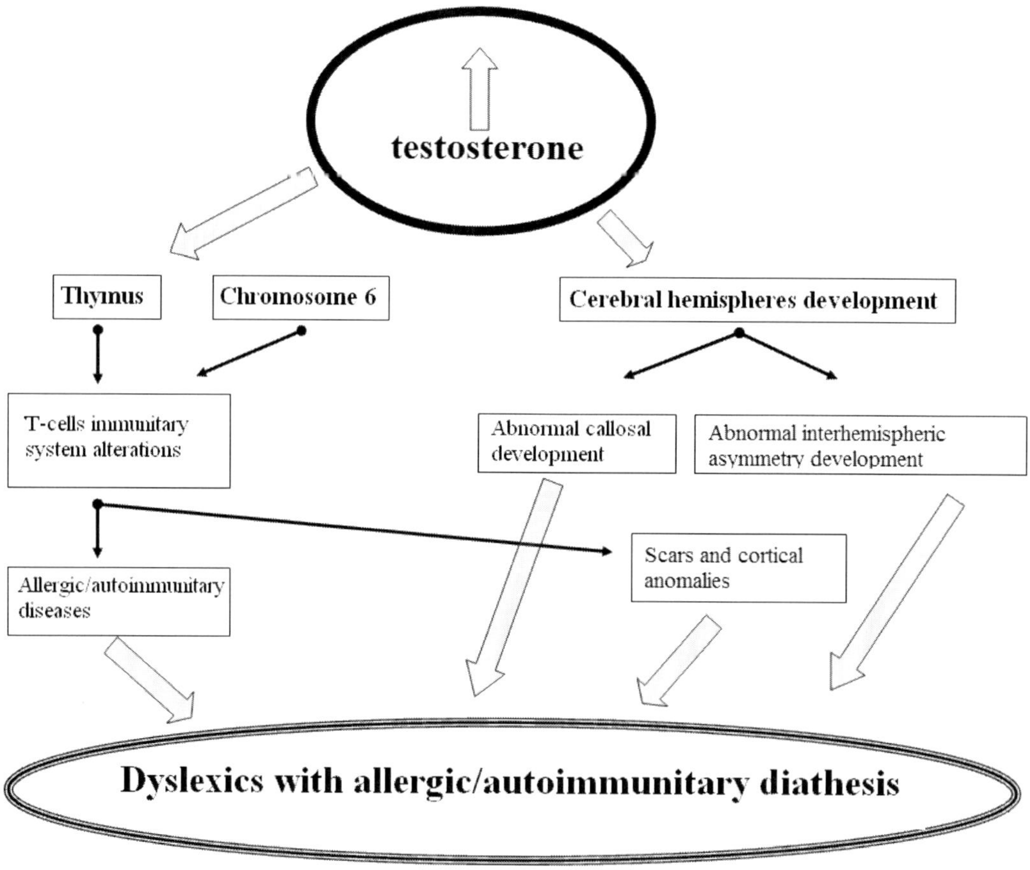

Figure 1. According to the *testosterone hypothesis* an increase in fetal testosterone during intrauterine life would hamper the normal development of the interemispheric asymmetry and promotes the onset of an immune environment that can affect the maturation of the cerebral cortex.

The theory of testosterone gave rise to a debate that reached its peak in the nineties. Some researchers sustained its legitimacy "in spite of a multitude of erroneous assumptions and failed predictions" [Previc, 1994], others maintained the model is not effectively supported by empirical evidence [Bryden et al., 1994].

Still, it has been underlined that an excess of fetal testosterone is not a requirement for the development of pathologies mediated by the T- immune system and in order to explain the association between developmental dyslexia and immunological diseases, an alternative model based on the histocompatibility factor HLA has been advanced [St-Marseille & Braum, 1994].

Actually, studies in animal models about the effect of testosterone on the brain development and immune system failed to show any correlation. Therefore, the major susceptibility of dyslexics to autoimmune diseases cannot be attributed to an abnormal serum concentration of testosterone: the hormone, if anything, would have a protective effect (sic!) [Denbung & Berenbaum, 1995].

Nevertheless, on the one hand the incidence of immune pathologies is higher among dyslexics, on the other hand lexical difficulties (especially the phonological ones) are more frequent among allergic subjects, as found by Tønnessen in a group of 32 asthmatics [Tønnessen et al., 1994][24].

In conclusion, the role of hormonal factors and in particular of testosterone is a controversial issue, whose implications have been dwarfed by the substantial equivalence of dyslexia in the two genders (therefore not more frequent in males, as previously stated). However, the involvement of the immune system is supported by experimental findings worthy of future investigations.

References

Berenbaum SA, Denburg SD. (1995). Evaluating the empirical support for the role of testosterone in the Geschwind-Behan-Galaburda model of cerebral lateralization: commentary on Bryden, McManus, and Bulman-Fleming. Brain Cognition, 27: 79-83.

Bryden MP, McManus IC, Bulman-Fleming MB. (1994). Evaluating the empirical support for the Geschwind-Behan-Galaburda model of cerebral lateralization. Brain Cognition, 26: 103-167.

Cardon LR, Smith SD, Fulker DW, Kimberling WJ, Pennington BF, Defries JC. (1994). Quantitative trait locus for reading disability on chromosome 6. Science, 266: 276-279.

Corriveau R, Huh G, Shatz C. (1998). Regulation of Class I MHC gene expression in the developing and mature CNS by neural activity. Neuron, 21: 505-520.

Crawford SG, Kaplan BJ, Kinsbourne M. (1994). Are families of children with reading difficulties at risk for immune disorders and non right handedness? Cortex, 30: 281-292.

Fisher S, Marlowe A, Lamb J, Maestrinin E, Williams D, Richardson A, Weeks D, Stein JF, Monaco A. (1999). A quantitative trait locus on chromosome 6p influences different aspects of developmental dyslexia. American Journal of Human Genetics, 64: 146-156.

[24] All the same, three years later Tønnessen, critically reviewed the theory of testosterone [Tønnessen, 1997].

Galaburda AM, Corsiglia J, Rosen GD, Sherman GF. (1987). Planum temporale asymmetry, reappraisal since Geschwind and Levitsky. Neuropsychologia, 25: 853-868.

Geschwind N. (1984). Cerebral dominance in biological perspective. Neuropsychologia, 22 : 675-683.

Geschwind N, Behan P. (1982). Association of left handedness with immune disease and developmental learning disorder. Proceedings of the National Academy of Science in the United States of America, 79: 5097-5100.

Geschwind, N, & Galaburda, A.M. (1985). Cerebral lateralization, biological mechanisms, associations, and pathology: I. A hypothesis and a program for research. Archives of Neurology, 42: 428–459.

Geschwind N, Galaburda AM. (1987). Cerebral Lateralisation: Biological Mechanisms, Associations and Pathology. MA; MIT Press Ed., Cambridge, UK.

Grigorenko EL, Wood FB, Meyer MS, Hart LA, Speed WC, Shuster A, Pauls DL. (1997). Susceptibility loci for distinct components of developmental dyslexia on chromosome 6 and 15. American Journal of Human Genetics, 60: 27-39.

Hugdahl K, Synnevåg B, Satz P. (1990). Immune and autoimmune diseases in dyslexic children. Neuropsychologia, 28: 673-679.

Humphreys P, Kaufmann WE, Galaburda AM. (1990). Developmental dyslexia in women: neuropathological findings in three patients. Annals of Neurology, 28: 727-738.

Moffat SD, Hampson E, Wickett JC, Vernon PA, Lee DH. (1997). Testosterone is correlated with regional morphology of the human corpus callosum. Brain Research, 767: 297-304.

Pennington BF, Smith SD, Kimberling WJ, Green PA, Haith MM. (1987). Left-handedness and immune disorders in family dyslexics. Archives of Neurology, 44: 634-39.

Previc FH. (1994). Assessing the legacy of the GBG model. Brain Cognition, 26: 174-180.

St-Marseille A, Braun CM. (1994). Comments on immune aspects of the Geschwind-Behan-Galaburda model and of the article of Bryden, McManus, and Bulman-Fleming. Brain Cognition, 26: 281-290.

Tønnessen FE. (1997). Testosterone and dyslexia. [Review]. Developmental Neurorehabilitation, 1: 51-58.

Tønnessen FE, Høien T, Lundberg I, Larsen JP. (1994). Immune disorders and dyslexia. Reading and Writing, 6: 151-160.

Vincent A, Deacon R, Dalton P, Salmond C, Bramire AM, Pendlebury S, Johansen-Berg H, Rajogopalan B, Styles P, Stein JF. (2002). Maternal Antibody mediated dyslexia? Evidence for a pathogenic serum factor in a mother of 2 dyslexic children shown by transfer to pregnant mice using behavioural and MRS studies. Journal of Neuroimmunology, 45: 87- 89.

Chapter IV

Inheritance

Undoubtedly, developmental dyslexia is a disease with hereditary features so that a genetic anomaly in one or both parents can be transmitted to the child, making him unable to read fluently [DeFries et al., 1987; Pennington & Smith, 1988; Scarborough, 1989; Snowling, 1991; Olson et al., 1994].

An important evidence for the genetic factor is provided by the analysis of the distribution of lexical performance in homozygous and heterozygous twins (of the twins only one is dyslexic), compared to the normal population [DeFries et al., 1987]. As a starting point, it is assumed that the frequency distribution peak referred to the reading ability of the homozygous twins of dyslexics localizes more on the left (i.e. worse) compared to the peak referred to heterozygous twins of dyslexics, which in turn is on the left compared to the peak of normal readers. When the mean lexical performance of the homozygous and heterozygous dyslexic twins is the same, a significant difference in the lexical function between the two populations composed by their respective twin brothers (homozygous and heterozygous, respectively) suggests a genetic influence in our clinical condition [DeFries et al., 1987].

A different approach is based on a multiple regression paradigm applied to the two classes. The model has been tested in 64 homozygote twins and 55 heterozygote twins and confirmed the presence of a hereditary component with a degree of penetrance of about 30% [DeFries et al., 1987]. For other authors, the percentage is higher and ranges from 40 to 80% [Pennington & Smith, 1988; Olson et al., 1989; Pennington, 1991; Olson, 2002; Plomin & Kovas, 2005].

Transmission modality is autosomal dominant, so that if one of the two parents is dyslexic, their children have 50% chance of inheriting the predisposition to the disease, which rises to 100% if both parents are affected [Stein & Talcott, 1999].

Indeed, familiarity is one of the most important risk factors: population studies estimated that 23% to 65% of dyslexic children are sons of a dyslexic [Scarborough, 1998] and that in 73% of cases they have one or more dyslexic relatives [Norn et al., 1969]. Moreover, the son of a dyslexic has an estimated risk of developing the disease of 40-60%: such a risk increases if there are other dyslexics in his/her family [Schumacher et al., 2007].

In addition, 40% of siblings of dyslexics are dyslexic and from 27% to 49% of the parents of affected children when subsequently examined would turn out to be dyslexic [Pennington & Gilger, 1996].

The most representative genetic studies based on samples of American, Canadian, British families and one German family focused on the short arm (*q*) of chromosome 6 [Cardon et al., 1994; Grigorenko et al., et al., 1997, 2000; Petryshen et al., 2001]. On the *q* arm of chromosome 6 at locus 22 are found two genes strongly suspected to be associated with the disease[25]: gene DCDC2 and gene K1AA0319. Interestingly, the first is widely expressed in cortical regions that show abnormal activation in patients, as the inferotemporal and the mediotemporal area [Horwitz et al., 1998; Shaywitz et al., 1998; Meng et al., 2005; Schumacher et al., 2006; Silanes et al., 2005]. Studies in rats showed that a depression of this genetic expression reduces neuronal migration [Meng et al., 2005], an event that would account for the reported ectopy in the brains of patients (see chapter 2). The same applies to the gene K1AA0319 [Paracchini et al., 2006]. It is noteworthy the finding on the chromosome 6 (locus p 21.3) of specific genes for the magnocellular system [Prasad et al., 1997]: indeed, magnocellular dysfunctions (as we will discuss hereinafter) are argued to be an aetiopathogenetical key factor of developmental dyslexia. Under particular surveillance are also chromosome 15 [Grigorenko et al., 1997; Schulte-Körne et al., 1998; Nopola-Hemmi et al., 2000], that seems to be involved in single words reading, chromosome 1 [Grigorenko et al., 2001], chromosome 2 [Fagerheim et al., 1999] and chromosome 3 [Knob-Hemmi et al., 2001] (Figure 1).

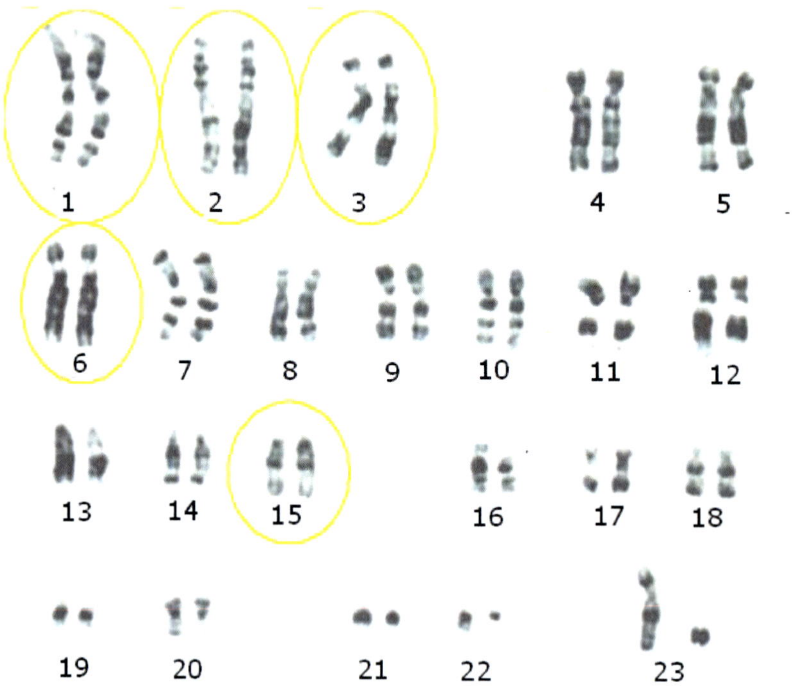

Figure 1. The human genome. In evidence are the chromosomes involved in the hereditary transmission of developmental dyslexia.

[25] According to Grigorenko, chromosome 6 is responsible only for the phonological performance [Grigorenko et al., 1997], while for Stein it accounts also for the orthographic function [Stein, 2001].

According to Stein, there are at least three genes responsible, one in charge for the phonological ability, another for the spelling ability, and the third for both [Stein, 2001]: this position supports those researchers who believe that dyslexic subjects have to be classified into subtypes with prevailing phonological, orthographic or mixed factors.

In conclusion, the genetic component is undoubtedly a major aetiological factor in developmental dyslexia; however, it seems to have more to do with the phonological aspects than with the visuoperceptive ones [Ho & Decker, 1988; Pennington & Smith, 1988; Scarborough, 1989; Castles et al., 1999].

It is likely that in some cases the familiarity for reading disabilities matches the familiarity for those slight alterations of visual perception that, as we will discuss hereinafter, have a role in a substantial proportion of patients.

References

Cardon LR, Smith SD, Fulker DW, Kimberling WJ, Pennington BF, Defries JC. (1994). *Quantitative trait locus for reading disability on chromosome 6.* Science, 266: 276-279.

Castles A, Datta H, Gayan J, Olson RK. (1999). *Varieties of developmental reading disorder: genetic and environmental influences.* Journal of Experimental Child Psychology, 72: 73-94.

DeFries J, Fulker DW, La Buda MC. (1987). *Evidence for a genetic aetiology in reading disability of twins.* Nature, 329 : 537-539.

Fagerheim T, Raeymaekers P, Tønnessen FE, Pedersen M, Tranebjaerg L, Lubs HA. (1999). *A new gene (DYX3) fpr dyslexia is located on chromosome 2.* Journal of Medical Genetics, 36 : 664-669.

Grigorenko EL, Wood FB, Meyer MS, Hart LA, Speed WC, Shuster A, Pauls DL. (1997). *Susceptibility loci for distinct components of developmental dyslexia on chromosome 6 and 15.* The American Journal of Human Genetics, 60: 27-39.

Grigorenko EL, Wood FB, Meyer MS, Pauls DL. (2000). *Chromosome 6p Influences on Different Dyslexia-Related Cognitive Processes: Further Confirmation.* The American Journal of Human Genetics, 66: 715-723.

Grigorenko EL, Wood FB, Meyer MS, Pauls JE, Hart LA, Pauls DL. (2001). *Linkage studies suggest a possible locus for developmental dyslexia on chromosome 1p.* American Journal of Medical Genetics, 105: 120-129.

Ho HZ, Decker SN. (1988). *Cognitive resemblance in reading-disabled twins.* Developmental Medicine & Child Neurology, 30: 99-107.

Horwitz B, Rumsey JM, Donohue BC. (1998). *Functional connectivity of the angular gyrus in normal reading and dyslexia.* Proceedings of the National Academy of Sciences of the United States of America, 95: 8939-8944.

Meng H, Smith SD, Hager K, Held M, Liu J, Olson RK, Pennington BF, DeFries JC, Gelernter J, O'Reilly-Pol T, Somlo S, Skudlarski P, Shaywitz SE, Shaywitz BA, Marchione K, Wang Y, Paramasivam M, LoTurco JJ, Page GP, Gruen JR. (2005). *DCDC2 in associated with reading disability and modulates neuronal development in the brain.* Proceedings of the National Academy of Sciences of the United States of America, 102: 17053-17058.

Nopola-Hemmi J, Taipale M, Haltia T, Lehesjoki AE, Voutilainen A, Kere J. (2000). *Two translocations of chromosome 15q associated with dyslexia.* Journal of Medical Genetics, 37: 771-775.

Nopola-Hemmi J, Myllyluoma B, Haltia T, Taipale M, Ollikainen V, Ahonen T, Voutilainen A, Kere J, Widén E. (2001). *A dominant gene for developmental dyslexia on chromosome 3.* Journal of Medical Genetics, 38: 658-664.

Norn MS, Rindziunski E, Skydsgaard H. (1969). *Ophthalmologic and orthoptic examinations of dyslectics.* Acta Ophthalmologica, 47: 147-160.

Olson KK, Wise B, Conners F, Rack J, Fulker D. (1989). *Specific deficits in component reading and language skills- genetic and environmental influences.* Journal of Learning Disabilities, 22: 339-348.

Olson RK. (2002). *Dyslexia: nature and nurture.* Dyslexia, 8: 143-159.

Olson RK, Forsberg H, Wise B. (1994). *Genes, environment, and the development of orthographic skills.* In The varieties of orthographic knowledge I: Theoretical and developmental issues. V.W.Bergingher Ed., Dordrecht: Kluwer.

Paracchini S, Thomas A, Castro S, Lai C, Paramasivam M, Wang Y, Keating BJ, Taylor JM, Hacking DF, Scerri T, Francks C, Richardson AJ, Wade-Martins R, Stein JF, Knight JC, Copp AJ, Loturco J, Monaco AP. (2006). *The chromosome 6p22 haplotype associated with dyslexia reduces the expression of K1AA0319, a novel gene involved in neuronal migration.* Human Molecular Genetics, 15: 1659-1666.

Pennington BF. (1991). *Reading Disabilities: Genetic and Neurological Influences.* Pennington Ed., Kluwer: Dordrecht.

Pennington BF, Smith SD. (1988). *Genetic influences on learning disabilities: An update.* Journal of Consulting & Clinical Psychology, 56: 817-823.

Pennington BF, Gilger JW. (1996). *How is dyslexia transmitted?* In: Developmental dyslexia: neural, cognitive, and genetic mechanisms. Chase, Rosen, Sherman Eds., Baltimore: New York Press, New York.

Petryshen TL, Kaplan BJ, Fu Liu M, de French NS, Tobias R, Hughes ML, Field LL. (2001). *Evidence for a susceptibility locus on chromosome 6q influencing phonological coding dyslexia.* American Journal of Medical Genetics, 105: 507-517.

Plomin R, Kovas Y. (2005). *Generalist genes and learning disabilities.* Psychological Bulletin, 131: 592-617.

Prasad SS, Chaudhuri A, Cynader MS. (1997). *Toward the identification of a dyslexia gene: defining magnocellular layer-specific genes within the 6P21.3 region of human chromosome 6* [Abstract]. Society of Neuroscience, 23: 1626.

Scarborough HS. (1989). *Prediction of reading disability from familial and individual differences.* Journal of Educational Psychology, 81: 101-108.

Scarborough, H. S. (1998). *Early identification of children at risk for reading disabilities: Phonological awareness and some other promising predictors.* In: Specific reading disability: A view of the spectrum, Shapiro, Accardo, & Capute Eds., Timonium, MD: York Press, New York.

Schulte-Körne G, Grimm T, Nöthen MM, Müller-Myhsok B, Cichon S, Vogt IR, P Propping P, Remschmidt H. (1998). *Evidence for linkage of spelling disability to chromosome 15.* The American Journal of Human Genetics, 63: 279-282.

Schumacher J, Anthoni H, Dahdouh F, König IR, Hillmer AM, Kluck N, Manthey M, Plume E, Warnke A, Remschmidt H, Hülsmann J, Cichon S, Lindgren CM, Propping P,

Zucchelli M, Ziegler A, Peyrard-Janvid M, Schulte-Körne G, Nöthen MM, Kere J. (2006). *Strong genetic evidence of DCDC2 as a susceptibility gene for dyslexia.* The American Journal of Human Genetics, 78: 52-62.

Schumacher J, Hoffmann P, Schmäl C, Schulte-Körne G, Nöthen MM. (2007). *Genetics of dyslexia: the evolving landscape.* Journal of Medical Genetics, 44: 289-297.

Shaywitz SE, Shaywitz BA, Pugh KR, Fulbright RK, Constable RT, Mencl WE, Shankweiler DP, Liberman AM, Skudlarski P, Fletcher JM, Katz L, Marchione KE, Lacadie C, Gatenby C, Gore JC. (1998). *Functional disruption in the organization of the brain for reading in dyslexia.* Proceedings of the National Academy of Sciences of the United States of America, 95: 2636-2641.

Silani G, Frith U, Demonet JF, Fazio F, Perani D, Price C, Frith CD, Paulesu E. (2005). *Brain abnormalities underlying altered activation in dyslexia: a voxel based morphometry study*. Brain, 128: 2453-2461.

Snowling M. (1991). *Developmental reading disorders*. Journal of Child Psychology & Psychiatry, 32: 49-77.

Stein JF, Talcott J. (1999). *Impaired neuronal timing in developmental dyslexia-the magnocellular hypothesis.* Dyslexia, 5: 59- 77.

Stein JF. (2001). *The magnocellular theory of developmental dyslexia.* Dyslexia, 7: 12-36.

Chapter V

The Revival of the Visuoperceptive Hypothesis

It is paradoxical that although developmental dyslexia was originally defined as *word blindness* and officially recognized as a clinical entity by two ophthalmologists, according to the arguments reported so far it looks as if it had little or nothing to do with the visual system [Frith & Frith, 1996; Shaywitz, 1996]: on the contrary, it seems to depend exclusively on linguistic deficits. Actually, the fact that eyes impairments do not hinder the ability to learn to read[26] [Norn et al., 1969; Hammemberg & Norn, 1972; Aasved 1987; Ygge et al., 1993a, b] gives evidence in favor of a phonological solution: for example children wearing contact lens after cataract surgery do not show reading problems with appropriate correction for close distance, as well as patients affected by congenital nystagmus [Lennerstrand &Ygge, 1992]. Refractive defects, too, are irrelevant: there are no differences in reading skills of myopic and hypermetropic children[27] followed since their birth [Williams et al., 1988], and simulating hyperopia by means of negative lenses may reduce the speed but not the accuracy of reading in normal volunteers [Garcia et al., 1989].

The prevalence of hyperopia is higher among dyslexics [Evans & Drasdo 1990], who in fact wear glasses with a double frequency compared to normal readers [Norn et al., 1969; Evans & Drasdo 1990]. However, this finding reflects the tendency of ophthalmologists to correct even small and insignificant refractive defects, when found in these patients [Norn et al., 1969]. In summary, no correlation between refractive defects and lexical performance has been proved in dyslexics [Norn et al., 1969; Aasved, 1987, 1988; Ygge et al., 1993a].

Results gathered from population studies exclude statistically significant differences in binocular function, visual acuity, convergence, accommodation, stereopsis, anisometropia, fusional amplitudes for far and close distance, color perception and eye's anterior segment anatomical alterations. [Norn et al., 1969; Helvestone, 1985; Aasved, 1988; Evans & Drasdo, 1990; Hall & Wick, 1991; Grisham et al., 1993; Ygge et al., 1993a,b; Evans et al., 1994; Lightstone & Evans, 1995; Olitsky & Nelson, 2003].

---

[26] Provided the characters print size is suitable for the discrimination capacity.
[27] Age: 7-11 years.

Norn found in a sample of 117 dyslexics a high rate of latent strabismus, in particular exophorias and hyperphorias[28], at near (30 cm). These conditions, however, are normalized by a considerable fusional power: therefore do not affect the lexical function [Norn et al., 1969].

No link is found between dyslexia and strabismus [Cassin, 1975]: on the contrary, the prevalence of dyslexia in children with strabismus is even lower than in normal population [Benton et al., 1965; Norn et al., 1969; Park & Barry, 1984].

Likewise, no connection is found between convergence deficiency on the one hand and lexical function or dyslexia on the other [Evans & Drasdo 1990; Eden et al., 1994; Morad et al., 2002]: therefore, dyslexics treated for concomitant binocular dysfunctions would improve as to these but not in their reading ability [Norn et al., 1969; Aasved, 1988].

Even if in dyslexics affected by phonological problems defective divergence of the visual axes is often reported, such an anomaly is not specific for dyslexia and can be present even in subjects with a reading delay associated with reduced IQ [Eden et al., 1994].

In confirmation of the lack of links between dyslexia and visual problems, after the latter have been cured the lexical function does not improve [Granet et al., 2006].

In contrast, great importance has been attributed to the linguistic-phonological mechanism, since a substantial proportion of dyslexics show signs of dysphasia or are not skilled in tasks that require rapid naming and speech articulation [Korhonen, 1995; Heilman et al., 1996]: and yet, it has to be explained why many dyslexics are not dysphasics and why many disphasics are not dyslexics [Habib, 2000].

Although many researchers believe that a phonological problem underlying our clinical condition can be detected in all patients, in certain cases (rare cases according to Pirozzolo and Rayner, 1988) visuoperceptive anomalies, far different from those commonly investigated in the clinical ophthalmological practice, are admitted being an aggravating factor [Trauzettel-Klosinski et al., 2002; MacKeben et al., 2004].

Indeed, despite the substantial negativity of the ophthalmological, orthoptic and refractive examinations, in many dyslexics the presence of visual symptoms and signs cannot be denied: for example, the sensation letters and words tangle with each other, overlap, and move. Moreover, the confusion between syllables and between mirror characters (as *p* and *q* or the *b* and *d*) is frequently reported. It has been therefore supposed that some patients, despite being clinically normal during an ophthalmologic examination, could conceal a fine visuoperceptive unbalance, too slight and specific to be discovered during a routine checkup.

In recent decades this possibility has renewed the interest for a visual approach of the disease so that, besides the traditional speculative line, which keeps on denying any neurophtalmological influence on the aetiopathogenetical level, a second current got developing, which instead suggests the roots of the disease to be placed even in the visual areas of the cerebral cortex.

In 1995 Cornelissen wrote on Vision Research that contrary to the opinions previously expressed by Vellutino and others, research in the last decade showed evidence that dyslexics behave differently from normal readers as regards visual tasks [Cornelissen et al., 1995].

Two years later, Stein and Walsh underlined that the phonological problems in dyslexics do not explain the plethora of other problems affecting children with specific reading

[28] Exophoria and hyperhoria refer to the tendency of the visual axes to diverge along the horizontal or vertical plane, respectively.

disability. In fact, such patients tend to transpose letters and to produce non-words (i.e. phonologically implausible strings of letters) that seem to stem from visual confusion [Stein & Walsh, 1997].

With these strong impressions, the novel speculative position has pinpointed the large amount of visuoperceptive alterations found in dyslexics and has ascribed them to a defect occurring in a particular cerebral ganglion system: the so-called magnocellular or M-system.

The Role of the Magno-and Parvocellular Image Processing

The image processing which begins in the retina and continues on the occipital cortex, is provided by two distinct cellular pathways: the *parvocellular system* or *P-system*, made of small ganglion cells arranged in receptive fields[29] of small size and the *magnocellular system* or *M system*, organized in wider receptive fields made of larger ganglion cells.

Magnocells make up the 10% of the total ganglion cell population [Shapley & Perry, 1986].

On the retina, parvocells localize mainly in the central region (the macular area) and serve for the recognition of stimuli that are directed to or immediately around the fixation point, while the magnocells are placed more peripherally [Hoffmann et al., 1972]. The topographical transition from one quota to another across the retina occurs in a progressive manner.

The overall amount of P cells, however, exceeds the amount of the M cells even in the periphery, constituting 90% of the total ganglion neurons on the retina [Silveira & Perry, 1991] but the receptive fields of the latter cover a retinal surface 10 times wider [Stein, 2003].

Each of these two systems project to specific regions in the lateral geniculate nucleus (LGN)[30].

In the LGN, parvocells synaptically connect with their correspondent ganglion neurons located in the four dorsal layers while the magnocells connect with the larger ganglion cells placed in the two most ventral layers (Figure 1).

The transmission of the visual input from the lateral geniculate body continues and reaches the complex and hypercomplex[31] cells of the striate cortex, keeping the information processed by each of the two systems as separate [Kaplan et al., 1990; Merigan & Maunsell, 1993], and from here to the extrastriate cortex.

From the area 17 (V1), the P- and M- systems projects via areas 18 (V2) and 19 (V3) to the inferotemporal region and the mediotemporal area (MT or V5), respectively. The

---

[29] The receptive field is the elementary functional entity of the primary sensory systems. In the retinal visual system, receptive fields are made of a number of photoreceptors that (indirectly, via bipolar cells) converge on a (usually) smaller number of ganglion cells. This functional entity subdivides the stimulus into its single features, emphasizing the contrast, and transfers them to the cerebral cortex. On the cortex, other and more complex receptive fields re-arrange the features and ensure the completion of the analysis.

[30] The lateral geniculate nucleus (or lateral geniculate body) is a relay station along the visual pathway, between the optic nerve and the visual cortex. The lateral geniculate body is made of receptive fields resembling those present in the retina.

[31] In particular, both the M- and P axons project to the lamina IV of the area17 (M- cells: lamina IVαc and IVb; P-cells: lamina IVa and IVcβ [Movshon & Newsome, 1996].

magnocellular pathways extends also to the posterior parietal cortex (PPC), considered an important visuo-attentive centre [Livingstone & Hubel, 1988; Vidyasagar, 1999: Figure 2].

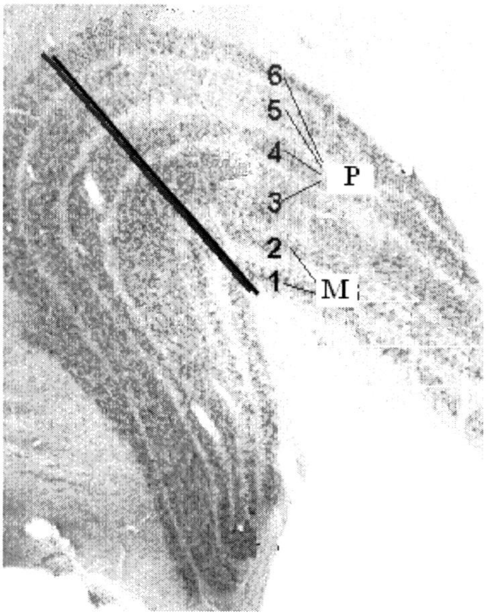

Figure 1. The lateral geniculate body. To be noted the division into six layers, the two more ventral are made up of M cells, the four more dorsal of P cells

The two systems are responsible for specific perceptive tasks that have been extensively investigated [Breitmeyer, 1975; Breitmeyer & Ganz, 1976; Stone et al., 1979; Breitmeyer, 1980; Livingstone & Hubel, 1987, 1988]:

- cells belonging to the P system are responsive for the whole duration of the stimulus. Since their axons are scarcely myelinated, parvocells show low conduction speed. For this reason the P system is referred to as "*sustained system*".
  Parvocells show best contrast sensitivity at high spatial frequencies and low temporal frequencies, especially in photopic conditions. This fact makes them suitable for the analysis of the details of images projected onto the foveal region and unsuitable for the detection of temporal changes (motion perception).
- on the contrary, the M system is responsible for the analysis of global configurations and in particular for motion perception. Especially under conditions of low luminance, in fact, the M system shows higher contrast sensitivity at low spatial frequencies and high temporal frequencies, which makes it less sensitive to details and highly sensitive to rapid changes over time [Purpura et al., 1988; Lee et al., 1997]. Due to their thick myelination, M-axons show high conduction speed. For

these reasons, the M system is defined "*transient system*"[32] and as such is particularly sensitive to motion detection and to the so-called visual persistence time[33].

M-cells show a peak of discharge when a light stimulus appears, followed by an abrupt drop of the response to its disappearance.

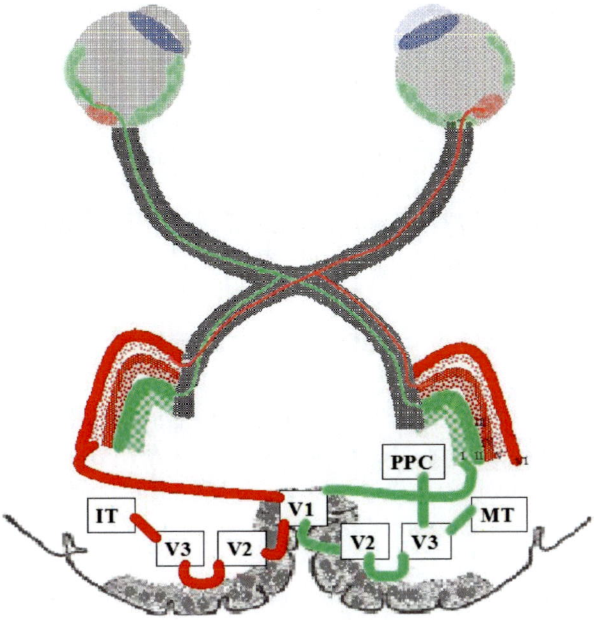

Figure 2. Schematic representation of the visual pathway. In red is the parvocellular system starting from the small retinal ganglion cells, mainly localized in the central region (the fovea), organized in receptive fields of small size and suitable for processing fine details of a stimulus. The fibers of each P cell are collected in the optic nerve and meet with those of the contralateral eye in the optic chiasm. Here, the outermost portion (temporal) continues its course in the homolateral optic tract while the remaining inner fibers (nasal) cross those of the other side (decussation) and then continue in the contralateral optic tract. At the end of the optic tract both nasal and temporal parvocellular axons project to the lateral geniculate body, a layered structure made up of P cells in the more dorsal portions (layer III, IV, V, VI). Here the transmission of the parvocellular input is transferred to the geniculate P cells and finally reaches the striate cortex, area V1, via the optical radiation. From V1 the stimulus continues in V2, V3 and eventually in the inferotemporal area.
In green is the magnocellular pathway beginning from big retinal ganglion cells, mainly localized in the peripheral areas, organized in large receptive fields and suitable to process the stimulus configuration as a whole and in particular movement perception.
The M projections are similar to those described for the P pathway: magnocellular fibers gather in the optic nerve, reach the chiasm where the nasal portion decussates while the temporal one remains on the same side and meets with those of the contralateral eye.
From the right and left optic tract, M fibers get to the more ventral layers of the lateral geniculate body (layer I-II). Here the impulse is elaborated by M geniculate receptive fields, along the optical radiations it reaches the striate cortex, area V1, then V2, V3 and finally the mediotemporal area (MT or V5) and the posterior parietal cortex (PPC).

[32] As pointed out by Skottun [2000], the terms *magnocellular* and *parvocellular* belong to the physiological field, whereas in psychophysics it would be preferable to refer to them as *sustained* and *transient*. However, the words *magnocellular* and *parvocellular*, introduced in the psychophysical literature on dyslexia in 1991 by Livingstone, are now customary.

[33] Visual persistence accounts for the apparent motion, which is the principle underlying the cinematography.

Even if the attention of researchers has focused on contrast, movement and visual persistence time, dyslexic are found to suffer even from other perceptual defects in charge of the transient system: for example stereopsis [Stein, 1988], illusory perception of edges [Hubel & Livingstone, 1987, 1988], figure-ground segregation [Livingstone & Coll, 1991], orientation discrimination between two lines [Eden et al., 1996], and spatial location [Stein et al., 1989, Solman & May, 1990].

Basically, the supporters of the visuoperceptive impairment in dyslexics pinpointed three defective functions pertaining to the transient pathway: reduced contrast sensitivity to low spatial frequencies and high temporal frequencies, deficit in motion perception and abnormally high visual persistence time. Such anomalies would be the sign that the M system of dyslexics is compromised so that their lexical difficulty[34] would be related to this malfunction.

On this basis the *theory of the deficit of the magnocellular system* has been formulated.

References

Aasved H. (1987). *Ophthalmological status of school children with dyslexia.* Eye, 1: 61-68.

Aasved H. (1988). *Øyenundersøkelser. Bergenprojektet III. Studier av barn med dysleksi og andre laerevansker.* Gjessing, Nygaard & Solheim Eds., Universitetsforlaget, Oslo.

Benton CD, McCann JW, Larsen M. (1965). *Dyslexia and dominance.* Journal of Pediatric Ophthalmology, 2: 53-57.

Breitmeyer BG. (1975). *Simple reaction time as a measure of the temporal response properties of transient and sustained channels.* Vision Research, 15: 1411-1414.

Breitmeyer BG. (1980). *Unmasking visual masking: a look at the "why" behind the veil of "how".* Psychological Review, 87: 52-69.

Breitmeyer BG, Ganz L. (1976). *Implications of sustained and transient channels for theories of visual pattern masking, saccadic suppression, and information processing.* Psychological Review, 83: 1-36.

Cassin B. (1975). *Strabismus and learning disabilities.* American Orthoptic Journal, 25: 38-45.

Cornelissen PL, Richardson AR, Mason A, Fowler MS, Stein JF. (1995). *Contrast sensitivity and coherent motion detection measured at photopic luminance levels in dyslexics and controls.* Vision Research, 35: 1483-1494.

Eden GF, Stein JF, Wood MH, Wood FB. (1994). *Differences in eye movements and reading problems in dyslexics and normal children.* Vision Research, 34: 1345-1358.

Eden GF, Stein JF, Wood HM, Wood FB. (1996). *Visuospatial judgement in reading disabled and normal children.* Perceptual and Motor Skills, 82: 155-177.

Evans BJW, Drasdo N. (1990). Review of ophthalmic factors in dyslexia. Ophthalmic & Physiological Optics, 10: 123-132.

[34] Even if the role of the M- and P systems during reading is still contradictory, it is revealing that reading a colored text on a (differently) colored isoluminant background (a condition enhancing the P-system activity, and minimizing the M-activity) generally is more difficult than in the ordinary codition (dark text on a white background) [Livingstone & Hubel, 1987].

Evans BJW, Drasdo N, and Richards IL. (1994). *Investigation of accommodative and binocular function in dyslexia.* Ophthalmic & Physiological Optics, 145: 5-20.

Frith C, Frith U. (1996). *A biological marker for dyslexia.* Nature, 382: 19-20.

Garzia RP, Nicholson SB, Gaines CS, Murphy MA, Kramer A, Potts J. (1989). *Effects of nearpoint visual stress on psycholinguistic processing in reading.* Journal of the American Optometric Association, 60: 38-44.

Granet DB, Castro EF, Gomi CF. (2006). *Reading: do the eyes have it?* American Orthoptic Journal, 56: 44-49.

Grisham JD, Sheppard MM, Tran WU. (1993). *Visual symptoms and reading performance.* Optometry & Vision Science, 70: 384-391.

Habib M. (2000). *The neurological basis of developmental dyslexia. An overview and working hypothesis.* Brain, 123: 2373-2399.

Hall S, Wick B. (1991). *The relationship between ocular functions and reading achievement.* Journal of Pediatric Ophthalmology & Strabismus, 28: 17-19.

Hammemberg E, Norn MS. (1972). *Defective dissociation of accommodation and convergence in dyslectic children.* Acta Ophthalmologica, 50: 651-654.

Heilman KM, Voeller K, Alexandew AW. (1996). *Developmental dyslexia: a motor-articulatory feedback hypothesis.* Annals of Neurology, 39: 407-412.

Helvestone ME. (1985). *Visual function and academic performance.* American Journal of Ophtalmology, 99: 346-355.

Hoffman KP, Stone J, Sherman SM. (1972). *Relay of receptive-field properties in dorsal lateral geniculate nucleus of the cat.* Journal of Neurophysiology, 35: 518-531.

Kaplan E, Lee BB,Shapley RM. (1990). *New views of primate retinal function.* Progress in Retinal Research, 9: 273-336.

Korhonen TT. (1995). *The persistence of rapid naming problems in children with reading disabilities: a nine-year follow-up.* Journal of Learning Disabilities, 28: 232-239.

Lee BB, Smith VC, Pokorny J, Kremers J. (1997). *Rod Inputs to macaque ganglion cells.* Vision Research, 37: 2813-2828.

Lennerstrand G, Ygge J. (1992). *Dyslexia: ophthalmological aspects 1991.* Acta Ophthalmologica, 70: 3-13.

Lightstone A, Evans BJW. (1995). *A new protocol for the optometric management of patients with reading difficulties.* Ophthalmic and Physiological Optics, 15: 507-512.

Livingstone M, Hubel D. (1987). *Psychophysical evidence for separate channels for the perception of form, color and movement, and depth.* The Journal of Neuroscience, 7: 3416-3468.

Livingstone M & Hubel D. (1988). *Segregation of form, color movement, and dept: anatomy, physiology, and perception.* Science, 240: 740-749.

Livingstone MS, Rosen GD, Drislane FW, Galaburda AM. (1991). *Physiological and anatomical evidence for a magnocellular defect in developmental dyslexia.* Proceedings of the National Academy of Sciences of the United States of America, 88: 7943-7947.

MacKeben M, Trauzettel-Klosinski S, Reinhard J, Dürrwächter U, Adler M, Klosinski G. (2004). *Eye movement control during single-word reading in dyslexics.* Journal of Vision, 4: 388-402.

Merigan WH, Maunsell JHR. (1993). *How parallel are the human visual pathways?* Annual Review of Neuroscience, 16: 369-402.

Morad Y, Lederman R, Avni I, Atzmon D, Azoulay E, Segal O. (2002). *Correlation between reading skills and different meauserements of convergence amplitude.* Current Eye Research, 25: 117-121.

Movs.hon JA, Newsome WT. (1996). *Visual response properties of striate cortical neurons projecting to area MT in macaque monkeys.* Journal of Neuroscience, 16: 7733-7741.

Norn MS, Rindziunski E, Skydsgaard H. (1969). *Ophthalmologic and orthoptic examinations of dyslectics.* Acta Ophthalmologica, 47: 147-160.

Olitsky SE, Nelson LB. (2003). *Reading disorders in children.* Pediatric Clinics of North America, 50: 213-224.

Park GE & Barry C. (1984). *Eye maturations and reading dificulties.* Journal of Educational Psychology, 12: 535-545.

Pirozzolo FJ, Rayner K. (1988). *Dyslexia, the role of eye movements in developmental reading disabilities.* In: Neuropsychology of Eye Movements. Johnston &.Pirozzolo EDS., Lawrence Eribaum Associates, Hillsdale, New Jersey.

Purpura K, Kaplan E, Shapley RM. (1988). *Background light and the contrast gain of primate P and M retinal ganglion cells.* Proceedings of the National Academy of Sciences of the United States of America, 85: 4534-4537.

Shapley R, Perry VH. (1986). *Cat and monkey retinal ganglion cells and their functional roles.* Trends in Neuroscience, 9: 229-235.

Shaywitz SE. (1996). *Dyslexia.* Scientific American, 275: 98-104.

Silveira LCL, Perry VH. (1991). *The topography of magnocellular projecting ganglion cells (M-ganglion cells) in the primate retina.* Neuroscience, 40: 217-237

Solman RT, May JG. (1990). *Spatial localization discrepancies: A visual deficiency in poor readers.* American Journal of Psychology, 103: 243-263.

Stein JF. (1988). *Aphasia.* Rose Ed., London.

Stein JF, Riddell PM, Fowler S. (1989). *Brain and Reading.* Von Euler, Lundberg & Lennerstrand Eds., Stockton, New York.

Stein JF, Walsh V. (1997). *To see but not to read: the magnocellular theory of dyslexia.* Trends in Neuroscience, 20: 147-152.

Stein JF. (2003). *Visual motion sensitivity and reading.* Neuropsychologia, 41: 1785-1793.

Stone J, Dreer B, Leventhal A. (1979). *Hierarchical and parallel mechanisms in the organization of the visual cortex.* Brain Research Reviews, 1: 345-349.

Trauzettel-Klosinski S, MacKeben M, Reinhard J, Feucht A, Dürrwächter U, Klosinski G. (2002). *Pictoral naming in dyslexic and normal children assessed by SLO.* Vision Research, 42: 789-799.

Vidyasagar TR. (1999). *A neural model of attentional spotlight: parietal guiding the temporal.* Brain Research Review, 30: 66-76.

Williams SM,, Sanderson GF, Share DL, Silva PA. (1988). *Refractive error, IQ and reading ability: A longitudinal study from age seven to 11.* Developmental Medicine & Child Neurology, 30: 735-742.

Ygge J, Lennerstrand G, Axelsson I, Rydberg A, Wijecoon S, Pettersson BM. (1993a). *Visual functions and oculomotor functions in a Swedish population of 9-year-old dyslexics and normal readers.* Acta Ophthalmologica, 71: 1-9.

Ygge J, Lennerstrand G, Rydberg A, Wijecoon S, Pettersson BM. (1993b). *Oculomotor functions in a Swedish population of dyslexic and normally reading children.* Acta Ophthalmologica, 71: 10-21.

Chapter VI

Contrast Sensitivity and Dyslexia

As discussed in the previous chapter, the anatomofunctional organization of the visual system is based on two cellular pathways: the M and P system.

The M system is in charge of the analysis of dynamic configurations: for this reason its contrast sensitivity is better for stimuli in the low spatial and high temporal frequency domain, especially at low luminance levels [Lee et al., 1997; Purpura et al., 1988]. An example of a stimulus suitable to the M system is a grating made of large dark and white bars, shifting in one direction or reversing alternatively their positions (*pattern reversal*).

On the contrary, the P system is aimed at processing details of static stimuli; contrast sensitivity of the parvocellular system, in fact, is at its best for stimuli in the high spatial and low temporal frequency domain, especially in photopic (high luminance) conditions. An example of a suitable stimulus to the P system is a static grating made of dark and white narrow bars.

Therefore, contrast sensitivity is usually measured by means of gratings. Luminance between adjoining bars is modulated by a sinusoidal function, as the luminance of a white bar is at its maximum along its central axis, decreases progressively towards its boundaries and reaches its minimum along the central axis of the black bar.

For this reason this kind of gratings, commonly used in psychophysics, are defined *sinusoidal gratings* and their spatial frequency is given as the number of cycles in the unit of space[35]. Keeping the size of the grating constant, the greater the number of cycles, the greater its spatial frequency (Figure 1).

The contrast of a grating characterized by a specific spatial frequency is expressed as the ratio between the difference of luminance of the darkest part of the black bars and the lightest part of the white bars divided by their sum (fraction of Michelson):

$$\text{contrast} = (L_{min} - L_{max}) / (L_{min} + L_{max}).$$

[35] A cycle corresponds to a pair of white/black bars. Since visual space is generally measured as angular value (deg or minarc), spatial frequencies are quantified in cycles per degree (c/deg).

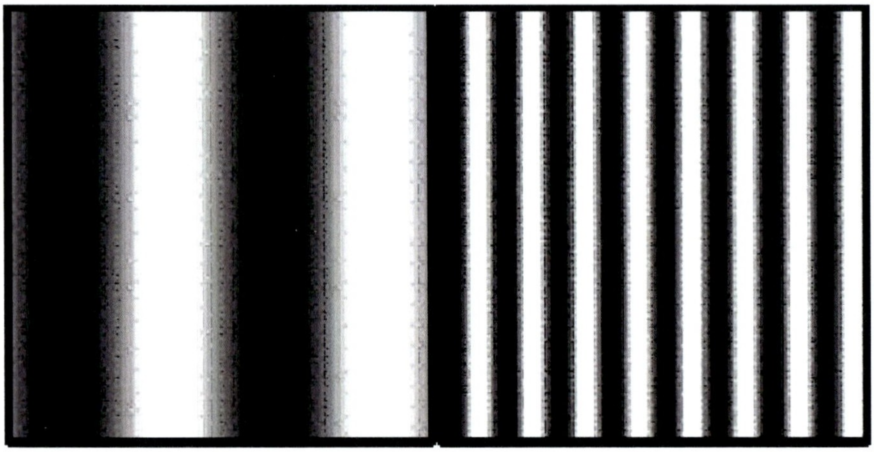

Figure 1. Two examples of sinusoidal grating. Left: low spatial frequency, right: high spatial frequency.

Contrast threshold at a given spatial frequency is the least amount of contrast needed for the individual bars of the grating to be recognizable.

Contrast sensitivity is the reciprocal of contrast threshold (1/contrast threshold) and the change of contrast sensitivity as a function of spatial frequency, called *contrast sensitivity function* (CSF) is shown in the left panel of Figure 2.

The curve depicted in figure 2 (left panel) is the result of the joined activity of the M system, mainly effective at the lowest spatial frequencies and of the P system, especially sensitive to the highest spatial frequencies. The cutoff from the P/M function in the spatial frequency domain is set around 1.5 cycles/degree [Legge, 1978][36]

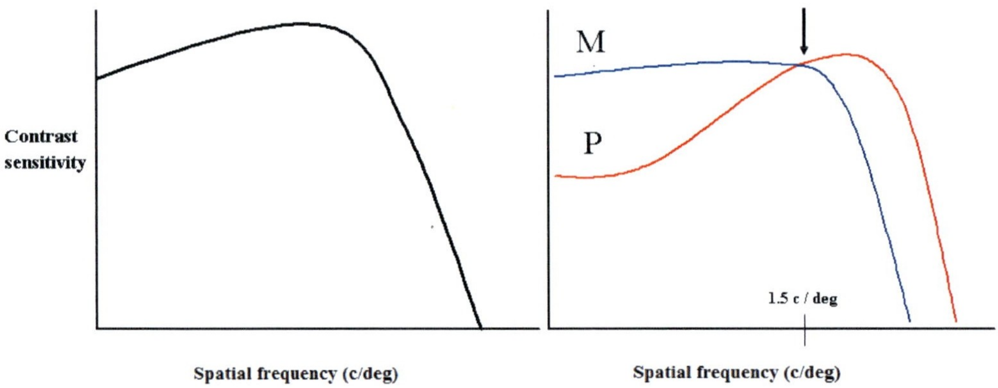

Figure 2. Left: CSF for spatial frequencies from 0.75 cycles/degree to 18 cycles/degree. Right: individual CSF of the M- and P system, sensitive to low and high spatial frequencies, respectively. The transition point is set around 1.5 cycles/degree and marked by the arrow. Above this value of spatial frequency, the P system is mainly active, under this value it depends on the M system (*Modified reprint from: Vision Research, Vol. 40, Issue 1, Skottun BC, The magnocellular deficit theory of dyslexia: the evidence from contrast sensitivity, pages 111-127, 2000, with permission from Elsewier).*

[36] Between 0.2 and 3.5 cycles/degree according to Tolhurst [1975].

Therefore, reduced contrast sensitivity at low luminance for gratings with spatial frequency below 1.5 cycles/degree suggests a malfunction mainly of the M system, because the P activity is weak in these conditions of stimulation. However, the result of the combined M+P functions shows that even when processing very low spatial frequencies the magnocellular system is joined by parvocellular activity to a certain amount. In fact, due to the large overlapping of the two functions, this cutoff must be considered as indicative. In order to isolate better the magnocellular alteration it is preferable to test spatial frequencies far lower.

In addition, the selectivity of the M system can be maximized if the stimulus instead of being stationary shifts or reverses at high temporal frequency, especially if the mean luminance level is reduced (scotopic and mesoscotopic conditions[37]).

M System and Deprivational Studies on Contrast Sensitivity

Important contribution for understanding the functions of the two ganglion subsystems has been provided mainly in the nineties, thanks to deprivational studies on the lateral geniculate body of the cat and monkey. The selective destruction of the ventral layers of the LGN, namely those pertaining to the M system, revealed reduced contrast sensitivity when serial configurations were displayed at very low spatial frequencies and high temporal frequencies [Merigan & Maunsell, 1990, 1993]: for example, 1 cycle/degree gratings flickering at 10 Hz [Merigan et al., 1991a]. In these experimental conditions a consistent isolation of the M pathway is expected, whereas presenting stationary or low temporal frequency gratings does not prevent from the concomitant stimulation of the P pathway, irrespective of the spatial frequency adopted.

The same applies to high temporal frequency gratings with spatial frequency not high enough [Merigan & Eskin, 1986; Schiller et al., 1990a, Merigan et al., 1991b].

A main reason why isolating the magnocellular function is difficult to obtain, is that the cumulative threshold activation of the parvocellular system is in general lower than the magnocellular one, therefore the former tend to respond to a broader spectrum of frequencies than expected by the CSF. Indeed, selective lesions of the P system reduce contrast sensitivity not only at the highest spatial frequencies, but to a certain extent even at the lowest (1 cycle/degree: Schiller et al., 1990a, b; 2 cycles/degree: Merigan et al., 1991b][38].

Merigan and Eskin found defective contrast sensitivity for low spatial frequencies[39], stationary gratings after selective destruction of the geniculate parvocellular layers. Such a

[37] In psychophysics the environmental luminance is referred to as *photopic* if it matches the brightness provided by artificial light or in daylight, *scotopic* if it corresponds to the night-gloom and *mesopic* if its level is in the middle.

[38] As pointed out by Skottun, the effect of the P pathway is overwhelming, so that its deprivation ends up to inhibit not only the response in its own domain but even in the magnocellular one. This finding, indeed, at first sight seems paradoxical, since the activation level of each P cell is lower compared to the M cells [Livingstone & Hubel, 1988; Shapley, 1990]. The solution lies in the probabilistic summation of the excitatory response so that the higher number of the P cells compared to the M neurons allows the P system as a whole to reach an activation level higher than the activation level of the antagonist system [Derrington & Lennie, 1984].

[39] Up to 0.5 cycles/degree.

finding confirms that even in the magnocellular frequency domain the P system takes part in the processing of the stimulus. The deficit, however, is shown to fade as the temporal frequency is increased. This finding suggests a further activation of the M pathway and a gradual reduction of the effect that the P system deprivation has on the cumulative response [Merigan & Eskin, 1986].

Since the response is saturated for spatial frequencies of about 1 cycle/degree and temporal frequency beyond 10 Hz, (with due caution) a grating with spatial frequency lower than 1 cycle/degree and temporal frequencies equal or higher that 10 Hz should be considered as the optimal combination to specifically measure the magnocellular activation.

Even (but not only) for these reasons, it is not surprising that the alteration of the M-mediated contrast sensitivity in dyslexics remains a controversial issue, to date.

Contrast Sensitivity in Dyslexics

As far as we know, the studies on contrast sensitivity in dyslexics began in the eighties. In 1980, patients were found to suffer from a contrast sensitivity deficit at low spatial frequencies, i.e.at 2 and especially 4 cycles/degree[40], when measured in mesoscotopic conditions (2.2 cd/m^2) [Lovegrove et al., 1980].

Two years later, a reduction of 0.1 log unit for spatial frequencies of 2 and 4 cycles/degree was observed in dyslexics even in presence of slightly higher luminance (10.3 cd/m^2) [Lovegrove et al., 1982]. At low luminance conditions, the reduction of sensitivity at low spatial frequencies seems to be amplified by presenting smaller stimuli: thus, by displaying gratings 2 degrees wide, patients' sensitivity lowered by about 0.2 log unit, provided the spatial frequency was below 4 cycles/degree or, better, 1 cycle/degree. However, when mean luminance was increased from 3.4 to 103 cd /m^2, contrast sensitivity reduction turned out to be less specific for the M system: in this case, in fact, it took place even at the highest frequencies tested, suggesting that a concurrent activation of the P system had occurred [Martin & Lovegrove, 1984].

Two years later, a selective deficit at low spatial frequencies was confirmed in 75% of patients. The defect was more evident at high temporal frequencies [Lovegrove et al., 1986]. The next year reduced contrast sensitivity was found in dyslexic children for flickering sinusoidal gratings (20 Hz) at a luminance of 11 cd/m^2. In this study, however, the loss was observed also at higher spatial frequencies[41] [Martin & Lovegrove, 1987].

The following year, Martin and Lovegrove published the results obtained with static stimuli presented at the same luminance level of their previous study[42]: contrast sensitivity was found reduced at 1, 2 and in particular 4 cycles/degree [Martin & Lovegrove, 1988].

A selective increase of contrast threshold at low spatial and high temporal frequencies in dyslexics was subsequently confirmed [Breitmeyer, 1989].

On the contrary, in a posterior study contrast sensitivity for 0.3, 6 and 11 cycles/degree gratings displayed at 20 Hz turned out to be impaired at the middle but not at the lower spatial

---

[40] The tested interval ranged from 2 to 16 cycles/degree.

[41] Range: from 0.5 to 12 cycles/degree.

[42] 11 cd/m^2.

frequency in a part of the recruited patients [Hill & Lovegrove, 1993]. After the luminance level was raised[43] any difference disappeared [Hill & Lovegrove, 1993].

Low sensitivity was observed in static conditions not only at 1.5 and 3 but also at 6 cycles/degree [Cornelissen, 1993]. Similar results come from the study of Mason et al. [1993][44].

Several other works have provided results often unequivocal.

Evans et al. [1994] for example, found reduced contrast sensitivity by presenting 1-8 cycles/degree stationary stimuli (maximum loss at 2 cycles/degree) and with flickering stimuli (10 Hz).

Instead, Walther-Müller [1995] did not report any difference between dyslexics and controls at 1 and 12 cycles/degree modulated at 16.8 Hz.

According to Gross-Glenn et al. [1995], reduced sensitivity in patients is found for tachistoscopic stimuli[45] presented at 12 but not at 0.6 cycles/degree.

Cornelissen et al. [1995] reported in dyslexics lower contrast sensitivity for gratings of 0.5 cycles/degree modulated at 20 Hz in photopic conditions[46]. Instead, no difference was found for static gratings with frequencies ranging from 0.5 to 6 cycles/degree.

The subsequent study of Hayduk et al. [1996] failed to find any difference in contrast sensitivity when measured with sinusoidal flickering gratings in patients (children as well as adults) compared to normal readers.

Demb et al.. [1998] reported reduced contrast sensitivity at low luminance for moving gratings[47], even if not statistically significant.

Finally, Borsting [Borsting et al., 1996] estimated contrast sensitivity in dyslexics after patients were classified into dyseidetics, dysphonetics, and dysphoneidetics according to the paradigm of Boder[48]. For spatial frequencies of 0.5 and 2 cycles/degree and temporal frequency of 10 Hz[49] the function turned out to be defective only in the dysphoneidetics. This result is noteworthy, since it suggests that contrast sensitivity may differ among different subtypes of dyslexics.

In his careful review based on 22 studies, Skottun [2000] concluded that only 4 investigations (that is: Lovegrove et al., 1982; Martin & Lovegrove 1984, 1988; Borsting et al., 1996] were consistent with a selective deficit of the M system, 11 showed deficits spread over a wide range of spatial frequencies, therefore equivocal, and eventually 7 are in contrast.

Indeed, as the activation cutoff of the M system is thought to be under 1-1.5 cycles/degree, reduced contrast sensitivity at spatial frequencies as low as 2 cycles/degree is not yet indicative. Nevertheless, such a result has been often judged as the evidence of a M-mediated selective defect [Skottun, 2000].

The majority of the reported investigations have dealt with the problem from the perspective of the spatial contrast, in other words evaluated contrast sensitivity in dyslexics

[43] From 11 cd/m^2 to 36 cd/m^2.

[44] In this experiment dyslexics were divided into two groups, one characterized by unstable ocular dominance as derived from the Dunlop test, the other by stable dominance (see chapter 10). The greater sensitivity deficit was recorded in the first group.

[45] Presentation time: 100 msec.

[46] 112 cd/m^2. However the result was not statistically significant.

[47] Luminance: 5 cd/m^2; spatial frequency: 0.4 cycles/degree, speed: 20.8 degrees/second.

[48] Boder, 1973: see chapter 14.

[49] Luminance: 22.6 cd/m^2.

taking as a main reference variable the spatial frequency in stationary conditions or at predetermined flickering frequency.

Other experiments focused on contrast sensitivity as a function of temporal modulation. These studies investigated the effect that increased temporal frequency of the stimulus has on contrast sensitivity, irrespective on its spatial frequency, that is to say keeping the spatial frequency constant.

A special way to assess the sensitivity to temporal contrast can be provided by the *critical fusion frequency,* i.e. the frequency threshold above which a flickering stimulus is perceived as steady.

In adult dyslexics, critical fusion frequency is lower by about 4 Hz compared to normal readers, suggesting reduced sensitivity to high temporal frequencies. This finding is particularly interesting since it is compatible with a magnocellular deficit and correlates with the lexical function ($r = 0.562$: Talcott et al., 1998).

At 2 cycles/degree[50], Martin and Lovegrove observed reduced contrast sensitivity in dyslexics when the temporal frequency was raised from 5 to 25 Hz. According to the authors, this finding supports a deficit of the M system [Martin & Lovegrove, 1987].

Contrast sensitivity was reduced in dyslexics when assessed by means of 4 cycles/degree gratings flickering at 6 Hz; increasing the temporal frequency up to 20 Hz, the defect extended at 8 and 12 cycles/degree [Martin & Lovegrove, 1988].

This finding would be confirmed eleven years later with 2 and 4 cycles/degree gratings presented in mesopic[51] conditions within a range of temporal frequencies from 4 to 16 Hz [Slaghuis & Ryan, 1999]. Even in this case the recruited dyslexics were previously been classified according to the Boder's paradigm. Defective contrast sensitivity was observed in dysphonetics and dysphoneidetics but not in dyseidetics. Substantially, this finding is in line with the reported study of Borsting.

In overall agreement with the two previous investigations of Martin and Lovergrove, Cornelissen showed some years later that the deficit, already present in static conditions at 1.5, 3 and 6 cycles/degree, worsened at a temporal frequency of 20 Hz [Cornelissen, 1993].

Even in the work of Mason et al. [1993] a loss at 20 Hz was observed in dyslexics, although not selective for the low spatial frequencies. In 1995 Felmingham and Jakobson confirmed a defect in the range of frequencies between 5 and 25 Hz with gratings of 2 c/deg.

Yet, the same year Walther-Müller [1995] failed to replicate the contrast sensitivity defects at high temporal frequencies (5 and 25 Hz) as reported in previous and contemporary works.

Also the group of Hayduk found no differences between adult dyslexics and controls [Hayduk et al., 1996]. One more counter evidence is provided by an Italian study [Spinelli et al., 1997] referred to a particular subtype of patients: those classified as *surface dyslexics* by Castles and Coltheart [Castles & Coltheart, 1993][52]. Indeed, the investigation failed to detect in most of these children any reduction in contrast sensitivity, if tested with sinusoidal gratings projected on the fovea and its surrounding region (*the parafovea*).

The inconsistency of the experimental findings is showed in figure 3. It can be noticed that results supporting a selective defect of the M system patients are a minority (16%).

[50] Luminance level: 11 cd/m^2.
[51] 24.7 cd/m^2.
[52] See chapter 14.

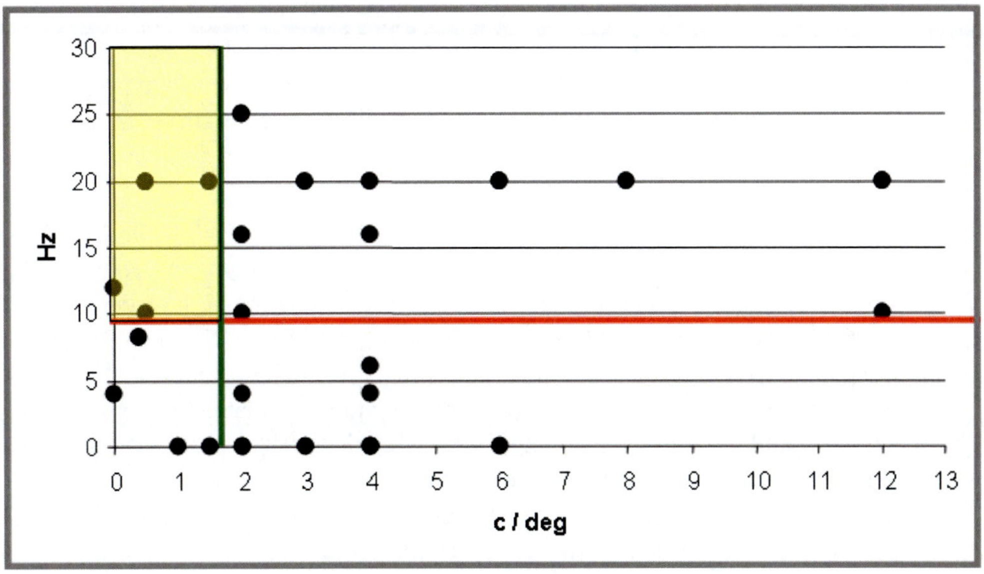

Figure 3. Global outcomes from the researches on contrast sensitivity in dyslexics reported in the text. Each study is marked by a black circle and is plotted as a function of the spatial (x-axis) and temporal (y-axis) frequency examined. The studies showing a deficit for spatial frequencies <1.5 cycles/degree and temporal frequencies > 10c/deg are considered suggestive of a defect of the magnocellular system and localized within the yellow area. Such evidence does not exceed 16%. The findings that meet the criterion for a deficit of the M system only on the basis of the spatial frequency localize to the left of the green line, those that agree only on the basis of the temporal frequency are placed above the red line.

It has already been postulated that one reason for such a lack of agreement is that the parvocellular system as a whole turns out to be more responsive than the magnocellular pathway, so that to a certain extent it may be activated even by configurations specifically devised for the transient system. Moreover, many experiments suffer from a procedural problem, i.e. the properties of the stimulus are not always adequate, since a stimulation considered selective for the M pathway may trigger the P-system as well. In other words (and in accordance with Skottun) an optimal survey ought to adopt stimuli unequivocally within the field of activation of the magnocellular system, for example sinusoidal gratings of spatial frequency below 1 cycle/degree displayed with temporal frequencies higher than 25 Hz[53] displayed at a very low luminance level (2-3 cd/m^2).

However, in dyslexics the deficit at low spatial frequencies and (at the same time) at high temporal frequencies measured at low luminance, suggestive of impaired M system, should combine with the absence of alterations at high spatial frequencies and low temporal frequencies (or static conditions) at photopic levels, so as to ensure the integrity of the complementary P system.

Moreover, to support the specific presence of a magnocellular deficit in dyslexics, apart from its presence in patients, the lack of any magnocellular impairment in normal readers is required, too. In many of the studies considered thus far, this point has not been clearly addressed.

---

[53] Even if a temporal frequency of 10Hz is believed to be enough to stimulate selectively the M system [Regan, 1983; Anderson & Burr, 1985; Merigan & Maunsell, 1990, Strasburger et al.,1993].

Apart from two exceptions, the recruitment of unclassified patients, therefore affected by a variable degree of phonological impairment, may contribute to bias the results.

Indeed, as we shall discuss hereinafter[54], whether are there different subtypes of dyslexia is an open question. Nevertheless, it is likely that different features in different patients tend to be ignored whereas the pattern of response to the contrast sensitivity may differ according to the type of patient.

In summary, contrast sensitivity at low spatial frequencies and high temporal frequency under mesoscotopic conditions[55] seems to occur in at least one subtype of dyslexic patients. Even though it remains a controversial issue, such an impairment is argued to be an expression of defective magnocellular system and could reveal as a visuoperceptual marker suitable to separate dyslexic subjects from normal readers [Cornelissen et al., 1995].

It is advanced that the alleged visuoperceptive alterations mediated by the M system are artifactual: they would be simply due to linguistic difficulties such as to require more time for the visual processing when administering the psychophysical tests.

On this subject, it is worth mentioning the recent study of Jordan and Patching [2005], which assessed contrast sensitivity in non-dyslexic subjects divided into good and poor readers. Compared to good readers, poor readers (even though non-dyslexic) showed reduced contrast sensitivity for spatial frequencies ranging between 2 and 6 cycles/degree, and the lower was the reading rate, the greater the contrast sensitivity reduction. Therefore, perceptual differences between better and worse readers can be disclosed even in normal subjects, and the visuoperceptive performance turns out to be correlated with reading rate. Now (apart from these specific findings), such a discrepancy has not been found using a linguistic task. Therefore, in this experiment the worse performance in poor readers cannot be due to linguistic factors and contrast sensitivity may be an indicator of the lexical function not only in dyslexics but even in normal readers.

Recently, the effect of contrast sensitivity on the lexical function has been assessed by measuring contrast threshold for the identification of single letters and words[56], [Martelli et al., 2009]. In dyslexics, contrast threshold for the recognition of single letters matched the threshold of normal readers[57], whereas for words made of 10 characters it turned out to be 0.3 log units higher. Adding noise (made of squares 2 pixels wide) made contrast threshold 0.7 log units higher in both groups. In summary, this study suggests that the problem in dyslexic deals with the *integration* of the letters that make up the words and not at the level of single letters processing. Moreover, such a finding is not related to reduced signal-to-noise ratio, since by adding noise the threshold in dyslexics and controls raises by the same amount. Therefore, the worsening in the signal-to-noise ratio in dyslexics, suggested in a previous study on motion perception [Talcott et al., 2000] [58], has been not confirmed in this more recent work.

In summary, the presence of a selective contrast sensitivity defect as a demonstration of a transient system damage in developmental dyslexia has probably been the most claimed

[54] See chapter 14.

[55] Even though slight and within 0.1-0.3 log units.

[56] Luminance: 28 cd/m^2, presentation time: 200 msec, size of the character: 1 degree.

[57] In accordance with a previous evidence [Barnard et al., 1998].

[58] See chapter 7.

visuoperceptual argument by the supporters of the M theory, but also the most debated[59]. Despite the inconsistency of many results, the positive findings cannot be ignored, suggesting the occurrence of a moderate depression of the magnocellular function, probably not ubiquitary but involving a particular type of patients.

Yet, what are its implications in the lexical disability remains a controversial point.

References

Anderson SJ, Burr DC. (1985). *Spatial and temporal selectivity of the human motion detection system.* Vision Research, 25:1147-1154.

Barnard N, Crewther SG, Crewther DP. (1998). *Development of a Magnocellular Function in Good and Poor Primary School-Age Readers.* Optometry and Visual Science, 75: 62-68.

Boder E. (1973). *Developmental dyslexia: a diagnostic approach based on three atypical reading-spelling patterns.* Developmental Medicine and Child Neurology, 15: 663-687.

Borsting E, Ridder WH, Dudeck K, Kelley C, Matsui L, Motoyama J. (1996). *The presence of a magnocellular defect depends on the type of dyslexia.* Vision Research, 36: 1047-1053.

Breitmeyer, BG. (1989). *A visually based deficit in specific reading disability.* The Irish Journal of Psychology, 10: 534-541.

Castles A, Coltheart M. (1993). *Varieties of developmental dyslexia.* Cognition, 47: 149-180.

Cornelissen P. (1993). *Fixation, contrast sensitivity and children's reading.* In: Facets of dyslexia and its remediation, Wright & Groner Eds., Elsevier, Amsterdam.

Cornelissen PL, Richardson AR, Mason A, Fowler MS, Stein JF. (1995). *Contrast sensitivity and coherent motion detection measured at photopic luminance levels in dyslexics and controls.* Vision Research 1995; 35: 1483-1494.

Demb JB, Boynton GM, Best M, Heeger DJ. (1998). *Psychophysical evidence for a magnocellular pathway deficit in dyslexia.* Vision Research, 38: 1555-1559.

Derrington AM, Lennie P. (1984). *Spatial and temporal contrast sensitivities of neurons in lateral geniculate nucleus of Macaque.* Journal of Psysiology (London), 357: 219-240.

Evans BJW, Drasdo N, Richards IL. (1994). *An investigation of some sensory and refractive visual factors in dyslexia.* Vision Research, 34: 1913-1926.

Felmingham KL, Jakobson LS. (1995). *Visual and visuomotor performance in dyslexic children.* Experimental Brain Research, 106: 467-474.

Gross-Glenn K, Skottun BC, Glenn W, Kushch A, Lingua R, Dunbar M, Jallad B, Lubs HA, Levin B, Rabin M, Parke LA, Duara R. (1995). *Contrast sensitivity in dyslexia.* Visual Neuroscience, 12: 153-163.

Hayduk S, Bruck M, Cavanagh P.(1996). *Low level visual processing skills of adults and children with dyslexia.* Cognitive Neuropsychology, 13: 975-1016.

Hill R, Lovegrove WJ. (1993). *One word at a time: A solution to the visual deficits in SRDs?* In: Facets of dyslexia and its remediation, Wright, Groner & Kauffman-Hayoz Eds., Elsevier, Amsterdam.

Lee BB, Smith VC, Pokorny J, Kremers J. (1997). *Rod Inputs to macaque ganglion cells.* Vision Research, 37: 2813-2828.

Legge GE. (1978). *Sustained and transient mechanisms in human vision: temporal and spatial properties.* Vision Research, 18: 69-81.

[59] See Skottun, 1997a, b; Skottun & Parke, 1998; Skottun, 2000.

Livingstone M & Hubel D. (1988). *Segregation of form, color movement, and dept: anatomy, physiology, and perception.* Science, 240: 740-749.

Lovegrove WJ, Bowling A, Badcock D, Blackwood M. (1980). *Specific reading difficulty: Differences in contrast sensitivity as a function of spatial frequency.* Science, 210: 439-440.

Lovegrove WJ, Martin F, Bowling A, Blackwood M, Badcock D, Paxton S. (1982). *Contrast sensitivity functions and specific reading disability.* Neuropsychologia, 20: 309-315.

Lovegrove WJ, Martin F, Slaghuis W. (1986). *A theoretical and experimental case for a visual deficit in specific reading disability.* Cognitive Neuropshychology, 3: 225-267.

Martelli M, Di Filippo G, Spinelli D, Zoccolotti P. (2009). *Crowding, reading, and developmental dyslexia.* Journal of Vision, 4: 14, 1-18.

Martin F, Lovegrove WJ. (1984). *The effects of field size and luminance on contrast sensitivity differences between specifically reading disabled and normal children.* Neuropsychologia, 22: 73-77.

Martin F, Lovegrove WJ. (1987). *Flicker contrast sensitivity in normal and specifically disabled readers.* Perception, 16: 215-221.

Martin F, Lovegrove WJ. (1988). *Uniform-field flicker maskimg in control and specifically-disabled readers.* Perception, 17: 203-214.

Mason A, Cornelissen P, Fowler S, Stein J. (1993). *Contrast sensitivity, ocular dominance and specific reading disability.* Clinical Vision Science, 8: 345-353.

Merigan WH, Eskin TA. (1986). *Spatio-temporal vision of macaques with severe loss of Pb retinal ganglion cells.* Vision Research, 26: 1751-1761.

Merigan WH, Maunsell JHR. (1990). *Macaque vision after magnocellular lateral geniculate lesions.* Visual Neuroscience, 5: 347-352.

Merigan WH, Byrne CE, Maunsell JHR. (1991a). *Does primate motion perception depend on the magnocellular pathway?* Journal of Neuroscience, 11: 3422-3429.

Merigan WH, Katz LM, Maunsell JHR. (1991b). *The effects of parvocellular lateral geniculate lesions on the acuity and contrast sensitivity of macaque monkeys.* Journal of Neuroscience, 11: 994-1001.

Merigan WH, Maunsell JHR. (1993). *How parallel are the human visual pathways?* Annual Review of Neuroscience, 116: 369-402.

Patching GR, Jordan TR. (2005). *Spatial frequency sensitivity differences between adults of good and poor reading ability.* Investigative Ophthalmology and Visual Science, 46: 2219-2223.

Purpura K, Kaplan E, Shapley RM. (1988). *Background light and the contrast gain of primate P and M retinal ganglion cells.* Proceedings of the National Academy of Sciences of the United States of America, 85: 4537-4537.

Regan D. (1983). *Spatial frequency mechanisms in human vision investigated by evoked potential recording.* Vision Research, 23: 1401-1407.

Schiller PH, Logothetis NK, Charles ER. (1990a). *Functions of the colour-opponent and broad-band channels of the visual system.* Nature, 343; 68-70.

Schiller PH, Logothetis NK, Charles ER. (1990b). *Role of the colour-opponent and broad-band channels in vision.* Visual Neuroscience, 5: 321-346.

Shapley R. (1990). *Visual sensitivity and parallel retinocortical channels.* Annual Review of Psychology, 41: 635-658.

Skottun BC. (1997a). *Some remarks on the magnocellular deficit theory of dyslexia.* Vision Research, 37: 965-966.

Skottun BC. (1997b). *The magnocellular deficit theory of dyslexia.* Trends in Neurosciences, 20: 397-398.

Skottun BC. (2000). *The magnocellular deficit theory of dyslexia: the evidence from contrast sensitivity*. Vision Research, 40: 111-127.

Skottun BC, Parke LA. (1998). *The possible relationship between visual deficits and dyslexia: examination of a critical assumption*. Journal of Learning Disabilities, 32: 2-5.

Slaghuis WL, Ryan JF. (1999). *Spatio-temporal contrast sensitivity, coherent motion, and visible persistence in developmental dyslexia*. Vision Research, 39: 651-668.

Spinelli D, Angelelli P, De Luca M, Di Pace E, Judica A, Zoccolotti P. (1997). *Developmental surface dyslexia is not associated with deficits in the transient visual system*. NeuroReport, 8: 1807-1812.

Strasburger H, Murray IJ, Remky A. (1993). *Sustained and transient mechanisms in the steady-state visual evoked potential: onset presentation compared to pattern reversal*. Clinical Vision Sciences, 8: 211-234.

Talcott JB, Hansen PC, Willis-Owen C, McKinnell IW, Richardson AJ, Stein J. (1998). *Visual magnocellular impairment in adult developmental dyslexics*. Neuroophthalmology, 20: 187-201.

Talcott JB,. Hansen PC, Assoku EL, Stein JF. (2000). *Visual motion sensitivity in dyslexia: evidence for temporal and energy integration deficits*. Neuropsychologia, 38: 935-943.

Tolhurst DJ. (1975). *Reaction times in the detection of gratings by human observers: a probabilistic mechanism*. Vision Research, 15: 1143-1149.

Walther-Muller PU. (1995). *Is there a deficit of early vision in dyslexia?* Perception, 24: 919-936.

Chapter VII

Motion Perception and Dyslexia

The magnocellular system is defined *transient* because it is mainly responsible for motion perception. The final stage of motion perception is the mediotemporal area, also called MT or V5 [Newsome & Parè, 1988; Newsome et al., 1995] and characterized by the large size of its magnocellular receptive fields. Studies in macaques showed that the cells of MT are tuned for the direction of dynamic configurations [Newsome & Parè, 1988], so that a selective lesion of the transient system on the cortex [Maunsell & van Essen, 1983; Newsome & Parè, 1988] or in the ventral layers of the lateral geniculate body [Maunsell et al., 1990; Merigan & Maunsell, 1990; Schiller et al.. 1990a, b; Merigan et al., 1991] makes the animal insensitive to dynamic stimuli [Merigan & Maunsell, 1993]. Schiller for example found a deep loss of motion perception after the selective ablation[60] of geniculate M neurons of the macaque but not after the destruction of geniculate P cells [Schiller et al., 1990a, b]. Similar results were reported two years earlier by Newsome and Paré [1988] after focal destruction of the magnocells in the mediotemporal cortical region.

These premises persuaded the researchers who had previously dealt with the contradictory findings obtained in contrast sensitivity to focus on motion perception and its possible impairment in dyslexic patients.

In humans, psychophysical and functional experiments have adopted two different paradigms: drifting sinusoidal gratings or, more often, random dot configurations.

Random dots look to be the most appropriate technique. The random dot paradigm measures the sensibility to the so-called *coherent motion*, i.e. the detection threshold for the joined (*coherent*) displacement of a clusters of dots embedded in a background of identical dots moving in random order. Threshold is expressed as the least number of coherent dots required to detect the moving cluster[61] (Figure 1).

---

[60] Obtained by injection of ibotenic acid.

[61] For the normative data on coherent motion perception see McKee et al. [1986] and Debruyn & Orban [1988].

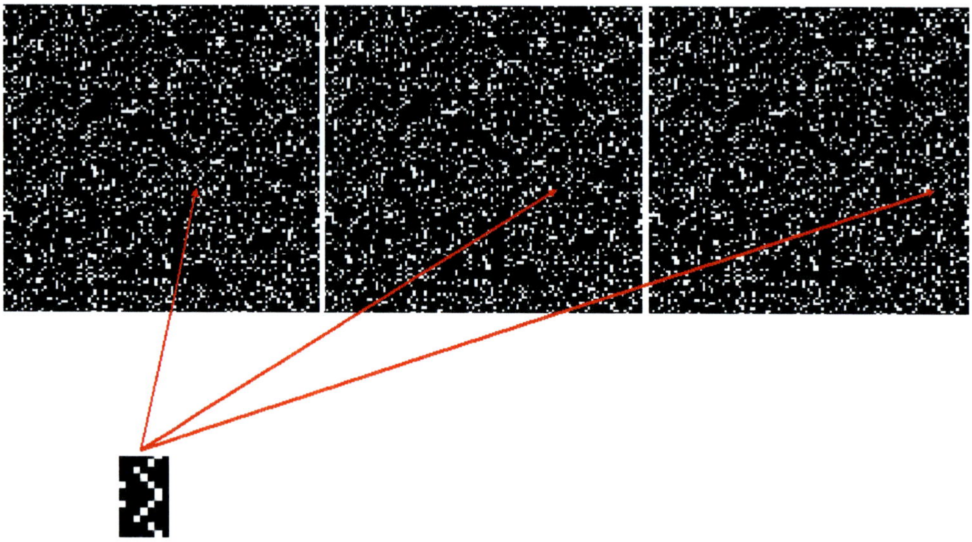

Figure 1. Coherent motion and the random dot paradigm. The cluster of coherently moving dots is shown enlarged in the small box at the bottom. The three displays are in temporal order. Among dots moving in random order, those belonging to the cluster drift consistently to the right. Their position in the three consecutive phases is indicated by the arrows.

The main advantage of this model is its selectivity for the magnocellular system, since differently from other types of configuration (i.e. sinusoidal gratings), random dots are free from high spatial frequencies: in fact, dots lack of shape or edges suitable to stimulate the parvocellular pool, thereby reducing the specificity of the test and spoiling the results[62].

Coherent motion threshold turned out to be 3-4% higher in 29 dyslexic children and 29 adults compared to normal age-matched readers[63]. Despite the considerable overlap in the two samples (due to the heterogeneity of the dyslexic group), in patients motion sensitivity was lower not only compared to the age-matched normal readers, but even to the younger normal readers of the same lexical level. This effect suggests that the impairment of motion detection can be causally related to the lexical disability [Cornelissen et al., 1995].

In a further investigation, the threshold of 10 dyslexic children in average turned out to be double compared to normal readers. The anomaly, evident in 6 subjects persisted the following year [Raymond & Sorensen, 1998].

In general agreement are Slaghuis and Ryan [1999][64], Talcott [Talcott et al., 1998, 2000a], Hansen (but in his experiment the luminance was considerably higher[65]: Hansen et al., 2001) and Pammer and Wheatley [2001].

Compared to contrast sensitivity, the relationship between motion perception and lexical disability is stronger: of the 26 studies published from 1999 to 2011 and recently reported by

[62] Yet, even random dots are not free from this drawback. In fact, the movement of the coherent pattern does not occur along a single axis but in different directions and this omnidirectional displacement is claimed to prevent from effectively isolating the response of the M system [Skottun, 2000]. Moreover, dot-shaped stimuli may reside in the domain of high spatial frequencies and as such are processed by the parvocellular system.

[63] Average luminance: 58.7cd /m 2, contrast: 99%.

[64] In mesopic luminance level: background : 0.4 cd/m2; random dots: 40.7 cd/m2.

[65] 130 cd/m^2.

Boets, 20 (77%) are consistent with a coherent motion deficit in dyslexics [Boets et al., 2011][66], while the same proportion referred to the contrast sensitivity does not exceed 16%.

Imaging techniques are a valuable contribution for investigating motion perception. Eden employed the functional magnetic resonance to measure the cortical response to coherent motion in MT and V1 areas in a group of patients and found that brain activity was virtually absent in MT but normal in V1[67] [Eden et al., 1996a, b]. Indeed, abnormal sensitivity to coherent motion reported without a concomitant deficiency of contrast sensitivity [Cornelissen et al., 1995; Demb et al., 1998b] may be explained in the light of this topographic dissociation: normal response in V1 with defective mediotemporal receptive fields [Eden et al., 1996a].

Lower sensitivity to motion perception in MT would stem from reduced density of the magnocellular receptive fields in this cortical area [Talcott et al., 2000a]. In the framework of the random dot paradigm, the defect is explainable as decreased signal-to-noise ratio: lower density of M cells in MT makes the detection of the coherently moving cluster more affected by the surrounding dots. In other words, the visual system is less efficient in isolating the dynamic component of the target.

Instead of random dots, other researchers preferred to use gratings for assessing motion perception.

By using two sinusoidal gratings moving at different speeds, Demb measured motion discrimination in 5 adult dyslexics[68] and compared the results with those obtained in 5 normal subjects [Demb et al., 1997, 1998a]. Demb integrated its psychophysical experiments studying the cortical metabolic activation by means of functional MRI: cortical activation in dyslexics turned out to be weaker not only in MT but even in V1 [Demb et al., 1997, 1998a][69].

In line with the other findings [Cornelissen et al., 1995, 1998a, b; Demb et al., 1998a, b; Talcott et al., 1998], the correlation between motion threshold and cortical metabolic activation proved to be significant in V1 and (especially) in MT ($r = -0.65$ and -0.79, respectively). Interestingly, a strong correlation was found even between cortical activation (MT) and reading speed ($r = 0.80$[70]: Demb et al., 1998b).

In summary, motion discrimination seems to be more reliable than contrast sensitivity as a marker of dyslexia, especially in adults. In addition, it is correlated with the metabolic activity in V1 and MT.

---

[66] See Boets et al. [2011], p.855, for a detailed list of these publications. In disagreement are three studies on German dyslexics. In these investigations motion threshold was similar or even better in patients than in controls [Kronbichler et al., 2002; Hawelka & Wimmer, 2005; Hutzler et al., 2006]. Other works which failed to find differences in the two samples are Amitay et al. [2002], Kim & Davis (in Korean hangul speaking dyslexics: 2004), White et al. [2006] and Tsermentseli et al. [2008].

[67] See Vanni et al. [1997] for a counter evidence at magnetoencephalography. (Magnetoencephalography [MEG] estimates fluctuations of the magnetic field generated by the brain's electrical activity).

[68] Mean age: 22.2 years, luminance: 5 cd / m^2. The spatial frequency of the two gratings was 0.4 cycles/degree, the speed of the reference grating was 20.8 degrees/sec, the speed of the test grating was always higher even if variable. To prevent the sample from discriminating the relative difference in speed by counting the moving bars, stimulus duration was systematically changed (interval: from 360 to 540 msec).

[69] The result is in disagreement with that obtained by Eden and reported above: the difference is probably due to the different contrast, to the type of stimulation (Eden made use of the random dot while Demb employed sinusoidal gratings) or to the recruited sample.

[70] Contrast: 30%.

Not only functional resonance but also electrophysiological techniques have provided important contribution for better understanding motion perception in dyslexics: the latency of visual potentials evoked from a drifting checkerboard-like stimulus appeared increased in 70% of patients [Kubova et al., 1995].

In a group of German dyslexic children, the global brain electrical activity (the so-called Global Field Power: GFP) recorded while presenting fast moving sinusoidal gratings[71] turned out to be depressed [Scheuerpflug et al., 2004]. On the other hand, the use of the random dot paradigm in the same experiment did not show any difference with normal readers. However, luminance was significantly lower for gratings than for random dots (12 vs. 86 cd/m^2) and since M system is effective for low luminance levels, the stimulation with random dots in this study probably was not enough specific for the transient function.

This explanation is supported by another German experiment that, in a sample of 12 patients, showed an attenuation of the two positive components P100 and P200[72] of the visual evoked potentials when presenting a field of moving random dots [Schulte-Körne et al., 2004a]. A month later, the same researchers replicated the observation after replacing random dots with sinusoidal gratings [Schulte-Körne et al., 2004b]: the study confirmed the reduced amplitude of the waves P100 and P200 in 8 dyslexics[73] compared to 14 age-matched normal readers[74].

The increased amplitude of the two components (especially the P200) as the stimulus drift was made faster was evident only in the control subjects; in patients, the lack of correlation between stimulus speed and response of the transient system is regarded as an indicator of magnocellular malfunctioning.

In summary, the results are consistent with reduced sensibility to motion perception in dyslexics.

Although researchers have found a link between motion perception and contrast sensitivity (motion perception improves as stimulus contrast increases[75]: Edwards & Badcock, 1994, 1995), motion perception is undoubtedly more reliable than contrast sensitivity as a marker of dyslexia. It is revealing, indeed, that motion perception (but not contrast sensitivity) is able to predict lexical ability both in dyslexics [Talcott et al., 1998] and in normal readers [Witton et al., 1998].

Combining psychophysical and functional results, scientists discovered both in dyslexics and in controls a relation among activation level of MT area, motion perception threshold and lexical performance.

In normal readers (both children and adults), the link between lexical skills and motion perception depends on the fact that motion perception would reflect how precisely letters are located and ordered [Cornelissen et al., 1998a, b, Talcott et al., 2000b]. Indeed, it is the orthographic and not the phonological skill when reading [Witton et al., 1998; Talcott et al.,

[71] Speed: 16 deg/sec.

[72] Visual potentials evoked from dynamic configurations are characterized by two positive waves, which, based on their latency from the beginning of the stimulation, are defined P100 (latency of 100-130 msec) and P200 (latency of about 230 msec). The P100 is recorded in the occipital area, the P200 in the parietal [Hoffmann et al., 2001; Hirai et al., 2003]. The amplitude of these two waves increases as a function of the speed of stimulus [Hoffmann & Bach, 1997].

[73] Mean age: 12.7 years.

[74] The stimuli were low spatial frequency (2cycles/ degree) vertical gratings with average luminance 12 cd/m2 and speed 2, 8 and 16 deg/sec, drifting horizontally.

[75] Up to 20%.

2000a, b] to be related to motion perception in reading. This relation confirms the role of the visual function in the development and in the alterations of the lexical skills, even if how this could happen and how abnormal motion perception could determine reading disability is still unclear.

It has been advanced motion perception to be one facet of a more generalized defect of signal integration in both the temporal domain and visual space: according to this perspective, not only motion perception *per se* but the overall ability to integrate the signal over time would be impaired in dyslexics [Raymond & Sorensen, 1998]: in fact, in patients motion perception is found normal when displaying only two random dots kinematograms[76] and impaired when the number of sequential kinematograms reaches seven[77] [Raymond & Soerensen, 1998]. This finding is in line with a previous experiment of Mikami, who showed in monkeys that neurons in MT are sensitive to motion when simulated by using a high number of presentations, while do not respond if only two kinematograms are displayed [Mikami et al., 1986].

Such an integration deficit in the temporal domain could extend to the spatial level: as will be discussed further, in dyslexics it is reported an abnormal ability to integrate contiguous characters due to increased lateral masking[78]. Therefore, to anticipate what will be clearer further, we can conclude that impaired motion perception and increased lateral masking, depending on a signal integration deficit, would both be ascribable to anomalous sequential processing.

In conclusion, the studies on motion perception have added an important piece to the complex puzzle that is developmental dyslexia. Nevertheless, to date, the causal link between reduced sensibility to dynamic stimuli and lexical disability remains unclear.

Perhaps another phenomenon dependent on the magnocellular system can be more illuminating: the visual persistence time.

References

Amitay S, Ben-Yehudah G, Banai K, Ahissar M. (2002). *Disabled readers suffer from visual and auditory impairments but not from a specific magnocellular deficit.* Brain, 125: 2272-2284.

Boets B, Vandermosten M, Cornelissen P, Wouters J, Ghesquiére P. (2011). *Coherent motion sensitivity and reading development in the transition from prereading to reading stage.* Child Development, 82: 854-869.

Cornelissen PL, Richardson AR, Mason A, Fowler MS, Stein JF. (1995). *Contrast sensitivity and coherent motion detection measured at photopic luminance levels in dyslexics and controls.* Vision Research, 35: 1483-1494.

Cornelissen PL, Hansen PC, Hutton JL, Evangelinou V, Stein JF. (1998a). *Magnocellular visual function and children's single word reading.* Vision Research, 38: 471-482.

[76] Compared to the first, in the second kinematogram the position of the cluster is shifted to a certain extent.

[77] The position of the cluster at the beginning and at the end of the movement and the cumulative duration of the stimulation is identical to the previous experimental condition.

[78] See chapter 13.

Cornelissen P, Hansen PC, Gilchrist I, Cormack F, Essex E, Frankish C. (1998b). *Coherent motion detection and letter position encoding.* Vision Research, 38: 2181-2191.

DeBruyn B, Orban GA. (1988). *Human velocity and direction discrimination measured with random dot patterns.* Vision Research, 12: 1323-1335.

Demb JB, Boynton GM, Heeger DJ. (1997). *Brain activity in visual cortex predicts individual differences in reading performance.* Proceedings of the National Academy of Sciences of the United States of America, 94: 13363-13366.

Demb JB, Boynton GM, Best M, Heeger DJ. (1998a). *Functional magnetic resonance imaging of early visual pathways in dyslexia.* The Journal of Neuroscience, 18: 6939-6951.

Demb JB, Boynton GM, Best M, Heeger DJ. (1998b). *Psychophysical evidence for a magnocellular pathway deficit in dyslexia.* Vision Research, 38: 1555-1559.

Eden GF, VanMeter JW, Rumsey JM, Maisog JW, Woods RP, Zeffiro TA. (1996a). *Abnormal processing of visual motion in dyslexia revealed by functional brain imaging.* Nature, 382: 66-69.

Eden GF, VanMeter JW, Rumsey JM, Zeffiro TA (1996b). *The visual deficit theory of developmental dyslexia [review].* Neuroimage, 4S: 108-117.

Edwards M, Badcock DR. (1994). *Global motion perception: interaction of the ON and OFF pathways.* Vision Research, 34: 2849-2858.

Edwards M, Badcock DR. (1995). *Global motion perception: No interaction between the first- and second-order motion pathways.* Vision Research, 35: 2589-2602.

Hansen PC, Stein JF, Orde SR, Winter JL, Talcott JB. (2001). *Are dyslexics' visual deficits limited to measures of dorsal stream function?* NeuroReport, 12: 1527-1530.

Hawelka S, Wimmer H (2005). *Impaired visual processing of multi-element arrays is associated with increased number of eye movements in dyslexic reading.* Vision Research, 45: 855-863.

Hirai MH, Fukushima H, Hiraki K. (2003). *An event related potentials study of biological motion perception in humans.* Neuroscience Letters, 344: 41-44.

Hoffmann MB, Bach M. (1997). *Motion onset VEPs: topographic distribution and dependence on stimulus velocity reveals two components.* Brain Topography, 10: 171.

Hoffmann MB, Unsöld AS, Bach M. (2001). *Directional tuning of human motion adaptation as reflected by the motion VEP.* Vision Research, 41: 2187-2194.

Hutzler F, Kronbichler M, Jacobs AM, Wimmer H. (2006). *Perhaps correlational but not causal: no effect of dyslexic readers'magnocellular system on their eye movements during reading.* Neuropsychologia, 44: 637-648.

Kim J, Davis C. (2004). *Characteristics of poor readers of Korean Hangul: auditory, visual and phonological processing.* Reading and Writing, 17: 153-185.

Kronbichler M, Hutzler F; Wimmer H. (2002). *Dyslexia: Verbal impairments in the absence of magnocellular impairments.* Neuroreport, 13: 617-620.

Kubovà Z, Zuba M, Pregrin J, Nováková V. (1995). *Visual Evoked potential evidence for magnocellular system deficit in dyslexia.* Physiological Research, 44: 87-89.

Martelli M, Di Filippo G, Spinelli D, Zoccolotti P.(2009). *Crowding, reading, and developmental dyslexia.* Journal of Vision, 4: 14, 1-18.

Maunsell JHR, Van Essen DC. (1983). *The connections of the middle temporal visual area (MT) and their relationship to a cortical hierarchy in the macaque monkey.* The Journal of Neuroscience, 3: 2563-2586.

Maunsell JHR, Nealey TA, Depriest DD. (1990). *Magnocellular and parvocellular contributions to responses in the middle temporal visual area (MT) of the macaque monkey.* The Journal of Neuroscience, 10:3323-3334.

McKee SP, Silverman GH, Nakayama K. (1986). *Precise velocity discrimination despite random dot variations in temporal frequency and contrast.* Vision Research, 26: 609-619.

Merigan WH, Maunsell JHR. (1990). *Macaque vision after magnocellular lateral geniculate lesions.* Visual Neuroscience, 5: 347-352.

Merigan WH, Maunsell JHR. (1993). *How parallel are the human visual pathways?* Annual Review of Neuroscience, 16: 369-402.

Merigan WH, Byrne CE, Maunsell JHR. (1991). *Does primate motion perception depend on the magnocellular pathway?* The Journal of Neuroscience, 11: 3422-3429.

Mikami A, Newsome WT, Wurtz RH. (1986). *Motion selectivity in macaque visual cortex. II. Spatiotemporal range of directional interactions in MT and V1.* Journal of Neurophysiology, 55: 1328-1339.

Newsome WT, Paré EB. (1988). *A selective impairment of motion perception following lesions of the middle temporal visual area (MT).* The Journal of Neuroscience, 8: 2201-2211.

Newsome WT, Shadlen MN, Zohary E, Britten KH, Movshon JA. (1995). *Visual Motion: linking neural activity to psychophysical performance.* In: The Cognitive Neurosciences, Gazzaniga Ed., MA: MIT, Cambridge.

Pammer K, Wheatley C. (2001). *Isolating the M(y)-cell response in dyslexia using the spatial frequency doubling illusion.* Vision Research, 41: 2139-2147.

Raymond JE, Sorensen E. (1998). *Visual motion perception in normal children with dyslexia: normal detection but abnormal integration.* Visual Cognition, 5: 389-404.

Scheuerpflug P, Plume E, Vetter V, Schulte-Koerne G, Deimel W, Bartling J, Remschmidt H, Warnke A. (2004). *Visual information processing in dyslexic children.* Clinical Neurophysiology, 115: 90-96.

Schiller PH, Logothetis NK, Charles ER. (1990a). *Functions of the color-opponent and broad-band channels of the visual system.* Nature, 343: 68-70.

Schiller PH, Logothetis NK, Charles ER. (1990b). *Role of the color-opponent and broad band channels in vision.* Visual Neuroscience, 5: 321-346.

Schulte-Körne G, Bartling J, Deimel W, Remschmidt H. (2004a). *Visual evoked potentials elicited by coherently moving dots in dyslexic children.* Neuroscience Letters, 357: 207-210.

Schulte-Körne G, Bartling J, Deimel W, Remschmidt H. (2004b). *Motion-onset VEPs in dyslexia. Evidence for visual perceptual deficit.* NeuroReport, 15: 1075- 1078.

Skottun BC. (2000). *The magnocellular deficit theory of dyslexia: the evidence from contrast sensitivity.* Vision Research, 40: 111-127.

Slaghuis WL, Ryan JF. (1999). *Spatio-temporal contrast sensitivity, coherent motion, and visible persistence in developmental dyslexia.* Vision Research, 39: 651-668.

Talcott JB, Hansen PC, Willis-Owen C, McKinnell IW, Richardson AJ, Stein J. (1998). *Visual magnocellular impairment in adult developmental dyslexics.* Neuroophthalmology, 20: 187-201.

Talcott JB, Hansen PC, Assoku EL, Stein JF. (2000a). *Visual motion sensitivity in dyslexia: evidence for temporal and energy integration deficits.* Neuropsychologia, 38: 935-943.

Talcott JB,. Witton C, McLean MF, Hansen PC, Rees A, Green GG, Stein JF. (2000b). *Dynamic sensory sensitivity and children's word decoding skills.* Proceedings of the National Academy of Sciences of the United States of America, 97: 2952-2957.

Tsermentseli ST, O'Brien JM, Spencer JV. (2008). *Comparison of form and motion coherence processing in autistic spectrum disorders and dyslexia.* Journal of Autism and Developmental Disorders, 38: 1201-1210.

Vanni S, Uusitalo MA, Kiesila P, Hari R. (1997). *Visual motion activates V5 in dyslexics.* Neuroreport, 8:1939-1942.

White S, Milne E, Rosen S, Hansen P, Swettenham J, Frith U, Ramus F. (2006). *The role of sensorimotor impairments in dyslexia: A multiple case study of dyslexic children.* Developmental Science, 9: 237-255.

Witton C, Talcott JB, Hansen PC, Richardson AJ, Griffiths TD, Rees A, Stein JF, Greef GGR. (1998). *Sensitivity to dynamic auditory and visual stimuli predicts nonword reading ability in both dyslexic and normal readers.* Current Biology, 8: 791-797.

Chapter VIII

Visual Persistence and Dyslexia

Visual persistence (VP) is defined by Haber and Standing [1970] as the response to a visual stimulation that continues after its disappearance and that is indistinguishable from the response occurred during its presence.

Due to the visual persistence, two targets displayed in rapid succession are perceived as a single image if their temporal separation is below a given limit.

Visual persistence depends on the time required by the M pathway to suppress the activity of the P cells completely. Indeed, such an inhibitory effect of the magnocellular system is in agreement with the finding that VP time increases with the spatial frequency of the target: in fact, the higher is the spatial frequency, the stronger is the activation of the P cells[79] [Lovegrove & Brown, 1978; Bowling & Lovegrove, 1980; Lovegrove & Heddle, 1980; Lovegrove et al., 1980a].

Therefore, increased VP would occur when the transient system is defective [Breitmeyer et al., 1981], and as such unable to effectively inhibit the sustained system. In this case, in fact, the visual system is expected to be less sensitive to rapidly changing stimuli, i.e. less effective in detecting as distinct two visual events separated by a minimum interval of time [Slaghuis & Lovegrove, 1984; Lovegrove et al., 1986][80].

Since the early seventies, visual persistence is found to be abnormally strong in dyslexics, so that the interval required to identify two sequential stimuli is up to 100 msec longer that in normal readers. [Stanley & Hall, 1973; Petersik & Pantle, 1979; Lovegrove et al., 1980a; Badcock & Lovegrove, 1981; Di Lollo et al., 1983; Slaghuis & Lovegrove, 1984, 1985, 1986; Williams et al., 1989; Winters et al., 1989; Lovegrove et al., 1990; Slaghuis et al., 1993; Slaghuis et al., 1996]. Slaghuis and Ryan [1999] made use of a particular paradigm, defined *apparent movement of Ternus.*[81], to confirm this finding.

---

[79] And the weaker is the activation of the magnocellular system.

[80] But see Burr et al. [1994] and Walther-Müller [1995] for a counter evidence.

[81] Antis [1978] defined the apparent movement as the phenomenon by which a stimulus in retinal projection, when flickered in adjoining retinal positions, is illusory perceived in motion. The apparent movement of Ternus [Ternus, 1938] makes use of the visual persistence phenomenon to evoke the sensation of motion in a row of three identical and equally spaced stimuli. The presentation consists of two triplets differing only in their relative position, as the second triplet is shifted to the right by the length of a stimulus. The two triplets are sequentially displayed with a minimum interval of time: if this interval is less than about 50 msec, the observer perceives an illusory movement to the right of the first and last element, while if it is higher the whole block

In agreement with a selective damage of the magnocellular pathway, in patients visual persistence time is found to be longer especially at low spatial frequencies [Lovegrove et al., 1980a, b; Badcock & Lovegrove, 1981; Slaghuis & Lovegrove 1984, 1985, 1986; Lovegrove et al., 1986; Slaghuis et al., 1993] and its amount to be related to the reading difficulty [Slaghuis et al., 1993]. In the lexical context, increased visual persistence time enables the syllables projected in the parafoveal area to interfere with the syllables on the fixation point.

This solution seems to fit some of the most typical symptoms of developmental dyslexia, as visual confusion and the subjective movement of the letters [Jackson, 1976; Slaghuis & Ryan, 1999]: thereby, it looks to be more suitable than contrast sensitivity and motion perception alteration. Visual persistence time deserves further consideration even in light of the results obtained in the studies on eye movements[82], as longer visual persistence time is expected to desynchronize the saccadic sequence when reading. All the same, its increase seems too small to be considered the pivotal visuoperceptive element in developmental dyslexia.

References

Antis SM. (1978). *Apparent movement.* In: Handbook of Sensory Physiology, Vol.8, *Perception*, Teuber, Held &. Leibowitz Eds., Springer-Verlag, New York.

Badcock DR, Lovergrove WJ. (1981). *The effect of contrast, stimulus duration and spatial frequency on visible persistence in normal and specifically disabled readers.* Journal of Experimental Psychology: Human Perception and Performance, 7: 495-505.

Bowling A, Lovergrove WJ. (1980). *The effect of stimulus duration on the persistence of gratings.* Perception and Psychophysics, 27: 574-578.

Breitmeyer B, G, Levi DM, Harweith RS. (1981). *Flicker masking in spatial vision.* Vision Research, 21: 1377-1385.

Breitmeyer, BG, Ritter A. (1986a). *Visual persistence and the effect of eccentric viewing, element size, and frame duration on bistable stroboscopic motion percepts.* Perception & Psychophysics, 39: 275-280.

Breitmeyer, BG, Ritter A. (1986b). *The role of visible persistence on bistable stroboscopic motion.* Vision Research, 26: 1801-1806.

Burr DC, Morrone MC, Ross J. (1994). *Selective suppression of the magnocellular visual pathway during saccadic eye movement.* Nature, 371: 511-513.

looks to jump towards the right the length of a stimulus. The first case is due to the activation of the M system, while the P system is responsible for the second [Petersik & Pantle, 1979; Breitmeyer & Ritter, 1986a, b]. Increased temporal thresold required to evoke the apparent movement, as found in dyslexics by Slaghuis and Ryan [1999], means increased visual persistence time, therefore, magnocellular impairment. Two triplets suitable for the Ternus paradigm are shown below:

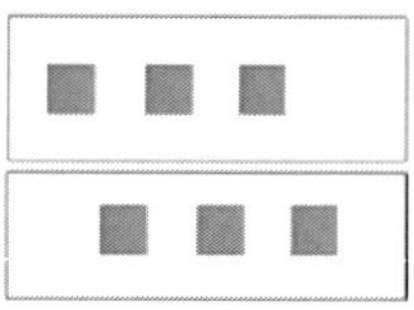

[82] Chapter 10.

Di Lollo V, Hanson D, McIntyre JS. (1983). *Initial stages of visual information processing in dyslexia.* Journal of Experimental Psychology, 9: 923-935.

Haber RN, Standing L. (1970). *Direct measures of the apparent duration of a flash.* Canadian Journal of Psychology, 24: 216-229.

Jackson M. (1976). *Reading disability, a case of reading malfunctioning: a program and therapy.* Australian Journal of Remedial Education, 8: 19-23.

Lovegrove WJ, Brown C. (1978). *Development of information processing in normal and disabled readers.* Perceptual & Motor Skills, 46: 1047-1054.

Lovergrove WJ, Heddle M. (1980). *Visual persistence as a function of spatial frequency and age.* Perception, 9: 529-532.

Lovergrove WJ, Heddle M, Slaghuis W. (1980a). *Reading disability: spatial frequency specific deficits in visual information store.* Neuropsychologia, 18: 111-115.

Lovegrove WJ, Bowling A, Badcock D, Blackwood M. (1980b). *Specific reading disability: Differences in contrast sensitivity as a function of spatial frequency.* Science, 210: 439-440.

Lovegrove WJ, Martin F, Slaghuis W. (1986). *A theoretical and experimental case for a visual deficit in specific reading disability.* Cognitive Neuropshychology, 3: 225-267.

Lovegrove WJ,Garzia RP, Nicholson SB. (1990). *Experimental evidence for a transient system deficit in specific reading disability.* Journal of the American Optometric Association, 61: 137-146.

Petersik JT, Pantle AJ. (1979). *Factors controlling the competing sensations produced by a bistable stroboscopic display.* Vision Research, 19: 143-154.

Slaghuis WL, Lovergrove WJ. (1984). *Flicker masking of spatial frequency dependant visible persistence and specific reading disability.* Perception, 13: 527-534.

Slaghuis WL, Lovergrove WJ. (1985). *Spatial-frequency-dependent visible persistence and specific reading disability.* Brain and Cognition, 4: 219-240.

Slaghuis WL, Lovergrove WJ. (1986). *The critical duration in spatial frequency dependent visible persistence and specific reading disability.* Bulletin of the Psychonomic Society, 24: 416-418.

Slaghuis WL, Lovergrove WJ, Davidson J. (1993). *Visual and Language Processing deficits are concurrent in dyslexia.* Cortex, 29: 601-615.

Slaghuis WL, Twell AJ, Kingston KR. (1996). Visual and language processing disorders are concurrent in dyslexia and continue into adulthood. Cortex, 32: 413-438.

Slaghuis WL, Ryan JF. (1999). *Spatio-temporal contrast sensitivity, coherent motion, and visible persistence in developmental dyslexia.* Vision Research, 39: 651-668.

Stanley G, Hall R. (1973). *Short term visual processing in dyslexics.* Child Development, 44: 841-844.

Ternus J. (1938). *The problem of phenomenal identity.* In: D.W.Ellis: A sourcebook of Gestalt psychology: Routledge & Kegan Eds., London.

Walther-Muller PU. (1995). *Is there a deficit of early vision in dyslexia?* Perception, 24: 919-936.

Williams MC, Molinet K, LeCluyse K. (1989). *Visual masking as a measure of temporal processing in normal and disabled readers.* Clinical Vision Sciences, 4 :137-144.

Winters RL, Patterson R, Shontz W. (1989). *Visual persistence and adult dyslexia.* Journal of Learning Disabilities, 22: 641-645.

Chapter IX

The Theory of the Deficit of the Magnocellular System: Lights and Shadows

According to the investigations reported in the previous chapters, a defect in the magnocellular visual pathway[83] is believed to take place in a substantial number of patients[84] [Lovergrove et al., 1980a,b; Lovergrove et al., 1986, Lovergrove et al., 1990; Livingstone et al., 1991; Lovergrove, 1991; Maddock et al., 1992; Breitmeyer, 1993; Galaburda & Livingstone, 1993; Stein & Walsh, 1997]. Indeed, this hypothesis does not rest just upon contrast sensitivity, motion perception and visual persistence time but even upon more complex visual tasks such as spatial localization [Solman & May, 1990][85]. The involvement of M-cells has been verified by Sperling et al.. [2003] with a specific paradigm developed by Rogers-Ramachandran & Ramachandran [1998][86] and confirmed by anatomopathological, electrophysiological and imaging studies[87].

In patients, the ventral layers of the lateral geniculate body are disorganized and geniculate magnocells in average are smaller by 27% compared to the size of normal readers. On the contrary, the size of the P-cells is normal [Galaburda et al., 1985; Livingstone et al., 1991].

[83] In 2001, Pammer and Wheatley found that the impairment affects a particular magnocellular subpopulation, the M(y) cells, and that the amount of this deficit is related to the delay in the acquisition of the lexical function.

[84] Up to 75% of patients according to Lovergrove [Lovergrove et al., 1990].

[85] See part II, chapter 5.

[86] The paradigm deals with the presentation of figures made up of black dots among white dots. The polarity of the pattern is reversed with increasing temporal frequency. The same applies to isoluminant colored dots (red and green). Beyond a certain level of frequency, the black dots become indistinguishable and only the contour of the figure remains defined. Since the first type of configuration (black and white dots) stimulates the M system, dots vanish and the contour of the figure is evident at the higher temporal frequencies. Instead, the second (red and green dots) is selective for the P system and the contour of the figure appears at lower temporal frequencies. Sperling has shown that with the first type of configuration dyslexics perceive the contour of the figure at a lower temporal frequency than normal subjects, while in the colored isoluminant condition no differences were found. These results reveal in dyslexics a selective deficiency of the M system, with normal parvocellular function [Sperling et al., 2003].

[87] But see the counter evidence [Victoret al., 1993; Johanneset al., 1996; Skottun, 1997; Ramuset al., 2003].

In spite of the considerable overlapping of the measurements in the two groups (figure 1), increased latency and reduced amplitude of the electrophysiological response to stimuli specific for the magnocellular system have been attributed to these anatomical anomalies [Livingstone et al., 1991; May et al., 1991, 1992; Maddock et al., 1992; Lehmkuhle et al., 1992, 1993; Kubova et al., 1995; Kuba et al., 2001, Romani et al., 2001].

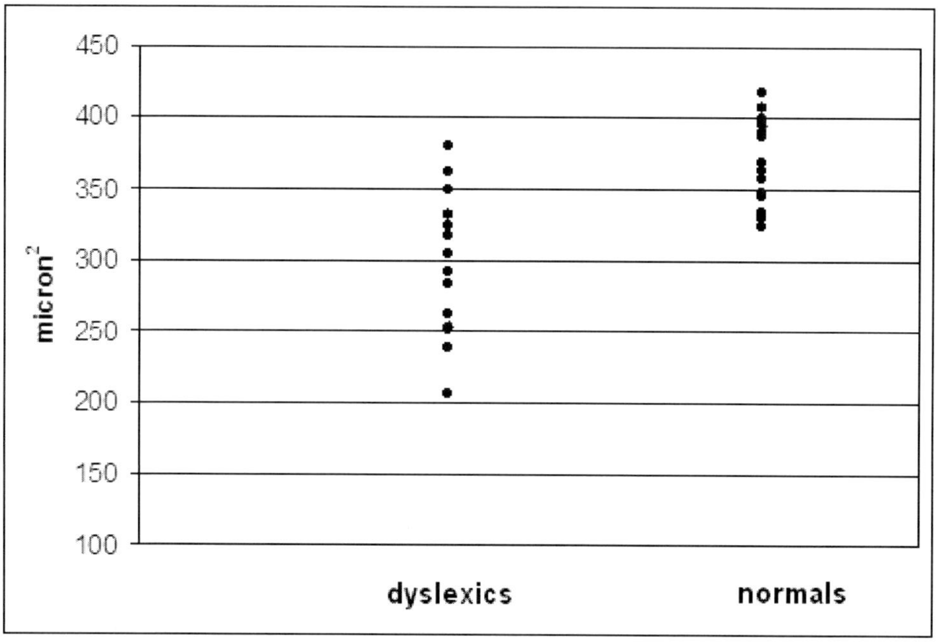

Figure 1. Size of M and P cells of the lateral geniculate body in normal and dyslexic subjects. Even if M cells in dyslexics are on average smaller than those of normal, the overlap in the respective measurements is consistent (data inferred from Livingstone et al., 1991).

In a small sample of dyslexic adults[88], Livingstone recorded the visual potentials evoked by the transient system by using a checkerboard pattern made of light and dark squares with low spatial frequency, contrast and luminance[89] [Livingstone et al., 1991] (an example is reported in figure 2).

By increasing the temporal frequency of stimulation (15Hz), the first peak turned out to be reduced in amplitude and delayed, making the record flattened.

Four years later Kubovà confirmed the electrophysiological depression of the response with transient stimulation and moving stimuli[90] [Kubova et al., 1995].

At the beginning of the nineties, Lehmkuhle measured VEPs in a group of 8 dyslexic children[91] using a sinusoidal grating at low spatial frequency (0.5 cycle/degree) and low contrast (0.1). The stimulus was displayed on a white field, before in a steady state and then flickering at high temporal frequency (12 Hz) [Lehmkuhle et al., 1993].

---

88 Mean age: 27.4 years.
89 Contrast: 0.02, luminance: 4 cd/m^2.
90 Counter evidence: Johannes et al. [1996].
91 Mean age: 10.6 years.

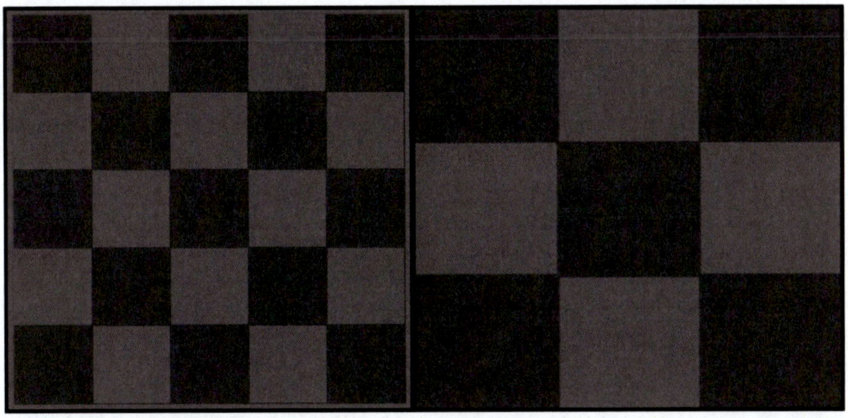

Figure 2. Example of a checkerboard pattern. Left: high spatial frequency. Right: low spatial frequency.

The latency of the first negative peak of the wave proved to be increased by 20-40 msec in patients: since this peak is an electrophysiological marker of the magnocellular function [Jones & Keck, 1978], it follows that M activity is reduced (figure 3).

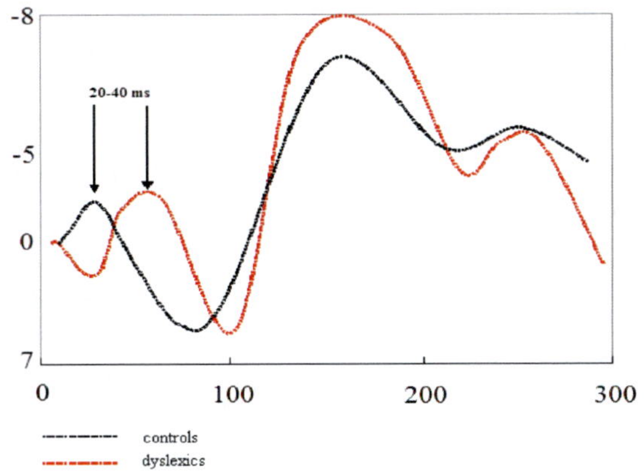

Figure 3. Simulation of the electrophysiological wave of visual potentials evoked in dyslexics compared with normal subjects. The latency of the first negative wave is shifted to the right in patients by about 40msec. In the abscissa are milliseconds.

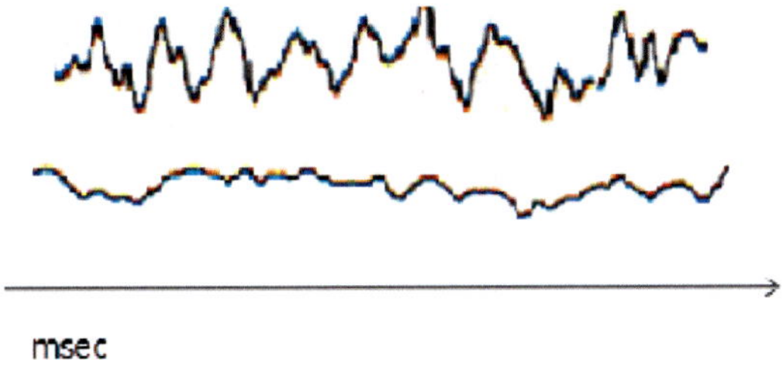

Figure 4. Simulation of VEPs in a normal (up) and in a dyslexic subject (down) on the occipital cortex during stimulation with flashing checkerboard patterns with low contrast and low luminance.

The use of a flickering background serves as a masking technique: in normal subjects, the flickering luminance of the background saturates the magnocellular function, reducing the electrophysiological response compared to the stationary condition (since in this way the response depends solely on the parvocellular system). On the contrary, when a malfunction of the M pathway takes place, such a stationary/flickering difference should be negligible.

In the stationary condition, the response recorded at 0.5 cycles/ degree in the dyslexic sample was weaker compared to controls but normalized at 4 cycles/ degree (i.e. in the parvocellular domain), in accordance with a defect of the magnocellular system. In the flickering condition, the lack of depression of the electrical response in the pathological group supports this finding [Lehmkuhle et al., 1993].

Some years later these results and the finding of delayed latency in 40-60% of patients with moving stimuli [Kuba et al., 2001] led to recommend to include VEPs with dynamic stimulations in the diagnostic protocols for dyslexia [Kuba et al., 2007].

As previously reminded, magnetic functional imaging (MRI) helps the anatomopathological and electrophysiological evidence to confirm the magnocellular impairment in dyslexics: Demb measured the cerebral response to sinusoidal moving gratings with low spatial frequency and low luminance [Demb et al., 1997, 1998] and discovered (especially in MT +) a significant correlation between the depression of the response and the reduction of the reading rate.

Since evidence seems favorable to the hypothesis of the deficit of the transient system, it has to be assessed whether the magnocellular defect occurs at a subcortical level (i.e. in the lateral geniculate body) or concerns mainly the cerebral cortex.

In the first case, results from psychophysical and functional imaging techniques, confirmed by histological [Galaburda et al., 1985; Livingstone et al., 1991] and deprivational studies [Maunsell et al., 1990; Schiller et al., 1990a, b; Merigan & Maunsell, 1990, 1993; Merigan et al., 1991], showed that the selective inactivation of subcortical magnocells reduces the response of the transient system on the cortex. Therefore, the depression of the cortical signal would depend on the loss of the M-neurons located at earlier stages of the visual pathway[92].

In the second case, it is more difficult to assess if an altered signal recorded on the cortex is selective for the transient system.

It has been reported that a cortical activation with relevant transient stimuli can result from the sum of the individual P cells, little responsive when taken individually but able to generate an appreciable cumulative response because of their high density[93] [Cornelissen et al., 1995]. Therefore, a putative depression of the magnocellular activity in the cortex can be due to a widespread reduction of the parvocellular function, "biasing" the specificity of the outcome.

Surprisingly, an Egyptian investigation found the P system and not the M system to be impaired in dyslexics [Farrag et al., 2002]. In this investigation, visual potentials evoked by a checkerboard-type stimulation were recorded in 52 Arab mother tongue patients (in Arabs the direction of reading is from right to left). Results were quite different from those reported in literature: in fact, the expected longer latency of the first negative wave in dyslexics was not evident at low spatial frequencies; on the contrary, it turned out to be reduced enough to make

[92] Abnormal magnocellular activation has been reported by Pammer & Wheatley [2001] even on the retina.

[93] See chapter 6.

the latency at the higher spatial frequencies longer than at the lowers. This finding would account for an impairment of the parvocellular (and not magnocellular) system. According to the authors, this finding would depend on the differences between Arabic and western languages: in fact, compared to the occidental scripts, reading in Arab requires a greater skill in the analysis of details; therefore, it needs a major involvement of the *sustained* system. For this reason a small disturbance of the parvocellular function, negligible by western readers, in Arab readers would help to make more evident a reading disability.

Yet, other studies focused on parvo-mediated functions (such as chromatic contrast or fine shape discrimination) deny any parvocellular impairment in patients [Chase & Jenner, 1993; Hayduket al., 1993].

A different question, elegantly faced by Skoyles and Skottun [2004], is the following: why not all those readers who suffer from a magnocellular deficit are dyslexics and vice versa? Indeed, despite a considerable amount of subjects is affected by anomalies in the transient system, the percentage of dyslexics (i.e., their prevalence *p*) is very low.

The consideration of the two scientists starts from the estimate of Lovegrove et al. [1986] that have quantified type M-defects in 75% of dyslexics and just in 8% of the normal population.

Based on these values, the number of patients affected by an M damage is given by *0.75p*, while in the rest of the population it is equivalent to:

$$NORM_M = (100-p) * 0.08$$

The ratio between the proportion of normal subjects with M damage and dyslexics with M damage is:

$$(100-p)0.08 / 0.75p$$

Based on the epidemiological studies of Rutter et al. [1970] and Duane [1974], *p* ranges between 4% and 15%.

Plotting the relation between normal readers with M damage and dyslexics with M damage as a function of the prevalence (*p*) of the patients in the population, the resulting function is shown in figure 5.

It is evident that if the prevalence of dyslexia is, for example, 4%, normal readers affected by M-damage are expected to be two and a half times more numerous than patients.

For higher prevalence values, this proportion decreases in favor of dyslexics so that for *p* of 9.6%, the number of normal readers and of patients with M-damage is the same.

So, paradoxically, a very high prevalence of the disease, nearly 10% of the population, implies an M damage equally distributed between patients and normal readers.

Assuming the prevalence of the disease to be higher than 9.6% implies a reversal of the relationship, which drops below the unity: for example for p= 15% the ratio is 0.6. Therefore, only from this hypothetical 9.6% of prevalence the overall amount of dyslexics that are affected by magnocellular impairment is larger than the normal readers who exhibit the same M-defect.

As a result, the M-damage could be considered as a marker of the disease if and only if the prevalence of our clinical condition were far higher than actually estimated.

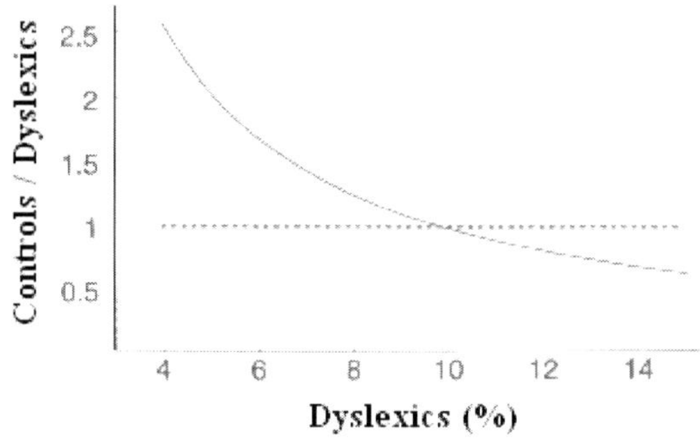

Figure 5. M-deficit as a marker of dyslexia. The intersection of the curve with the dotted line is the expected prevalence of the disease in order to make the number of patients with M-deficit and of normal readers with M-deficit equivalent. *(Reprint from: Brain and Language, Vol. 88, Issue 1, Skoyles J, Skottun BC, On the prevalence of magnocellular deficits in the visual system of non-dyslexic individuals, pages 79-82, 2004, with permission from Elsevier).*

The same can be applied to the hypothesis of fixation instability, which we will be discussed in chapter 10. Based on the data derived from the studies of Stein & Fowler [1981] and Stein [1986], fixation instability would affect 65% of patients and only 20% of the normal population. The ratio between the normal population with fixation instability and dyslexics with fixation instability is:

(100-p) 0. 2/(0.65p)

Plotting the relation between normal readers with fixation instability and dyslexics with fixation instability versus the prevalence of patients in the population, the resulting function is shown in figure 6.

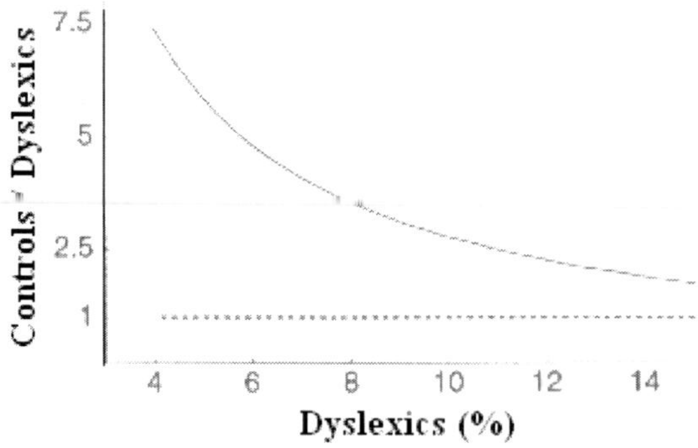

Figure 6. Fixation instability as a marker of dyslexia. The curve intercepts the equivalence line (number of patients with M damage equal to the number of normal readers with the same deficiency) for a prevalence of the disease of 23.5% (not shown in the graph). *(Reprint from: Brain and Language, Vol. 88, Issue 1, Skoyles J, Skottun BC, On the prevalence of magnocellular deficits in the visual system of non-dyslexic individuals, pages 79-82, 2004, with permission from Elsevier).*

In this case patients with fixation instability would match normal readers with the same defect if the prevalence of the disease were 23.5%. Hence, instable fixation would become a reliable marker only if the prevalence were well above 23.5%.

In summary, this argument aims at emphasizing that although the percentage of subjects with impaired magnocellular system or M-derived unstable fixation is much higher among dyslexics compared to normal readers, the absolute value is too low in patients and, at the same time, too high in the normal population. For this reason, M-deficits shows to be inadequate as a reliable marker of dyslexia.

The correlation between the magnocellular function and the lexical ability, even if statistically significant, does not exceed r = 0.45 [Stein, 2003], revealing that the former (as detected by the experimental techniques employed so far[94]) accounts for no more than 20% - 25% of the variance of the reading ability in the general population.

Probably, such a limit depends on the ability to accurately measure the magnocellular function [Talcott et al., 1998; Witton et al., 1998; Stein, 2003], so that more specific and sensitive tests could allow the function of figure 5 to converge on the dotted line more on the left along the x-axis.

For this purpose, the combination of different tests aimed at measuring the M-function could be a solution: for example, the performance referred to coherent motion perception joined to that obtained using the critical fusion frequency are found to increase the sensitivity up to 72.2% and the specificity up to 83.3%, and shows a strong correlation with the lexical ability when reading non-words ($r = 0{,}691$, $p \leq 0.001$) [Talcott et al., 1998].

Even the assessment of fixation stability might turn out to be a more effective marker of dyslexia, when aimed at detecting a specific typology of dyslexic and therefore, after a suitable classification has excluded subjects with a clear phonological origin.

Apart from these considerations, on this bases the theory of the deficit of the magnocellular system seems unable to explain the reading difficulties of dyslexics. To date, in spite of the use of different techniques and approaches, the investigations focused on the detection and characterization of the magnocellular deficit in patients have failed to address the question of how a malfunction of the M-cells along the visual pathway could actually interfere with the lexical ability [Chase etal,2005]. Still, it is unclear how motion perception alteration, decreased contrast sensitivity or prolonged visual persistence could prevent from reading fluently. As an example, a study has failed to show a correlation between coherent motion threshold and the oculomotor function (in particular the number of fixations required to read a series of non-words) in a group of 11 dyslexic children[95] [Hutzler et al., 2006].

With regard to contrast sensitivity, it has been advanced that defective contrast sensitivity in patients reduces the perceived contrast of the letters, so as to make them difficult to recognize. In fact, in order to halve the reading rate of a normal subject his/her contrast sensitivity has to be lowered by at least 1 log unit [Law et al. 1987]: and yet, contrast sensitivity in dyslexics is found to be reduced no more than 0.1 log units for stationary stimuli and 0.3 log units for stimuli flickering at high temporal frequency.

In addition, when found, the contrast sensitivity impairment is observed at low luminance levels (below about 10 cd/m2) and not in the ordinary reading photopic conditions (beyond 30-40 cd/m2) [Martin & Lovegrove, 1984; Cornelissen et al., 1995].

---

[94] In particular those based on motion perception.

[95] Age: 13 years.

The relationship between reading and visual persistence seems more reliable. As reported in chapter 8, increased visual persistence time is expected to generate confusion and the sensation of moving letters. Indeed, in dyslexics the interval of time required to detect two sequential stimuli is up to 100 milliseconds longer than in normal readers. This finding has been confirmed by Winters [Winters et al., 1989] and ten years later by Slaghuis & Ryan [1999] by using the apparent movement of Ternus. Still, the duration of a fixation is higher than 100 milliseconds, being usually about 180 milliseconds but sometimes raising up to 450 msec [McConkie & Zola, 1989]. Therefore, even if visual persistence time is longer than normal in dyslexics, it is not longer enough. From the beginning of a fixation to the next one, the elapsed interval of time is up to 4 times longer than the visual persistence time in dyslexics; so, by the time the fixation spends to move to the next letter, the phantom image of the previous letter induced by the delayed visual persistence is disappeared.

In conclusion, the arguments of the supporters of the visual theory seem to be confined to a sterile epiphenomenal level, unable to overcome the gap that divide it from the aetiopathogenetical one.

To support the causal implication of the transient system in developmental dyslexia, the remaining alternative is to show that magnocells carry one more function. A function closer to the lexical task compared to motion perception, visual persistence or contrast sensitivity.

This function is the oculomotor pattern in reading. To avoid the collapse of the theory of the deficit of the magnocellular system, the possible involvement of the M system even (and especially) in the programming and triggering of the fine eye movements has to be investigated.

References

Breitmeyer, BG. (1993). *The roles of sustained and transient channels in reading and reading disabilities.* In: Facets of dyslexia and its Remediation, Wright & Groner Eds., Elsevier, Amsterdam.

Chase C, Jenner AN. (1993). *Magnocellular visual deficits affect temporal processing of dyslexics.* Annals of the New York Academy of Sciences, 682: 326-329.

Chase C, Ashourzadeh A, Kelly C, Monfette S, Kinsey K. (2003). *Comment on letter to the editor: magnocellular reading and dyslexia.* Vision Research, 45: 135-136.

Cornelissen PL, Richardson AR, Mason A, Fowler MS, Stein JF. (1995). *Contrast sensitivity and coherent motion detection measured at photopic luminance levels in dislexics and controls.* Vision Research, 35: 1483-1494.

Demb JB, Boynton GM, Heeger DJ. (1997). *Brain activity in visual cortex predicts individual differences in reading performance.* Proceedings of the National Academy of Sciences of the United States of America, 94: 13363-13366.

Demb JB, Boynton GM, Best M, Heeger DJ. (1998). *Functional magnetic resonance imaging of early visual pathways in dyslexia.* The Journal of Neuroscience, 18: 6939-6951.

Duane DD. (1974). A neurological overview of specific language disability for the non neurologist. Bulletin of the Orton Society, 24: 5-36.

Farrag AF, Khedr EM, Abel-Naser W. (2002). *Impaired parvocellular pathway in dyslexic children.* European Journal of Neurology, 9: 359-363.

Galaburda AM, Livingstone M. (1993). *Evidence for a magnocellular defect in developmental dyslexia.* Annals of the New York Academy of Sciences, 682: 70-82.

Galaburda AM, Sherman GF, Rosen GD, Aboitiz F, Geschwind N. (1985). *Developmental dyslexia: four consecutive patients with cortical anomalies.* Annals of Neurology, 18: 222-233.

Hayduk S, Bruck M, Cavanagh P. (1993). *Do adult dyslexics show low level visual processing deficits?* Annals of the New York Academy of Sciences, 682: 351-353.

Hutzler F, Kronbichler M, Jacobs AM, Wimmer H. (2006). *Perhaps correlational but not causal: no effect of dyslexic readers'magnocellular system on their eye movements during reading.* Neuropsychologia, 44: 637-648.

Johannes S, Kussmaul CL, Munte TF, Mangun GR. (1996). *Developmental dyslexia: passive visual stimulation provides no evidence for a magnocellular processing defect.* Neuropsychologia, 34: 1123-1127.

Jones R, Keck, MJ. (1978). *Visual evoked response as a function of grating spatial frequency.* Investigative Ophthalmology & Visual Science, 17: 652-659.

Kuba M, Szanyi J, Gayer D, Kremlacek J, Kubová Z. (2001). *Electrophysiological testing of dyslexia.* Acta Medica (Hradec Kralove), 44: 131-134.

Kuba M, Kubovà Z, Kremlacek J, Langrova J. (2007). Motion-onset VEPs: characteristics, methods, and diagnostic use. Vision Research, 47: 189-202.

Kubovà Z, Kuba M, Peregrin J, Nováková V. (1995). *Visual Evoked potential evidence for magnocellular system deficit in dyslexia.* Physiological Research, 44: 87-89.

Legge GE, Rubin GS, Luebker A. (1987). *Psychophysics of reading-V. The role of contrast in normal vision.* Vision Research, 27: 1165-1175.

Lehmkuhle S, Garzia RP, Turner L, Hash T, Baro JA. (1992). *The effects of uniform-field flicker on visual evoked potential in children with reading disability.* Investigative Ophthalmology & Vision Science, 33: 718.

Lehmkuhle S, Garzia RP, Turner L, Hash T, Baro JA. (1993). *A defective visual pathway in children with reading disability.* New England Journal of Medicine, 328: 989-996.

Livingstone MS, Rosen GD, Drislane FW, Galaburda AM. (1991). *Physiological and anatomical evidence for a magnocellular defect in developmental dyslexia.* Proceedings of the National Academy of Sciences of the United States of America, 88: 7943-7947.

Lovergrove WJ, Heddle M, Slaghuis W. (1980a). *Reading disability: spatial frequency specific deficits in visual information store.* Neuropsychologia, 18: 111-115.

Lovegrove WJ, Bowling A, Badcock D, Blackwood M. (1980b). *Specific reading disability: Differences in contrast sensitivity as a function of spatial frequency.* Science, 210: 439-440.

Lovegrove WJ, Martin F, Slaghuis W. (1986). *A theoretical and experimental case for a visual deficit in specific reading disability.* Cognitive Neuropshychology, 3: 225-267.

Lovegrove WJ, Garzia RP, Nicholson SB. (1990). *Experimental evidence for a transient system deficit in specific reading disability.* Journal of the American Optometric Association, 61: 137-146.

Lovergrove WJ. (1991). *Spatial frequency processing in dislexic and normal readers.* In: Vision and Visual Dyslexia, Stein Ed., CRC Press, Boca Raton, FL.

Maddock H, Richardson A, Stein JF. (1992). *Reduced and delayed visual evoked potentials in dyslexics.* Journal of Physiology, 459: 130P.

Martin F, Lovegrove WJ. (1984). *The effects of field size and luminance on contrast sensitivity differences between specifically reading disabled and normal children.* Neuropsychologia, 22: 73-77.

Maunsell JHR, Nealey TA, Depriest DD. (1990). *Magnocellular and parvocellular contributions to responses in the middle temporal visual area (MT) of the macaque monkey.* The Journal of Neuroscience, 10: 3323-3334.

May JG, Lovergrove WJ, Martin F, Nelson P. (1991). *Pattern-elicited visual evoked potentials in good and poor readers*. Clinical Vision Sciences, 6: 131-136.

May JG, Dunlap WP, Lovergrove WJ. (1992). Factor scores derived from visual evoked potentials latencies differentiate good and poor readers. Clinical Vision Sciences, 7: 67-70.

McConkie GW, Zola D. (1989). *Some characteristics in readers' eyes movements.* In: Brain and reading. Von Euler, Lundberg & Lennerstrand Eds., Macmillian Press, London.

Merigan WH, Maunsell JHR. (1990). *Macaque vision after magnocellular lateral geniculate lesions*. Visual Neuroscience, 5: 347-352.

Merigan WH, Byrne CE, Maunsell JHR. (1991). *Does primate motion perception depend on the magnocellular pathway?* The Journal of Neuroscience, 11: 3422-3429.

Merigan WH, Maunsell JHR. (1993). *How parallel are the human visual pathways?* Annual Review of Neuroscience, 16: 369-402.

Pammer K, Wheatley C. (2001). *Isolating the M(y)-cell response in dyslexia using the spatial frequency doubling illusion.* Vision Research, 41: 2139-2147.

Ramus F, Rosen S, Dakin SC, Day BL, Castellote JM, White S, Frith U. (2003). *Theories of developmental dyslexia: insights from a multiple case study of dyslexic adults.* Brain, 126: 841-865.

Rogers-Ramachandran DC, Ramachandran VS. (1998*). Psychophysical evidence for boundary and surface systems in human vision.* Vision Research, 38: 71-77.

Romani A, Conte S, Callieco R, Bergamaschi R, Versino M, Lanzi G, Zambrino CA, Cosi V. (2001). *Visual evoked potential abnormalities in dyslexic children.* Functional Neurology, 16: 219-229.

Rutter M. Tizard J, Whitmore K. (1970). *Education Healt and Behavior*. Longman Ed., New York.

Schiller PH, Logothetis NK, Charles ER. (1990a). Functions of the colour-opponent and broad-band channels of the visual system. Nature, 343: 68-70.

Schiller PH, Logothetis NK, Charles ER. (1990b). *Role of the colour-opponent and broad band channels in vision.* Visual Neuroscience, 5: 321-346.

Skoyles J, Skottun BC. (2004). *On the prevalence of magnocellular deficits in the visual system of non-dyslexic individuals.* Brain and Language, 88: 79-82.

Skottun BC. (1997). *Some remarks on the magnocellular deficit theory of dyslexia.* Vision Research, 37: 965-966.

Slaghuis WL, Ryan JF. (1999). *Spatio-temporal contrast sensitivity, coherent motion, and visible persistence in developmental dyslexia.* Vision Research, 39: 651-668.

Solman RT, May JG. (1990). *Spatial localization discrepancies: A visual deficiency in poor readers.* American Journal of Pshychology, 103:243-263.

Sperling AJ, Lu Z, Manis FR, Seidenberg MS. (2003). *Selective magnocellular deficits in dyslexia: a "phantom contour" study*. Neuropsychologia, 41: 1422-1429.

Stein JF, Fowler S. (1981). *Visual Dyslexia.* Trends in the Neurological Sciences, 4: 77-80.

Stein J. (1986). *The Dunlop test and reading in primary school children.* British Journal of Ophthalmology, 70: 317-320.

Stein JF. (2003). *Visual motion sensitivity and reading.* Neuropsychologia, 41: 1785-1793.

Stein JF, Walsh V. (1997). *To see but not to read: the magnocellular theory of dyslexia.* Trends in Neurosciences, 20: 147-152.

Talcott JB, Hansen PC, Willis-Owen C, McKinnell IW, Richardson AJ, Stein J. (1998). *Visual magnocellular impairment in adult developmental dyslexics.* Neuroophthalmology, 20: 187-201.

Victor JD, Conte MM, Burton L, Nass R. (1993). *Visual evoked potentials in dyslexics and normals: failure to find a difference in transient or steady-state responses.* Visual Neuroscience, 10: 939-946.

Winters RL, Patterson R, Shontz W. (1989). *Visual persistence and adult dyslexia.* Journal of Learning Disabilities, 22: 641-645.

Witton C, Talcott JB, Hansen PC, Richardson AJ, Griffiths TD, Rees A, Stein JF, Greef GGR. (1998). *Sensitivity to dynamic auditory and visual stimuli predicts nonword reading ability in both dyslexic and normal readers.* Current Biology, 8: 791-797.

Chapter X

Eye Movements and Dyslexia

Under a perceptual perspective, we can imagine the lexical function based on the subsequent decoding of characters arranged sequentially in the visual space.

For this purpose, it is essential not only to recognize the symbol, but even its position with respect to the previous and next one.

This requirement is common to all types of writing: the alphabetical writing of the western countries in which the development of the text is from left to right, the Hebrew idiom in which the direction is opposite, and finally the pictographic systems such as Chinese in which the symbols consist of ideograms and their arrangement is vertical.

In every case, reading is made of two fundamental stages: fixations and saccades.

To be correctly recognized, a letter or syllable must fall on the central region of the retina, *the fovea*. In fact, the anatomical and functional characteristics of the foveal region are the only one that fit the purpose. For this reason, the fovea is even called the *region of the sharp vision*.

However this is not enough: the configuration must remain on the fovea for an adequate period of time: not too short, otherwise the visual system would fail to complete the processing of the character, and not too long, otherwise the lexical decoding rate would turn out to be too slow.

This moment is defined *fixation*: during the fixation, part of a word is kept projected on the fovea for the time required to be correctly decoded.

The duration of each fixation is not always the same but depends on the difficulty of the text and ranges from 30-40 msec to 450 msec [McConkie & Zola, 1989], being in average 180 msec. Fixations placed at the end of the line tend to be shorter than the central ones [Abrams & Zuber, 1972].

Since letters and words have to be processed sequentially, fixation has to shift along the string at an even pace. Each repositioning of the fixation is not a smooth movement but it is sort of leaping and it is defined *saccade* (or *FEM, Fast Eye Movement*).

So, saccades are rapid eye movements that from time to time move the fixation along the sentence from one letter/syllable to the next. The direction of the scanning follows the arrangement of the text, so that when reading in western languages the majority of the saccades move from left to right and are referred to as *forward* saccades.

In average, forward saccades are 2 degrees wide[96], encompassing about 8 characters [McConkie & Zola, 1989]. However, forward saccades tend to shorten when facing with particularly difficult texts: therefore, the increased overall number of eye movements required to complete the analysis of the sentences[97] ends up to affect the fluency of reading, slowing down the lexical speed [Kowler & Anton, 1987].

In a small percentage of cases, saccades move in the opposite direction: these *regression saccades* or *backward saccades* are aimed at bringing back the fixation every time the lexical (words, letters or syllables) processing has not been satisfactory. Backward FEMs are shorter than forward sacccades, measuring about 1 degree, that is 4 letters. Although backward saccades are usually only 15% of the total FEMs[98] [Rayner, 1978; McConkie & Zola, 1989], their frequency increases when reading demanding or unfamiliar texts [Jones & Stark, 1983; Rayner & Pollatsek, 1987; McConkie & Zola, 1989].

In summary, when reading a demanding page *forward* and *backward* FEMs are increased in number and the former are reduced in size: it follows that, compared to an easier passage, reading time[99] becomes longer.

Once the fixation/saccade sequence reaches the end of the line, a wide regression movement, called *return sweep*, repositions the fixation at the beginning of the next line and the process starts again[100] (Figure 1). The position of the fixation depends on the landing point of the saccade at the end of its saltatory movement. This zone is defined *landing site* and in normal readers localizes between the beginning and the middle of the word [Rayner, 1979] or, according to McConkie [McConkie et al., 1988][101], on the third letter of the word. This is the position which minimizes the fixation time, and is therefore called *convenient viewing position* [O'Regan, 1981] or *preferred viewing location* [Rayner, 1979]. The term *perceptive centre-of-gravity* or *optimum viewing location* [O 'Regan & Jacobs, 1992], theorized under the name of *optical centre* of *gravity* [Findlay, 1982; Ottes et al., 1984] and further studied by Crawford and Higham [2001], refers to the theoretical position that would allow the best processing of the word, and that is localized at its midpoint[102].

Evidently, the correct positioning of the fixation depends on adequate saccadic movements: too short or too long saccades drag the fixation on the one side or on the other side of the optical centre -of-gravity, preventing from correctly processing the text.

Since the early eighties, a number of investigations have centered on the dynamics underlying eye movements during reading. In substance, three main speculative currents will be considered: the first refers to the cognitive theories, the second to oculomotor strategies, the third to the so-called *pull and push* theory, that is the closest to the hypothesis of the deficit of the magnocellular system.

---

96 At the usual reading distance (33 cm).

97 In addition, the number of forward saccades required to process a word depends on its length [MacKeben et al., 2004].

98 5-20% according to Eden et al. [1994].

99 90-95% of the reading time is made of fixations and the remaining 5-10% is used by the saccadic movements [Eden et al., 1994].

100 The return sweep is modulated by the cerebellum [Stein, 2001].

101 Often in very short and simple words (like articles and prepositions) the landing site is missing. Therefore, short words are not fixated but tend to be automatically "derived" from the meaning of the text or processed from the the parafoveal region (i.e. the retinal area just on the right of the fixation point). On the contrary, long words are often provided with two landing sites, the one proximal and the other distal [Dunn-Rankin, 1978; Rayner,1979].

102 For further details and references see Radach et al., 2004, pp. 28-29.

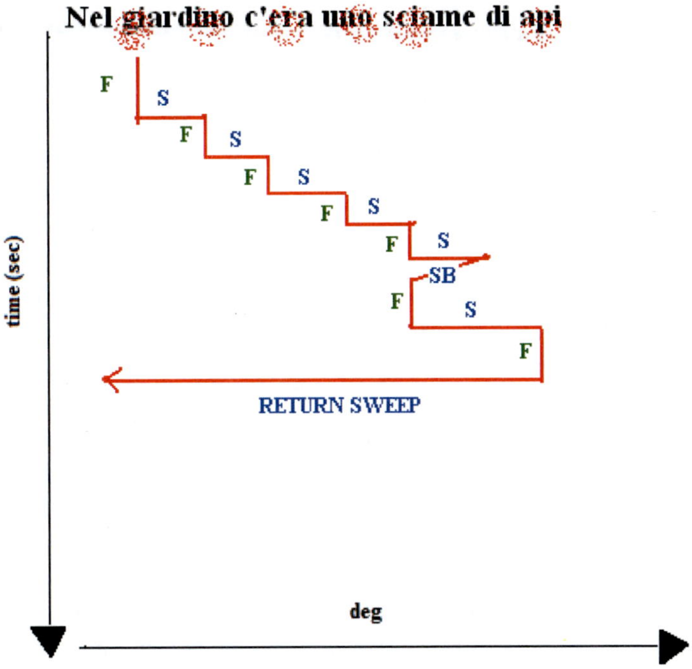

Figure 1. Schematic representation of the eye movements when reading a line of text ("*In the garden there was a swarm of bees"*). In abscissa is the amplitude of the saccades that move sequentially along the string, in ordinate is the (fixation) time. The line represents the alternation of fixations and saccades. Near the end of the sequence, a backward saccade (SB) goes back to the previous fixation. At the end, a wide return sweep moves the gaze back to the beginning of the next line. The dotted spots along the string represent the landing site that in normal readers match the convenient viewing position.

According to the cognitive theories, the fixation lingers on the word for the time required for its comprehension, and then it is suppressed by the saccadic movement which provides for its repositioning to the next preferred viewing location [Just & Carpenter, 1980].

The oculomotor strategy hypothesis explains the saccadic pattern according to stereotyped models refined with the experience. The effect of the strategy is modulated via more and more precise corrective movements based on the acquired experience of the characteristics of the visuoperceptive afferent inputs (i.e. on the properties of the words).

The theory advanced by Levi-Schoen and O'Regan [1987] belongs to this area. According to the authors, the saccadic strategy aims at locating the fixation near the optical centre-of-gravity of the word and if the result is not as accurate as expected, a re-fixation movement would correct the positional error.

A paradigm that does not rule out (rather complements) the oculomotor strategy, considers the saccades activation time as a probabilistic event. The features of a stimulus (for example a word), has an effect on the parameters that modulate the probabilistic distribution of the saccadic activation [McConkie & Dyre, 2000][103]. According to this conjecture, reading

[103] The time taken by the lexical stimulus to reach the visual areas and to activate the reflex that triggers the saccade is approximately 90 msec. So, for very short fixations (less than 90 msec), the triggering of the next saccade occurs before the retinal image has reached the visual areas [McConkie & Zola, 1989]. This timing discrepancy seems to imply that the saccade activation is an automatic process, not dependent on the reflex of fixation, on the processing of the lexical stimulus and on the cognitive factor.

experience would increase the probability for a saccade to be triggered after a time *t* by a given type of stimulus and after a time t_l by a second, different one[104], therefore optimizing the progression of the oculomotor sequence.

All the same, the paradigm that seems to fit better the current positions on the pathogenetical mechanisms of developmental dyslexia in the visuoperceptive domain is based on the studies of Findlay and Walker [1999] and defined the *pull-and-push model.* According to the pull-and-push model, the saccade-fixation sequence is not driven by a cognitive or probabilistic process but depends on an interactive-competitive system between two cerebral centers acting both at the oculomotor and visuoperceptive level[105].The alternate success of the center responsible for the fixation and of the center in charge for the saccadic activation, dictates the rhythm of the fixation-saccade-fixation sequence during reading.

It is likely the cognitive influence to play a modulatory role by increasing the latency of the saccadic activation in order to help prolonging the fixation[106]: this subject would explain why reading is slower with demanding texts.

Nevertheless, the same effect on the saccades' latency may depend also by visuoperceptive difficulties. Actually, three types of saccades can be distinguished based on their latency: early saccades and normal saccades, both insensitive to the informational and linguistic content, and late saccades [Yang & McConkie, 2001]. Late saccades occur when the informational content of the stimulus (for example the perception or the comprehension of a word) is not clear: in this case, the planned normal saccade is cancelled and replaced by a late saccade. This change leads to increased ratio between the two movements in favor of the second. Since the activation of late saccades depends also on the lexical comprehension, late saccades would be the only ones liable to be modulated by the cognitive process.

Yang and McConkie have formulated a modified version of the push-and-pull theory, the *competition-interaction theory* [Yang & McConkie, 2001].

In short, the duration and the release of the fixation is affected by the result of the competition between a so-called *central vision-related fixate-center*, whose activation promotes the fixation and supports its stability, and a *peripheral vision-related move-center*, whose activation triggers the saccadic movement. The two centers would be competitively linked so that the activation of the one leads to the inhibition of the other. A stimulus that falls on the peripheral visual field (or outside of the fixation area) leads to a progressive activation of the peripheral vision-related move-center and a gradual inhibition of the central vision-related fixate center. When the activation level of the central vision-related fixation center falls below a threshold value, the fixation is suppressed and the saccadic movement occurs, so that the eyes move towards the next preferred viewing location[107]. During the saccadic shift, the progressive re-activation of the central vision-related fixation center gradually inhibits the peripheral movement center. When the activation level of the peripheral movement center

[104] If the second stimulus (i.e. the second word) is more complex than the first one, then t_l will be longer than *t*.

[105] In the visuoperceptive domain, this competitive interaction acts so that when the P-system is activated (by processing a foveal target) and at the same time the M-system is elicited by the onset of a stimulus at the periphery of the visual field, the former is immediately inhibited. The ecological value of such a mechanism, which obliges to pay attention to what occurs in the suburbs before keeping on processing the foveal stimulus, is intuitive.

[106] The same applies to visual attention (see chapter 11).

[107] During the saccadic movement, the M-system suppresses the perception of the stimulus in order to avoid the occurrence of visual confusion [Campbell & Wurtz, 1978].

falls below a cut off value, the saccade finally "lands" and a new fixation takes place. It is possible however that the cognitive function affect this competitive circuit.

This hypothesis fits well the theory of the deficit of the magnocellular system: the P system, responsible for the fixation and therefore identifiable as the *central-vision-related fixate-center,* is mostly represented in the foveal region; on the contrary, the M system, responsible for the saccadic triggering[108] and therefore identifiable as the *peripheral-vision-related move center*, localizes mainly in the parafoveal and peripheral region.

The theory of the competition-interaction is enriched by a series of additions: first, when the activation level of the central vision-related fixation center drops below the threshold value, the latency of the forthcoming saccade is a random interval which follows a Poisson[109] distribution. Moreover, the gradual (not abrupt) fading of the inhibition of the fixation at the end of the saccadic activation helps the establishment of a refractory period useful to avoid an undesired, untimely FEM activation. Therefore, this refractory phase prevents premature saccadic activation through the maintenance of a sort of "fixation tone". The mechanism, however, if on the one hand is aimed at preventing untimely saccades, on the other hand predisposes to visual confusion. Visual confusion, indeed, would take place when a fixation "hypertone" persists during the subsequent eye movement, causing interference between the syllable processed by the previous fixation and the forthcoming perception of the next group of letters.

In figure 2 is represented the competitive interaction of the saccade-fixation system.

The lapse of time immediately before the saccade triggering, shown in figure 3, is crucial: as mentioned, immediately after the landing of the FEM, its level activation is at its minimum since it is inhibited by the P-mediated fixation center (figure 2, lower panel, point I).

However, as a dynamic process, during the fixation the CVRFC-driven inhibitory effect gradually decreases at the same pace with the raise of the saccadic potential.

After about 125 msec [Yang & McConkie, 2001], this trend becomes faster until it reaches a *plateau.* At the *plateau,* the programming of the saccade is completed and the forthcoming time of its trigger is a random interval that depends on the instant the fluctuation of the activation state would cross the threshold.

Yang &McConkie [2001] have highlighted the importance of the *plateau* and it is noted that its position is variable not only from subject to subject, but also in the same reader, depending on the difficulty of the lexical material: on the one hand; the interindividual variability of the *plateau* would explain the differences in reading rate in the population, regardless of cultural, cognitive or linguistic elements. On the other hand, the intra-individual variability aims at optimizing the rhythm of the saccadic sequence, modulating the accessibility of the lexical material. Therefore, for simple texts the *plateau* tends to localize higher, allowing faster saccadic activations, while for a more demanding reading it settles lower, allowing on the contrary longer times of fixation (in order to help the comprehension of the word).

---

108 The role played by the M system in generating the saccadic movements is testified by its projection to the superior colliculus. The superior colliculus, a structure placed in the midbrain, is of great importance in the oculomotor planning and execution.

109 Introduced for the first time by the French mathematician SD Poisson (1781-1840), the distribution that bears his name describes the relative frequency of a number of rare events that (in case of saccades) occur in the unit of time. Refer to statistics texts for details.

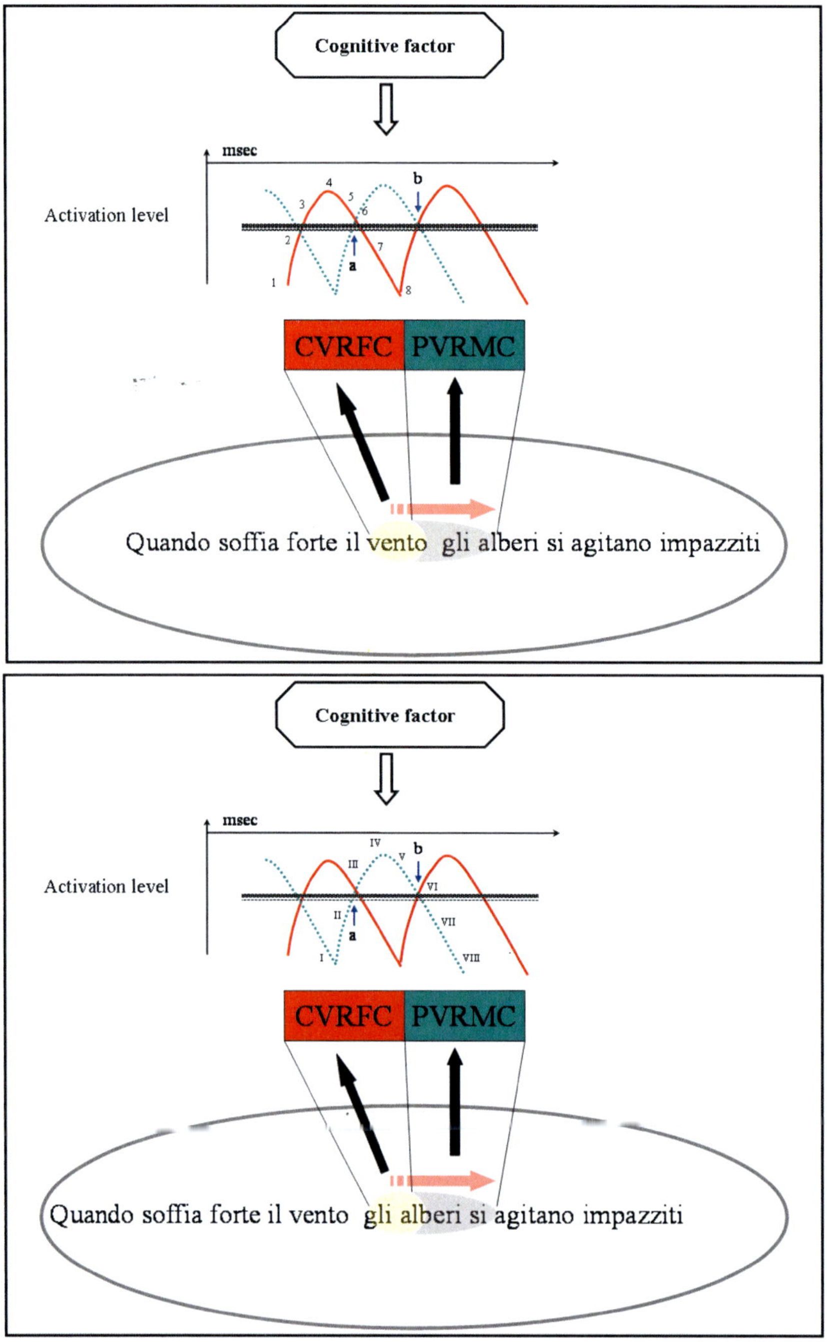

Figure 2. The saccade-fixation sequence according to the competition-interaction theory (revised). Top panel: progression from the viewpoint of the fixation. Lower panel: progression from the viewpoint of the saccadic movements. In the lower part of the two panels a line of Italian text ("when the wind blows hard the trees toss crazily") is shown, together to the fixation (yellow circle) and the region where the subsequent saccadic movement is expected to occur (gray area). The fixation is promoted and maintained by the central-vision-related fixate center (CVRFC) while the peripheral-vision-related move center (PVRMC) is in charge for the eye movement. In the upper part is depicted the mutual integration of the activation of the two programming stations (red line: CVRFC; green dotted line: PVRMC).
Top: The CVRFC activation increases gradually (1, 2), reaching and then exceeding the level of the PVRMC

activation (thick horizontal bar) (3). This way, the CVRFC promotes the fixation and, growing further (4), stabilizes it on the landing site. The fixation is maintained, despite the activation level of CVRFC is fading progressively (5) until it reaches (6) and then drops below the PVRMC activation level (7), which in the meantime is rising. At this point the effect of the saccadic center prevails and the fixation interruption is impending (a). When the CVRFC activation is reduced to the minimum (8) and at the same time the activation of the PVRMC is at its maximum, the saccade is triggered and its movement lasts until the CVRFC has returned to an energy level able to counter the PVRMC (b), making finally the saccade land.
Bottom: the PVRMC activation increases gradually (I, II), reaching and then exceeding the level of the CVRFC activation (a), represented by the thick horizontal bar (III). Growing up to a maximum level (IV), the PVRMC promotes the triggering of the saccadic movement. The movement continues despite the level of the PVRMC activation shows a progressive decay (V) until it reaches (VI) and then drops below the CVRFC activation level (VII), which in the meanwhile is rising. At this point, the effect of the central vision related-fixation center prevails and the saccade progressively loses momentum (b). When the PVRMC activation is reduced to the minimum (VIII) and at the same time the activation of the CVRFC is at its maximum, the saccade lands and the fixation takes place. The fixation lasts until the PVRMC has returned to an energetic level able to counter the CVRFC, triggering a new saccade directed toward the next landing site.
The influence of the cognitive element in this model is admitted.

Although the modulatory effect of the cognitive function takes place before the completion of the saccadic programming, i.e. before the function has reached the plateau, in some situations it could occur later. In both cases, the result is prolonged cumulative fixation time and increased frequency of backward and late saccades[110].

In summary, if we assume the oculomotor pattern in reading is driven by the antagonist interaction and the alternate activation of the M- and P cells along the visual pathway, the push-and-pull theory can be adopted in a more neurophysiological[111] context.

Obviously, the synchronization of these two systems must be extremely accurate.

If for any reason such a delicate balance between the two cellular pathways should be troubled, a disarticulation of the sequence saccade-fixation would take place. In particular, if the M-driven saccadic activation were weak, it would be expected:

- A delay in saccadic activation.
- An incomplete inhibition of fixations, so that the persistence of a residual activity of the P-system during the saccadic movement leads to a superimposition of the syllables processed in two subsequent fixations, that is visual confusion.

---

[110] To date, the cerebral structure responsible for late saccades is unknown. The frontal eye fields (FEF) may be involved [Schall, 1991].

[111] The balanced cooperation between M-system and P-system recruits anatomical structures not necessarily placed along the retinocortical pathway pathway. The superior colliculus is an example. Mohler and Wurtz [1976] found that in some neurons of this region the discharge rate raises immediately before the saccadic activation. The authors refer to these special cells as *visually triggered movement cells (VTMC).* The VTMCs localize at the boundary between the superficial and intermediate layers of the superior colliculus and integrate the visual (retinal) information directed to the superficial layers with the motor programming of the saccadic events that rely on the cells of the intermediate layers. This way, the VTMCs inform the motor programming neurons of the intermediate layers about the optimal parameters of the saccade as a function of the perceptive characteristics of the target: indeed, such a link between sensory subsystem and oculomotor subsystem results in a downright visuomotor integration complex [Sparks, 1986]. From the superior colliculus, the integrated information is then transmitted to the frontal cortex (in particular the frontal eye fields, that is the oculomotor planning center) and to the parietal cortex that re-checks the pre-estimated value of amplitude and direction. This information is then transferred to the brain stem. Here, the oculomotor nuclei trigger the gauged impulse for the eyes movement. In this circuit, which involves not only the superior colliculus [Sparks, 1986] and the parietal cortex [Stein, 1992] but even the cerebellum [Rae et al., 1998], the right parietal cortex plays a key role as suggested by the association between lesions in this area and deficits of fixation, of vergence as well as slow eyes movement (SEM) impairment [Fowler et al.,1991] (See further).

- FEMs inaccuracy and reduced amplitude with a consistent discrepancy between the landing site and the optimal viewing position.

It is argued, thereby, these defects to be responsible for the reading problems in dyslexics [Breitmeyer, 1980]. Still, this point of view, which supports the theory of the deficit of the magnocellular system applied to the oculomotor side, has to be confirmed by looking for such abnormalities in patients during the lexical task.

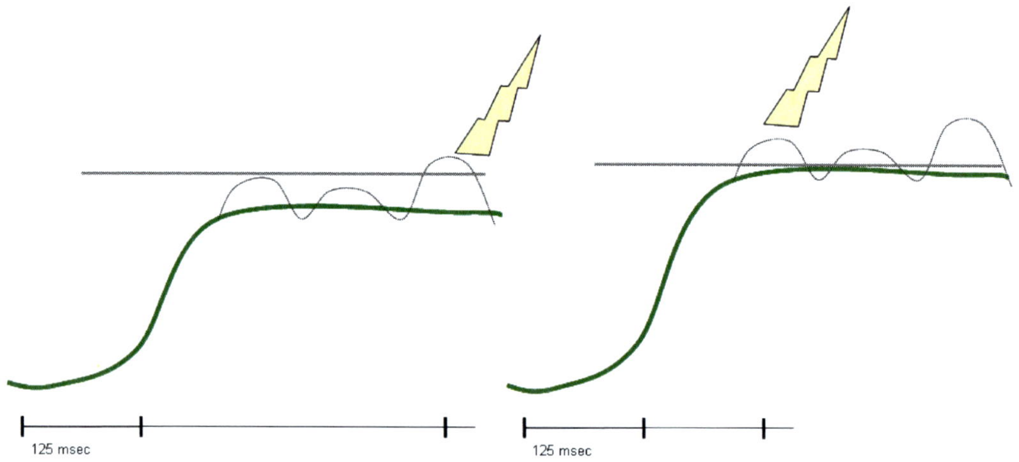

Figure 3. The saccadic activation. During each fixation, the saccadic activation level is at its minimum and increases gradually. After about 125 milliseconds, the progression becomes faster until a *plateau* is reached. At this level of stabilization the programming of the following saccade is completed: the forthcoming time of its trigger is a random interval that depends on the instant the fluctuation of the activation state will cross the threshold (upper horizontal line). The inter-individual variability of the plateau accounts for the reading rate differences in the population. The intra-individual variability depends on the characteristics of the text. For simpler texts, the plateau would be placed closer to the activation threshold (right figure), favoring the probabilistic event that leads to the saccadic activation, therefore speeding up the lexical processing: for more difficult passages, it would be placed lower, making fixation time longer in order to help the lexical comprehension.
In figure 2, this graph would localize in the lower panel at the point II.

Eye Movements in Dyslexic Subjects

Since the fifties, a growing body of evidence has been showing that eye movements during the lexical task are impaired in dyslexics. This oculomotor alteration would be partly responsible for their inaccurate and slow reading [Tinker, 1958; Ruby & Minden, 1973; Elterman et al., 1980; Rayner, 1978, 1985].

Yet, reduced reading rate is common even in inexpert readers, since their lexical function relies on an oculomotor system not yet fully developed. In these children the oculomotor pattern is characterized by:

- Increased number of fixations (double or threefold per line compared to skilled readers).
- Longer fixation time (in average 300-450 msec vs. 180 msec in normal readers).

- Reduced size of forward saccades (up to half than the saccades length of normal readers).
- Increased number of backward saccades: in the beginner more than one fixation over four takes place after a backward saccade.

As the child develops, the situation tends to normalize and around the tenth year of age lexical ability is about 2/3 compared to adult normal readers.

During this period, the improvement is mainly due to a reduction of the number and length of fixations [Rayner, 1986].

Later on, the completion of the lexical development relies on the improvement of the saccadic function, mainly due to the progressive reduction of the number of backward saccades [McConkie & Zola, 1989].

According to some researchers, the oculomotor pattern in dyslexic children reminds the pattern of the beginners [Olson et al., 1991, Hyönä & Olson, 1995]. This resemblance has led to believe that in patients the alteration of saccades and fixations instead of having a causal role are simply the result of linguistic problems [Pirozzolo, 1979, Kowler & Martins, 1982, Rayner, 1985, 1986]. In fact, when dyslexic children are asked to read material appropriate for their chronological age but not for their lexical age, their eye movements do not differ from those of their normal reader peers [Pirozzolo, 1979]. On the contrary, when normal readers are asked to read lexical material too difficult for their age, their oculomotor pattern closely resembles that observed in dyslexics [Rayner, 1986].

Yet, although the saccadic development in dyslexics is free from qualitative differences compared to the beginners, it is delayed, and as such has to be considered pathological. Moreover, this oculomotor maturation retardation would have a role in causing the lexical disability, irrespective of linguistic problems [Biscaldi et al., 1994]. Therefore, abnormal fixation time and shorter saccades in patients would not depend on the difficulty of the text, so that (at least for these two parameters) a linguistic influence can be ruled out [Trauzettel-Klosinski et al., 2010].

As a matter of fact, in dyslexics, a defective oculomotor control during reading has been confirmed in many studies and can be summarized as follows:

- higher number of fixations [De Luca e al, 1999; Hutzler & Wimmer, 2004; Trauzettel-Klosinski et al., 2010; Hatzidaki et al., 2011; Jainta & Kapoula, 2011; Kuvač Kraljević & Palmović, 2011].
- longer fixation time[112] [Zangwill & Blakemore, 1972; Adler-Grinberg & Stark, 1978; Olson et al., 1991; Biscaldi et al., 1994; De Luca et al., 1999; Zoccolotti et al., 1999; De Luca et al., 2002; Hutzler & Wimmer, 2004; MacKeben et al., 2004; Trauzettel-Klosinski et al., 2010; Hatzidaki et al., 2011; Jainta & Kapoula, 2011; KuvačKraljević & Palmović, 2011], that matches the fixation time of beginners[MacKeben et al., 2004] and is not due to poor comprehension of the text[113].

[112] See of Rubino and Minden [1973] and Olson et al. [1983, 1991] for counter evidence.

[113] Effectively, patients do not show problems when reading single words even when made difficult to process because displayed tachistoscopically, i.e. for a very short period of time [Zangwill & Blakemore, 1972].

- reduced amplitude of the forward saccades [Olson et al., 1991; De Luca et al., 1999; Zoccolotti et al., 1999; De Luca et al., 2002; MacKeben et al., 2004; Trauzettel-Klosinski et al., 2010], that when reading long words is halved compared to normal readers[114].
- higher number of forward saccades [Adler-Grinberg & Stark, 1978; De Luca et al., 1999; Zoccolotti et al., 1999; MacKeben et al., 2004, Hawelka & Wimmer, 2005[115]; Trauzettel-Klosinski et al., 2010].
- increased amplitude of backward saccades[116] [Tinker, 1958; Gruber, 1962; Zangwill & Blakemore, 1972; Rayner, 1978; De Luca et al., 2002; Hawelka & Wimmer, 2005; Trauzettel-Klosinski et al., 2010; Jainta & Kapoula, 2011; KuvačKraljević & Palmović, 2011][117].
- Presence of the so-called "*Reversed staircase pattern*" [Zangwill & Blakemore, 1972; Elterman et al., 1980]: the *return sweep,* that is the wide regression saccade which normally shifts the fixation to the beginning of the next line, is replaced by a sequence of small backward saccades (Figure 4).

Moreover, some dyslexics show a high prevalence of saccades with very short latency (80-135 msec), therefore called *express saccades* [Fischer & Weber, 1990]. Subsequent investigations have identified a subgroup of patients able to trigger only express saccades (*express saccades-makers*[118]: Fischer et al., 1993; Biscaldi et al., 1994]. The over activation of express saccades would be due to the hyperactivity of a particular type of neurons in charge of the fixations (named *fixation neurons:* Biscaldi et al., 1996; Cavegn & Biscaldi, 1996]. Since abnormal visual attention can prevent from stable fixation causing irregular saccadic triggering [Cavegn, 1996], the *scenario* suggests the express saccades-makers to be affected by a visuo-attentional[119] defect [Biscaldi et al., 1998].

[114] See Jainta & Kapoula [2011] for counter evidence.

[115] According to these authors, forward saccades are about twice compared to normal readers.

[116] According to this finding, dyslexics would read better in the opposite direction. In some patients, indeed, reading rate and the saccadic pattern improves to quasi-normal level when the text is presented backwards [Ciuffreda et al., 1985].

[117] Despite the overall raise of the number of backward saccades, for the concomitant increase of the forward saccades the proportion of the regression FEMs on the overall FEMs in patients is similar to normal readers [De Luca et al., 1999; Hutzler & Wimmer, 2004] or only slightly increased [Trauzettel-Klosinski et al., 2010].

[118] Although to a less extent, *express saccade-makers* are found even in the normal population [Biscaldi et al., 1996].

[119] Generally, express saccades occur when the fixation is disrupted before the onset of a second stimulus. An example is the appearance and disappearance of a target that is repeated after a given interval of time: if visual attention on the fixation of the previous target is released before the next one appears, express saccades are triggered [Fischer & Boch, 1983]. In 1998, the oculomotor pattern in a group of 185 young subjects between 8 and 25 years of age has been evaluated. Their reading skills followed a Gaussian frequency distribution, ranging from normal to impaired, with the cutoff (normal readers/ dyslexics) set by the operational definition of the disease. This study, which made use of a non-lexical paradigm, showed a high percentage of express saccades (even more than 30% of the total) in many dyslexics [Biscaldi et al., 1998]. So, it has been suggested the increase in the number of express saccades in dyslexic patients to be related to a defect in engaging and disengaging the fixation, in turn linked to attentional problems [Sakata et al., 1980; Goldberg et al., 1986; Fischer & Weber, 1990; Munoz & Wurtz, 1993]. In fact, visual attention impairment can interfere with the fixation maintenance, allowing an abnormal and irregular saccadic activation [Cavegn, 1996]. In chapter 11 the evidence in support of a visuoattentive defect in dyslexics will be reported.

The fixation neurons are arranged in the frontal eye fields (FEF) [Sakata et al., 1980; Goldberg et al., 1986]. The main afferent stimuli to the frontal eye fields come from the area V4 and MT, from the inferoparietal lobe and from the area 46 and project extensively to the middle layers (but even to the

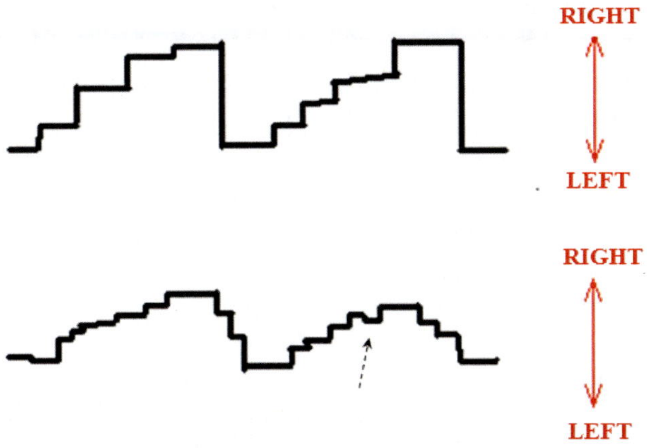

Figure 4. Top: oculographic pattern simulation of the eye movements in a normal adult subject. The left-to-right reading direction involves a series of forward saccades interspersed by moments of pause corresponding to the fixations. At the end of the line, the eye comes back at the beginning of the next one with a wide backward movement (*return sweep*). Bottom: oculographic pattern of a dyslexic subject: forward saccades are shorter and more frequent. The arrow refers to a backward saccade. Note the return sweep has changed into a reversed staircase pattern, made of three backward saccades.

This argument is crucial, since the connection between a visuoperceptive function like visual attention and the oculomotor aspect of the express saccades suggests that the alteration of the eye movements in patients would not be primitive but to some extent due to visuoperceptive anomalies.

Apart from the presence and from the putative role of the express saccades, the impaired oculomor pattern in dyslexics during the lexical task in recent years has received further confirmations.

In a German study published in 2004, eye movements when reading single words [MacKeben et al., 2004] have been monitored in a group of German dyslexic children (age ranging between 11 and 16 years) by means of LASER scanning ophthalmoscopy[120].

Results confirm that patients suffer from an anomalous oculomotor pattern. In particular:

- Longer fixations[121], which are independent from the length of the previous forward saccade and from the extent of the word. However, as an inverse correlation between this parameter and reading rate is missing, it has been argued that increased fixation

superficial ones) of the superior colliculus, both directly and via the basal ganglia. Other projections involve the pontine gaze center, the intralaminar nucleus and the medial pulvinar in the thalamus [Goldberg & Segraves, 1989]. It is stated that more than 50% of the FEF cells activity concerns the saccadic movements. Indeed, some of these cells discharge at a high rate when the appearance of an extrafoveal stimulus requires a rapid fixation displacement (i.e. the triggering of a saccade), some cells show an activation timing independent from this reflex and others discharge in both situations. It has to be noticed that the chemical deactivation of the fixation neurons in macaques prevents fixations to remain stable on a target and a salvo of reflected saccades is recordable all around it. Yet, the abnormally high number of express saccades in dyslexics would not be a reliable marker, as express saccades are found to be increased even after aspecific FEF impairment.

[120] The LASER scanning ophthalmoscopy (SLO) is a technique suitable to project a visual stimulus such as a letter or a part of a word onto the fovea with high degree of precision (spatial resolution <5 minarc). More recently, another German investigation with the SLO in dyslexics has been published by Trauzettel-Klosinski [Trauzettel-Klosinski et al., 2010].

[121] Median: 297 msec vs. 250 msec in controls.

time in dyslexics is not directly responsible for their slow reading but reflects the need for a more prolonged attentional process [Hari et al., 1999].

- Unexpectedly, saccadic accuracy as well as fixation stability was normal: therefore, the landing site and the oscillation of the fixation around the character in the patients matches those observed in the normal readers122. Evidently, this finding does not support the theory of the fixation instability, which will be discussed further on.
- Increased number of backward saccades when reading words made of at least 7 letters and proportional to their length.
- Shorter forward saccades (by up to 50% than the normal width for words long at least 10 letters[123]).
- Increased number of forward saccades (and therefore of fixations, as Hyönä and Olson pointed out almost ten years earlier: Hyönä & Olson, 1995) when reading words of more than 4 letters, whereas for shorter words no difference was found compared to normal readers (figure 5). However, in dyslexics the overall higher number of saccades is not related to an increase of their activation frequency (i.e. the number of events per time unit), that in fact is slightly less than two events per second, like in the normal readers.

In summary, according to this investigation, reduced reading rate in dyslexics is due mainly to increased number of regression saccades and shorter amplitude of forward FEMs without a substantial concomitant increase of their activation frequency. Longer fixation time would results from raised attentional demand.

Precursors of these findings since the fifties and even more in the seventies, some researchers argued a *primitive* alteration of the fine eye movements during reading to be the causal factor of the disease [Mosse & Daniels, 1959; Zangwill & Blakemore, 1972, Rubino & Minden, 1973, Pirozzolo & Rayner, 1978, Elterman et al., 1980].

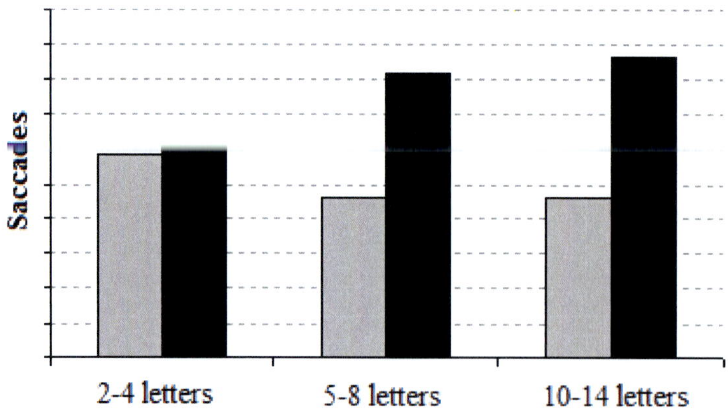

Figure 5. Number of forward saccades as a function of word length. Gray: normal readers; black: dyslexics (data inferred from MacKeben et al., 2004).

[122] Fixation fluctuates on average by ± 0.135 degrees in patients and ± 0.097 degrees in normal readers: a not significant difference.

[123] For example, for words made of 14 characters the median size is about 68 minarc in dyslexics, 106 minarc in controls.

Yet, in order to maintain that the oculomotor alteration is a *primitive/causal* factor and as such directly responsible for the reading disability, it is not enough to document in patients saccadic anomalies when reading: indeed, in addition, it has to be shown that these changes persist even *outside of* the lexical task.

The claim that defective FEMs are the primary (and therefore causal) alteration in developmental dyslexia, stems from some evidence of saccadic alterations not only during reading but even when patient are required to perform extra lexical tasks. Actually, in some investigations when dyslexics were asked to look steadily at a target jumping horizontally from right to left and from left to right, an oculomotor perturbation with a consistent number of FEM not aimed at the target but in the opposite direction has been documented [Pavlidis, 1978, 1981a,b, 1983; 1985a,b; Elterman et al., 1980].

The assessment of a substantial agreement of these extra lexical results with the findings reported during reading [Zangwill & Blakemore, 1972; Griffin et al., 1974; Ciuffreda et al., 1976; Pirozzolo & Rayner, 1978; Elterman et al., 1980], has lead to the conclusion that eye movements are the primary cause of the disease. Accordingly, the oculomotor defect would be an early indicator of dyslexia. However, even if a poor quality of fixation and anomalous forward saccades for non-lexical tasks in dyslexics have been confirmed in some later investigations [Biscaldi et al., 1994; Eden et al., 1994], many other studies failed to replicate these results. As an example, oculographic eye movements records in 5 dyslexic children[124] and 2 normal subjects provided contradictory elements: in one patient FEMs were normal both during reading and when presenting a string of symbols, in others a *reversed staircase pattern* was evident, with difficulty in restarting the oculomotor sequence on the next line [Elterman et al., 1980]. In some patients this anomalous behavior was observed only when processing string of symbols (extra lexical task), in others only when reading, and sometimes in both conditions. Therefore, a primitive alteration of the eye movements as a causal factor can be advanced only in those subjects who showed saccadic anomalies even in the extra-lexical conditions, i.e. when scanning the string of symbols.

Nevertheless, it is arguable that processing a string of symbols is not so different compared to a string of letters: hence, the discovery of eye movement deficiencies during such a non-lexical task does not seem so crucial to demonstrate that a *primitive* (i.e. independent from the reading task) oculomotor alteration occurs in dyslexics.

On the contrary, in the last thirty years the position of many other researchers was categorical:

there are no significant differences in the saccadic pattern between normal readers and dyslexics when recorded outside of the lexical task [Adler-Grinberg and Stark, 1978; Brown et al., 1983a, b; Stanley et al., 1983a, b;, Black et al., 1984a, b; Rayner, 1985; Olson et al., 1983, 1991; Crawford and Higham, 2001]. This conclusion remains unchanged even after having classified patients as surface dyslexics[125]: in an Italian investigation the oculomotor function of 10 surface-dyslexics[126] has been tested both during reading and with extra-lexical stimuli and results were compared to those obtained from normal subjects (De Luca et al., 1999]. In agreement with the previous studies, during the lexical task patients showed longer

[124] Age: 7 years.
[125] See chapter 14.
[126] Mean age; 12.6 years.

fixations (290 vs. 234 msec), shorter and more frequent forward saccades and increased number of backward saccades[127] compared to normal readers.

Yet, outside of the lexical task the study revealed no differences between the two groups.

In summary, and in agreement with Lennerstrand & Ygge [1992], the oculomotor control of children with developmental dyslexia in tasks requiring sequential saccadic activations is similar to the performance of normal children. Thus, a visual test looking for anomalies of FEMs would be of no value for the early diagnosis of dyslexia.

Hutzler more recently confirmed this opinion, showing the lack of fixation/saccadic impairment during a non-lexical task, namely the so-called *string processing tasks*[128] [Hutzler et al., 2006]. The string processing task is similar to the lexical task but is lacking in language content. Still, the string processing task is conceived within a lexical context and therefore requires the sequential activation of saccades and fixations.

On the contrary, when reading *non-words*[129] patients showed an anomalous oculomotor pattern with a higher number of fixations and a longer permanence of the gaze on the target.

Therefore, children with surface dyslexia show an altered oculomotor pattern when reading. In contrast, their ability to gaze firmly and to make saccadic movements toward a non-linguistic stimulus is substantially spared. This is the reason why it has been claimed that eye movements' impairment in surface dyslexia does not depend on oculomotor dysfunctions but it is secondary to a defect in the visual processing of the linguistic material [De Luca et al., 1999].

Even Farmer and Klein a few years before maintained that the oculomotor anomalies in dyslexics cannot be considered the primary reason for their lexical difficulty [Farmer & Klein, 1995].

Unstable Dominance and Fixation Deficit

And yet, a primitive oculomotor defect can be examined under a different perspective: rather the saccadic transfer of the fixation, the defect would affect the fixation itself.

In order to adequately process a visual stimulus, stable fixation is required: each syllable has to remain steadily projected onto the fovea until its processing is completed. In developmental dyslexics the fixation could not to be stable enough.

Eden compared the fixation stability of a group of 26 patients[130] with a sample of 39 normal children of the same age. In the experiment, subjects were asked to look steadily at a stimulus displayed for a few seconds at the center of a monitor. In the meantime, the involuntary oscillations of their eyes were recorded by an infrared tracking system. In one

[127] Despite the overall increased number of backward saccades, their proportion over the total FEMs in dyslexics does not differ from the proportion measured in the control group; moreover, their length turns out to be shorter (0.9 degrees in dyslexics vs. 1.6 degrees in normal readers), in agreement with Zangwill and Blakemore [1972] and Biscaldi [Biscaldi et al., 1998].

[128] I n the string processing task, short strings of letters are presented to the child. In some of these strings there are two adjacent identical letters, which are the target: for example HMMD, BCRR. The subject is required to detect (when present) the target in each string.

[129] Non-words are series of consonants and vowels arranged to form non-sense words. By using non-words instead of words, the linguistic processing is prevented.

[130] Mean age: 11.6 years.

fourth of dyslexics the slight deviations from the target were wider than in controls[131]. The phenomenon has been referred to unstable binocular fixation.

Now, the requirement for binocular fixation stability is a good motor control, i.e. a perfect synchrony in the movements of the two eyes [Eden et al., 1994; Stein & Walsh, 1997].

At close distance (for example when reading a book), each eye converges on the target to maintain the fixation on the same letter or syllable: in other words, the aim of the binocular convergence is to make sure the same character projects to the fovea of the two eyes. To achieve such a perfect retinal correspondence, binocular cooperation must be precise. Yet, the occurrence of slight differences in the direction of the two visual axes may lead to occasional perceptual discrepancies so that a letter is projected onto the fovea of one eye and the adjacent character falls on the fovea of the fellow eye. To avoid the onset of binocular rivalry, the visual system is expected to assign to one of the two eyes the role of "gaze director", making it the dominant eye [Stein & Fowler, 1984]. This way, the position of the letters on the page is time after time encoded by the dominant eye that guides the fixation of the fellow eye.

Therefore, the presence of a stable ocular dominance while reading enables to neutralize the slight positional differences of the two visual axes, when present, preserving the correct processing of the stimulus during the fixation: the stronger the dominance, the more steady and effective is the fixation of the target.

This is the expected *scenario* in normal readers.

Interestingly, in many dyslexics the ocular dominance is found to be weak or absent, so that when reading fixation tends to be unstable. Fixation instability would make the visual axes oscillate around the letter, hampering its processing and its positional encoding [Riddell et al., 1987a,b, 1988; Stein & Fowler, 1993]. Indeed, visual confusion and the other perceptive symptoms like the sensation of merging, moving and jumping letters with frequent exchange in their position[132] would stem from this anomalous situation.

In 1982 this hypothesis has been tested after assessing the ocular dominance in dyslexics and normal readers by means of a modified version of the Dunlop[133] test. In a group of 80

---

131 In addition, the authors found an anomaly of the final stage of the saccadic movement (close to the landing site). Even this impairment could be related to fixation instability.

132 Reading monocularly is argued to be easier, since fixation instability worsens in binocular conditions [Stein, 2001].

133 The Dunlop test makes use of a synoptophore, a tool able to project two images onto the foveal region of the two eyes. It is made of two spyglasses, each of which shows a complementary image: for example a lion and a cage. If the lion falls on the fovea of one eye and the cage on the fovea of the other eye, the scene seen by the child would be a lion into a cage. If the lion appears out of the cage, by adjusting appropriately the angle of the two telescopes the child will be able to see the two complementary images (lion and cage) as merged into a single one (lion into the cage). The degree of adjustement depends on the amount of latent deviation of the two visual axes. On the contrary, if the technician increases the angle between the two telescopes when the subject is observing the two figures merged into a single one (the lion in the cage), within a given angular interval the child would still manage to perceive a single image. Beyond this tolerance interval, visual fusion is disrupted and the two figures are seen as separate (the lion out of the cage). The tolerance interval expressed as degrees or prismatic dioptres varies from subject to subject and is defined *fusional amplitude*.

Instead of the fusional amplitude, in the Dunlop test the synoptophore is used to asses the ocular dominance. In the original studies, a house with an arrow-shaped stake on the left side of the door was presented to the right eye while the same house with a paddle-shaped stake on the right side of the door was projected onto the fovea of the left eye. The angle between the two telescopes allows the fusion of the two images, so that the child sees a house with an arrow-shaped stake on the left and paddle-shaped stake on the right of the entrance door. Hence, the angle between the two telescopes is slowly increased. At the beginning, the child would manage to perceive the image thanks to its fusional amplitude but at a certain point he would have the impression that one of the two stakes moves toward the house. The procedure is repeated ten times. A child with a stable dominance should (almost) always report the shift of the same stake. If the perceived dyslexic children[134], dominance was found to be unstable in 63% of the cases whereas in the controls (except one) it proved to be stable [Stein & Fowler, 1982].

Therefore, patients showing unstable dominance have been defined *visual dyslexics*.

A few years later the finding was confirmed in a larger sample, made of 148 patients[135]: in 65% of the cases the dominance was unstable [Stein & Fowler, 1985] compared to 30% in the normal age-matched population[136] [Stein et al., 1986]. It was estimated that even in the normal (i.e. not diagnosed as dyslexic) sample, when present, the fixation instability due to unstable dominance may lower the lexical age of about 6.3 months.

Crossed dominance[137] was found in less than the half of the patients compared to normal readers (18% vs. 41%)[138], in disagreement with the opinion that crossed dominance is prevalent in dyslexics [Dunlop et al., 1973], and in line with a population study dating back 1969 [Norn et al., 1969].

In the eighties, some other laboratories confirmed the defective ocular dominance in many dyslexics: in a small sample of patients[139] dominance turned out to be unstable in 64% of cases (versus 21% of controls: Bigelow & McKenzie, 1985). A further study of Masters is in line with this finding [Masters, 1988].

So, what would distinguish the visual dyslexics from the normal readers is unstable dominance responsible for fixation instability, and not crossed dominance: as a matter of fact, fixation instability is due to an impairment of the right posterior parietal cortex[140] [Breitmeyer, 1989; Fowler et al., 1989; Stein et al., 1989] and of the cerebellum [Miall et al., 1993], two regions found to be deficient in dyslexics.

Since fixation instability is found also in dyslexics without evident phonological defects, the possibility that this imbalance depends on linguistic problems is ruled out [Eden et al., 1994], whereas it can be related to the abnormal saccadic pattern: in a Japanese study, the effect of ocular dominance on the saccadic movements has been evaluated during the lexical task by means of video-oculography[141]. The saccades of the dominant eye were found to be faster compared to the fellow (non-dominant) eye [Oishi et al., 2005], suggesting a relation between dominance instability and saccadic alteration during reading.

As an indirect confirmation of the effect unstable dominance has on the lexical function, a monocular occlusion prescribed for several months and aimed at fostering the consolidation

---

movement is referred to the same stake at least 8 times out of 10, then the dominance can be regarded as stable [Cornelissenet al., 1991,1992]. In the technique adopted by Stein, instead of the two stakes were presented two trees of different height. Ocular dominance assessed in this way is closely related to fixation stability. In fact, in the non-dominant eye unstable fixation would cause the sensation the stake (or the tree) projected onto its fovea moves toward the house. Instead, stable fixation that characterizes the dominant eye makes the respective stake to stand still. For further detailson the Dunlop test refer to the original article [Dunlop, 1972].

[134] Age: 10 years.

[135] Age: 7-11 years.

[136] Interestingly, in normal readers (753 children) the prevalence of subjects with unstable dominance decreased with age: from 49% in 5 years old children to 11% in children aged 10.

[137] Dominance is referred to as crossed if the dominant eye is the contralateral with respect to the dominant hand (i.e. the hand normally used for writing or drawing).

[138] This result could be a biased estimation, since in the majority of the recruited dyslexics the dominance was unstable and as such neither direct nor crossed. Yet, even among patients with stable dominance the proportion of crossed dominants was not significantly higher compared to the controls.

[139] 14 subjects.

[140] Since patients with lesions of the right posterior parietal cortex are prevented from converging their visual axes onto small stimuli, they suffer also from defective stereoscopic vision [Fowler et al., 1989].

[141] In videooculography, an infrared ray system is employed to map in real time eye movements during visual tasks as following a moving target on a monitor or reading.

of the dominance in the uncovered eye is found to improve reading ability in dyslexic children with unstable ocular dominance [Stein & Fowler, 1985; Stein et al., 1987, 1988].

Therefore, unstable dominance would be one of the causes and not simply a consequence of a lexical difficulty: as a matter of fact, dyslexics' ocular dominance is weaker compared not only to normal readers of the same chronological age (age-matched), but even of the same lexical age (reading-matched)[142] [Stein et al., 1987; Riddell et al., 1990].

Interestingly, subjects with unstable dominance as assessed at the Dunlop test were found to be more sensitive to the size of the characters, and their reading was more accurate in monocular rather than in binocular conditions[143]. Visual confusion due to unstable fixation would account for the first finding: in presence of unstable fixation, indeed, visual confusion would worsen when the size of the letter is below a given value[144]. Even the second finding would be related to fixation instability, as fixation instability is enhanced by the mutual interference of the two eyes when reading in binocular conditions [Cornelissen et al., 1991, 1992]. These two factors are therefore indicative of the potential role of the dominance stability on the lexical function.

To better investigate this crucial point, the stability of fixation in dyslexics during reading has been evaluated by means of an infrared registration system [Cornelissen et al., 1993]. In the study, the stability of fixation was measured as the *standard deviation* of the mean convergence angle, so that the higher is this value, the more unstable is the fixation. When reading single words, the standard deviation of the convergence angle turned out to be on average 0.11 degrees in normal children and 0.08 degrees in normal adults[145]. Now, the results obtained from two age-matched groups of dyslexic children[146], respectively with normal or abnormal dominance stability[147], were compared with these normative data. Contrary to what expected, this study failed to show any abnormal deviation of the convergence angle during fixation in patients, no matter whether they were classified as stable or unstable dominant[148]. Results were unchanged when comparing the data obtained from the older dyslexic children with those coming from the younger normal readers with the same reading level. A possible explanation has been provided: even when the physiological variation of the convergence angle during fixation is the same in normal readers and in unstable dominant dyslexics, in the first case it is somehow compensated, in the second it is not. In fact, the visual system of normal subjects is tolerant to the physiological variation in the convergence angle during fixation. Therefore, even if sometimes the letter or the syllable projected onto the fovea of the dominant eye does not fall exactly on the fovea of the fellow eye, sort of *sensory fusion* takes place all the same and visual confusion is avoided. This"flexibility" would be missing in patients.

According to this solution, the basic problem would not concern the fixation instability *per se* but an anomalous *sensory fusion*: the visual fusion in children who fail the Dunlop Test

[142] That is to say not only compared to normal readers of the same age, but even compared to younger normal (non-dyslexic) subjects, whose lexical level, therefore, matches that of the patients.

[143] In binocular conditions, patients made more errors and were prone to transform words into non-words.

[144] According to the authors, a text printed in lowercase Helvetica and single-spaced ordinary font size (12 points) can be affected by unstable dominance.

[145] Age of the sample: 9-11 years and 24-36 years.

[146] 10 subjects in both cases.

[147] As assessed at the Dunlop test.

[148] Standard deviation in normal readers, in stable dominant dyslexics and in unstable dominant dyslexics: 0.115, 0.111 and 0.129 degrees, respectively.

would not be effective enough to compensate adequately for the axes disparity, leading to visual confusion.

Therefore, the alteration in visual dyslexics does not rest just (or mainly) on the motor fusion but even (or mainly) on such a sensory fusion.

Provided not only the motor fusion, but even the sensory fusion depends on ocular dominance, then the motor and sensory aspect of the ocular dominance should be considered separately.

In summary, the perceptual compensation of the variation of the convergence angle during fixation involves even the sensory dominance that, if weak, would contribute to account for the dyslexics'visual symptoms in a more incisive manner than unstable motor dominance *per se*. Since the Dunlop test is greatly influenced by the motor component of dominance, a technique able to assess separately motor and sensory dominance is desirable.

In 1989, the shortcomings regarding the Dunlop test and the hypothesis of unstable dominance in dyslexics were published on the *British Journal of Ophthalmology* [Bishop, 1989].

Despite the reported experimental evidence, it has been maintained that the investigations focused on the Dunlop test are not suitable to assess a real link between unstable dominance and reading difficulty[149], since for less intelligent children the Dunlop test would be too difficult to be performed correctly [Bishop et al., 1979]. Due to this bias, many patients would be positive at the Dunlop test not because their dominance is unstable but simply for a misunderstanding of the examination. In addition, it has been inferred ocular dominance to be more stable in older subjects[150]. Therefore, the Dunlop test would be influenced both by the cognitive and chronological age and, as such, would not be specific.

Moreover, dominance is found to be unstable not only in a group of patients but also in a consistent number of normal subjects (about 30%: Stein et al., 1986): it would follow that dominance *per se* is not enough to determine the lexical impairment.

It was argued that dyslexics with unstable dominance (the "visual dyslexics") make more visual errors when reading than the other dyslexics do [Stein & Fowler, 1982]. However, exact criteria to allow a definition of the term "visual dyslexia" would not be provided. It has been remarked that the validity of the distinction between "visual errors" (i.e.: loss of the mark along the line, reverse sequence of letters, syllables, or their rotation) and "not visual errors" (i.e. difficulty to find the rhyme or the alliteration for common words, difficulty to name the days of the week or the months of the year) is an open issue. In addition, this classification is claimed to be arbitrary, too categorical and as such biased by the cases of mixed forms, and eventually inapplicable to a condition that has to be conceived as the tail of a distribution of lexical abilities.

Finally, it has been highlighted that the proof of the existence of such visual difficulties outside of the lexical task would be lacking, and there would be no evidence that in visual dyslexics a phonological deficit is absent or slighter as compared to non-visual dyslexics [Bishop, 1989].

These arguments have been punctually and readily rebutted [Stein, 1989]. For example, the effect of IQ on the Dunlop test would be biased by the type of method used for its

[149] Newman in particular failed to found in his large sample (323 children, mean age 8.5 years) an association between dominance stability and reading ability [Newman et al., 1985a, b].

[150] 52% of stable dominance at 5 years of age, 90% at 10 years of age [Stein et al., 1986]

measurement: the WISC. As a matter of fact, results from WISC would penalize poor readers disproportionately, so that the lower IQ obtained at WISC in patients with positive Dunlop's test would reflect their poor reading condition rather than their true intellective quotient [Stein, 1989]. Therefore, claiming that patients were positive at the Dunlop test not for their unstable dominance but simply for a misunderstanding of the examination would not be tenable.

Besides, the mixed forms would not bias the visual/non visual classification of developmental dyslexia, as they simply stem from the association of defective dominance and phonological alterations. Moreover, the visuoperceptive difficulties of visual dyslexics are detectable even in extra lexical tasks, since children with weak dominance are worse even in dot localization tasks[151] [Riddel et al., 1987]. Finally, even if direct evidence of reduced or absent language deficits in visual dyslexia is missing, it is revealing that the phonological rehabilitation is not so frequently administered in this kind of patients.

No doubt that the theory of unstable dominance in dyslexic remains a controversial issue. Despite the reported results, a body of evidence has failed to confirm that dyslexics suffer from unstable dominance or unstable fixation [Rubino & Minden, 1973; Olson et al., 1983; Olson et al., 1991; Evans et al., 1994; Goulandris et al., 1998; De Luca et al., 1999] and is unquestionable that further research testing the theory of dominance instability in dyslexics with a properly controlled double-masked study is desirable.

It should be assessed that dyslexics the same age and the same IQ (measured using techniques other than the WISC scale) who make visual errors are *unstable dominant.* In this regard, a test suitable to estimate the ocular dominance both on its motor and sensory side should be adopted. In turn, it should be ascertained that all *unstable dominant* dyslexics the same age and the same IQ make mainly visual errors, and that all *stable dominant* dyslexics the same age and the same IQ make predominantly non-visual errors.

The possibility that the ocular dominance reinforcement allows reading better remains to be confirmed and the positive effect of the monocular occlusion on the lexical performance it is stated to be an optimistic and not proved consideration [Bishop, 1989].

Whatever it be, this line of research has helped to move the terms of the problem from the oculomotor point of view toward a more visuoperceptive domain. Interestingly, in dyslexics a correlation between unstable dominance and visuoperceptive deficit has been advanced: contrast sensitivity, for example, has been measured in a sample of patients with stable dominance and in another sample with unstable dominance, both of the same chronological age. A reduction of 0.15 log units in the second group compared to the first one has been observed[152] [Mason et al., 1993].

When repeating the experiment selecting the stable and unstable dominant sample so as to be of the same lexical age, the result did not change and contrast sensitivity of the unstable dominants was reduced by 0.15 log units compared to the other group.

It is worth noting that the hypothesis of fixation instability looks to be in contrast with the theory of the deficit of the magnocellular system: in fact, since according to the competitive interaction theory fixation depends on the parvocellular activity, if the fixation is unstable, then the P system and not the M pathway is expected to be impaired. Nevertheless, it is

[151] Personal communication at the St Bartholomew's Hospital Meeting of the Association of British Neurologists.

[152] The authors used sinusoidal gratings ranging from 0.5 to 6 cicles/degree, stationary or flickering at 20 Hz and presented in low luminance conditions (3.8 cd/m2).

argued the transient system to play a major role *even* in stabilizing the vergence, that is to say, the fixation, and not only in the saccadic triggering [Mowforth et al., 1981][153].

A recent strand of research has considered this conflicting dualism between saccadic alterations and fixation instability in a novel perspective. It is documented that when reading the saccadic, conjugate movements of the two visual axes (called *versions*) are not perfectly synchronized: indeed, the eye in abduction takes a broader and more rapid movement than the eye in adduction[154]. As a result, a slight, fleeting discrepancy (*disconjugation*) between the two visual axes takes place. Normally, this difference is counterbalanced in about 50-100 milliseconds by an opposite vergence shift, which brings the visual axes to meet on the landing site [Bucci et al., 2008; Kapoula & Vernet, 2009] [155].

This saccadic disconjugation is found to be wider in dyslexic compared to normal readers when asked to perform a lexical task made of both isolated words [Bucci et al., 2008] or complete sentences [Jainta & Kapoula, 2011]. So, in patients the compensatory movement has to be wider than normal. Yet, this is not the case and the expected correspondence between the visual axes disconjugation and the subsequent corrective movement is lacking. Therefore, when reading, on the one hand the patient suffers from abnormal disconjugation of the visual axes during the saccadic version, on the other hand he/she fails to perform a suitable opposite compensatory movement: the result is an imprecise retinal correspondence of the stimulus (the syllable) in the two eyes and unstable binocular fixation. In summary, these findings disclose a relationship between impaired saccadic pattern during reading and unstable fixation as reported in dyslexic subjects.

To date, despite the acquisition of such new elements, the alteration of the oculomotor structure in dyslexics, be this impairment related to saccadic perturbation or consequent to fixation instability, needs to be clarified. Indeed, the contradictory nature of the results is difficult to explain. Maybe, due to the randomization criteria, in most of the studies the pathological sample happened to be made of dyslexics suffering from abnormal eye movements only during reading together to dyslexics with abnormal FEMs even in non-lexical tasks [Pollatsek, 1983; Rayner, 1985]. Therefore, different findings would depend on the different proportion of these two subtypes of patients in the sample: in case results were consistent with a primitive abnormal oculomotor pattern, then the recruited sample would be made mostly of subjects belonging to the second group, otherwise to the former.

In conclusion, the existence of a dichotomy between abnormal eye movements during reading and normal oculomotor pattern when required to perform extra lexical tasks, contributes to discredit the causal role of the oculomotor imbalance in developmental dyslexia. In dyslexics, this semeiological fracture may depend on the different way visuoperceptive impairment affects the written text compared to non-lexical stimuli.

[153] As far as we know, only one study supports the presence of a parvocellular rather than a magnocellular anomaly in dyslexics [Farrag et al., 2002].

[154] The eye in abduction is the eye moving far from to the nose: (the right one in the left-to-right reading systems). The eye in adduction is the eye moving toward the noise. (the left one in the left-to-right reading systems).

[155] For further details on this subject, see Jainta & Kapoula [2011].

The Possible Involvement of the Slow Eye Movements (SEM)

Although, during reading, the role of the *slow eye movements* or *SEMs*[156] is negligible compared to the FEMs, nonetheless in dyslexics the former seem disrupted by saccadic intrusions[157] [Adler-Grinberg & Stark, 1978; Stark et al., 1990]. The phenomenon[158] would take place in 25% of the patients, so that its assessment has been judged important for the early diagnosis of the disease [Black et al., 1984c]. A similar finding reported by Eden et al. [1994] in 31% of her dyslexic sample (and only 18% of the control subjects) has been attributed to malfunctioning of the parietal cortex[159], therefore related to an attentional deficit[160].

SEM and fixations would be closely related because both are aimed at maintaining the target firmly projected on the foveal region: so, a concurrent alteration of the SEMs would be further evidence in support of the fixation instability in disabled readers [Stein & Alcott, 1999].

However, the current state of our knowledge does not allow making further remarks on the role SEMs may have in developmental dyslexia: compared to the interest for saccades and fixations, the involvement of slow eye movements is a topic that remains on a second plane.

In conclusion, to date it is neither excluded nor admitted an oculomotor alteration to occur in at least a subgroup of patients. Yet, if confirmed, this alteration is hardly compatible with the theory of the deficit of the magnocellular system in its original formulation. If the defect of the large ganglion cells would directly and primarily affect the saccadic pattern, this alteration should be independent of the lexical task and experimentally replicable in other experimental conditions: that is to say that the symptoms and the signs should be omnipresent. Actually, since many investigations do not convey on the presence of oculomotor anomalies in extra lexical conditions, for the moment it is not possible to maintain that anomalous saccades are the *primum movens* (in its aetiological sense) of developmental dyslexia.

On the contrary, the oculomotor anomalies may depend on the linguistic/phonological difficulties that seem to affect all patients, even if to a different degree[161]: Indeed, on the one hand the saccadic pattern of dyslexics tends to normalize when patients are presented with reading suited for their lexical age (Pirozzolo, 1979), on the other hand FEMs of normal readers seem to match those of dyslexics when asked to read tasks too difficult for their chronological age [Rayner, 1986].

In an aforementioned investigation [Hutzler et al., 2006], patients showed no oculomotor problems when tested with the *string-processing task*, a task considered to be similar to the lexical task but free from any linguistic content, whereas differences were found when

---

[156] SEMs are smooth and conjugate shifts of the eyes that take place during the observation of a slowly moving target. Their function is to keep the moving stimulus steadly projected on the fovea, so to allow its adequate processing.

[157] This anomalous oculomotor pattern is said *cog*-wheeling.

[158] Evaluated using a target moving horizontally at constant speed of 5 deg /sec.

[159] In particular a malfunctioning of the mediotemporal (MT) and medial superior temporal (MST) area [Pierrot-Deseilligny et al., 1997].

[160] See chapter 11.

[161] Pirozzolo [1979], Kowler and Martins [1982], Rayner [1985, 1986].

required to read non-words (thereby, passages resembling a text with an extremely complex linguistic content). Thereby, the eye movement alteration of dyslexics would depend on a phonological-linguistic difficulty, ruling out the visuoperceptive one.

However, an aspect must be taken into account: as already pinpointed, the string-processing task seems to be more similar to a visual search task than to the lexical function. On the contrary, non-words require a true processing of the analytical configuration, as expected during reading. In the *string-processing task,* in fact, it is asked to detect a couple made of two identical characters embedded in short alphabetic sequences, whereas in order to decode non-words each letter has to be processed in sequence. This operation is performed via analysis, deconstruction of the non-word in order to extract the single graphemes and then reassemble them: the difference is obvious, since the second is much more demanding. Therefore, it is wrong to believe that the string processing assesses the same visuoperceptive function of the non-word presentation, and that the two tests differ since the phonological component is absent in the former. In other words, in the opinion of the author, it is wrong to believe that the string-processing task differs from the lexical one only because it is devoid of linguistic content. As a matter of fact, it is far different and the lack of differences between cases and controls in this test confirms once more the lack of saccadic deterioration out of the lexical activity in the dyslexic patient.

Finally, the lexical oculomotor pattern could be driven by the orthographic features of the different languages: as an example, German dyslexics make more fixations per word compared to English patients. When coping with especially difficult lexical contents, the former react increasing their saccadic frequency while the latter tend to prolong the fixation time [Trauzettel-Klosinski et al., 2010).

This fact makes the interpretation of the results gathered from the international studies even more puzzling. In addition, it implies that dyslexics of transparent languages such as German and Italian tend to rely on the *sublexical route,* which is to say on the decomposition of the word and subsequent letter-per-letter processing, an operation that requires increased saccadic frequency. On the contrary, dyslexics speaking non-transparent languages (like English)[162] prefer to use the *lexical way* which provides the reading of the word as a whole, as a global configuration; for this purpose they do not need more saccades but longer fixation time. This is a perspective that matches well with the preponderance of the linguistic-phonological impairment reported in the English speaking dyslexics. Compared to the dominant phonological component in Anglophone patients, this difference makes more likely a visuoperceptive involvement in transparent dyslexics.

In summary, the role that the abnormal saccade/fixation pattern have in the pathogenesis of developmental dyslexia rather than directly causative is probably secondary to a peculiar visuoperceptive alteration. This alteration, however, is expected to be other from contrast sensitivity, motion perception or visual persistence, i.e. the functions whose impairment would be suggestive of a magnocellular deficit.

In an attempt to understand how perceptive and oculomotor aspects interact within the framework of the magnocellular theory, is worth investigating the way dyslexics perceive the visual space: in particular the way the spatial relationship of the single elements making up a shape (thereby a character) are estimated. We have called this function *spatial relationship perception.*

---

[162] And in general dyslexics speaking a language with a low grapheme-phoneme correspondence.

An alteration of the spatial relationship perception in dyslexics, that is to say a distortion of their visual space along the cardinal axes, could be able to account for the reported impaired M-mediated visual functions, for the abnormal oculomotricity when reading as well as for the signs and symptoms complained by the patients.

In this perspective, the saccadic pattern would be betrayed by a global visual distortion along the cardinal axes, which affects the perceived spatial relationship of the adjoining letters and syllables arranged in the sentence.

Upon this basis, to some extent developmental dyslexia would be *even* a visuoperceptive problem: a problem of spatial vision, according to its original definition of *word blindness*. To clarify this new speculative line, it is necessary to understand insight the way dyslexics see, process, perceive the shape of the words and of their elementary constituents.

References

Aasved H. (1988). *Øyenundersøkelser. Bergenprojektet III. Studier av barn med dysleksi og andre laerevansker.* H-J Gjessing, HD Nygaard and R Solheim. Universitetsforlaget, Oslo.

Abrams SG, Zuber BL. (1972). *Some temporal characteristics of informational processing during reading.* Reading Research Quaterly, 8: 40-51.

Adler-Grinberg D, Stark L. (1978). *Eye movements, scan paths, and dyslexia.* American Journal of Optometry and Physiological Optics, 55: 557-570.

Bigelow ER, McKenzie B. (1985). *Unstable ocular dominance and reading ability.* Perception, 14: 329-335.

Biscaldi M, Fischer B, Aiple F. (1994). *Saccadic eye movements of dyslexic and normal reading children.* Perception, 23: 45-64.

Biscaldi M, Fischer B, Stuhr V. (1996). *Human express-saccade makers are impaired at suppressing visually-evoked saccades.* Journal of Neurophysiology, 76: 199-214.

Biscaldi M, Gezeck S, Stuhr V. (1998). *Poor saccadic control correlates with dyslexia.* Neuropsychologia, 36: 1189-1202.

Bishop DV. (1989). *Unfixed reference, monocular occlusion, and developmental dyslexia-a critique.* British Journal of Ophthalmology, 73: 209-215.

Bishop DV, Jancey C, Steel AM. (1979). *Orthoptic status and reading disability.* Cortex, 15: 659-666.

Black JL, Collins DW, De Roach JN, Zubrick S. (1984a). *Dyslexia: saccadic eye movements.* Perceptual & Motor Skills, 58: 903-910.

Black JL, Collins DW, de Roach JN, Zubrick S. (1984b). *A detailed study of sequential saccadic eye movements for normal- and poor-reading children.* Perceptual & Motor Skills, 59: 423-434.

Black JL, Collins DW, de Roach JN, Zubrick S. (1984c). *Smooth pursuit eye movements in normal and dyslexic children.* Perceptual & Motor Skills, 59: 91-100.

Breitmeyer BG. (1980).*Unmasking visual masking: a look at the "why" behind the veil of "how".* Psychological Review, 87: 52-69.

Breitmeyer BG. (1989). *A visually based deficit in specific reading disability.* The Irish Journal of Psychology, 10: 534-541.

Brown B, Haegerstrom-Portnoy G, Adams AJ, *Yingling CD, Galin, D, Herron J, Marcus M. (1983a). Predictive eye movements do not discriminate between dyslexic and control children.* Neuropsychologia, 21: 121-128.

Brown B, Haegerstrom-Portnoy *G*, Yingling CD, Herron J, Galin, D, Marcus M. (1983b). *Tracking eye movements are normal in dyslexic children.* American Journal of Optometry and Physiological Optics, 60: 376-383.

Bucci MP, Bremond-Gignac D, Kapoula Z. (2008). *Poor binocular coordination of saccades in dyslexic children.* Graefes Archive for Clinical and Experimental Ophthalmology, 246: 417-428.

Campbell FW, Wurtz RH. (1978). *Saccadic omission-why we do not see a grey out during saccades.* Vision Research, 18: 1297-1303.

Cavegn D. (1996). *Bilateral interactions in saccade programming: A saccade latency study.* Experimental Brain Research, 109: 312-332.

Cavegn D, Biscaldi M. (1996). *Fixation and saccade control in express-saccade maker.* Experimental Brain Research, 109: 101-116.

Ciuffreda KJ, Bahill AT, Kenyon RV, Stark, L. (1976). *Eye movements during reading: Case studies.* American Journal of Optometry & Physiological Optics, 53: 389-395.

Ciuffreda KJ, Bahill AT, Kenyon RV, Stark L. (1985). *Eye movements during reading: further case reports.* American Journal of Optometry& Physiological Optics, 62: 844-852.

Cornelissen P, Bradley L, Fowler S, Stein JF. (1991). *What* children *see affects how they read.* Developmental Medicine & Child Neurology, 33: 755-762.

Cornelissen P, Bradley L, Fowler S, Stein JF. (1992). *Covering one eye affects how some children read.* Developmental Medicine and Child Neurology, 34: 296-304.

Cornelissen PL, Munro N, Fowler S, Stein J. (1993). *The stability of binocular fixation during reading in adults and children.* Developmental Medicine & Child Neurology, 35: 777-787.

Crawford TJ, Higham S. (2001). *Dyslexia and the centre of-gravity effect.* Experimental Brain Research, 137: 122-126.

De Luca M, Di Pace E, Judica A, Spinelli D, Zoccolotti P. (1999). *Eye movements patterns in linguistic and non-linguistic tasks in developmental surface dyslexia.* Neuropsychologia, 37: 1407-1420.

De Luca M, Borrelli, Judica A, Spinelli D, Zoccoletti P. (2002). *Reading words and pseudo-words: an eye movement study of developmental dyslexia.* Brain and Language, 80: 617-626.

Dickinson CM, Abadi RV. (1985). *The influence of nystagmoid oscillation on contrast sensitivity in normal observers.* Vision Research, 25: 1089-1096.

Dunlop P. (1972). *Dyslexia. The orthoptic approach.* Australian Orthoptic Journal, 12: 16-20.

Dunlop DB, Dunlop P, Fenelon B. (1973). *Vision-laterality analysis in children with reading disability: the results of new techniques of examination.* Cortex, 9: 227-236.

Dunn-Rankin P. (1978). *The visual characteristics of words.* Scientific American, 238: 122-130.

Eden GF, Stein JF, Wood MH, Wood FB. (1994). *Differences in eye movements and reading problems in dyslexics and normal children.* Vision Research, 34: 1345-1358.

Elterman RD, Abel LA, Daroff RB, Dell'Osso LF, Bornstein JL. (1980). *Eye movement patterns in dyslexic children.* Journal of Learning Disabilities, 13: 16-21.

Evans BJW, Drasdo N, and Richards IL. (1994). *Investigation of accommodative and binocular function in dyslexia.* Ophthalmic and Physiological Optics, 145: 5-20.

Farmer ME, Klein RM. (1995). *The evidence for a temporal processing deficit-linked to dyslexia.* Psychonomic Bulletin Review, 2: 460-493.

Farrag AF, Khedr EM, Abel-Naser W. (2002). *Impaired parvocellular pathway in dyslexic children.* European Journal of Neurology, 9: 359-363.

Findlay JM. (1982). *Global vision processing for saccadic eye movements.* Vision Research, 22: 1033-1045.

Findlay JM, Walker R. (1999). *A model of saccade generation based on parallel processing and competitive inhibition.* Behavioral & Brain Sciences, 22: 661-721.

Fischer B, Boch R. (1983). *Saccadic eye movements after extremely short reaction times in the monkey.* Brain Research, 260: 21-26.

Fischer B, Weber H. (1990). *Saccadic reaction times of dyslexic and age-matched normal subjects.* Perception, 19: 805-818.

Fischer B, Weber H, Biscaldi M, Aiple F, Otto P, Stuhr V. (1993). *Separate populations of visually guided saccades in humans: reaction times and amplitudes. Experimental Brain Research,* 92: 528-541.

Fowler MS, Munro N, Richardson A, Stein JF. (1989). *Vergence control in patients with posterior parietal lesions.* Journal of Physiology, 417: 92.

Fowler MS, Richardson AJ, Stein JF. (1991). *Orthoptic investigation of neurological patients undergoing rehabilitation.* British Orthoptic Journal, 48: 2-7.

Goldberg ME, Bushnell MC, Bruce CJ. (1986). *The effect of attentive fixation on eye movements evoked by electrical stimulation of the frontal eye fields.* Experimental Brain Research, 61: 579-584.

Goldberg ME, Segraves MA. (1989). *The visual and frontal cortices.* In: The neurobiology of saccadic eye movements, Wurtz & Goldberg Eds., Elsevier,. Amsterdam.

Goulandris N, McIntyre A, Snowling M, Bethel J-M, Lee JP. (1998). *A comparison of dyslexic and normal readers using orthoptic assessment procedures.* Dyslexia, 4: 30-48.

Griffin DC, Walton HN, Ives V. (1974). *Saccades as related to reading disorders.* Journal of Learning Disabilities, 7: 52-58.

Gruber E. (1962). *Reading ability, binocular coordination and the ophthalmograph.* Archives of Ophthalmology, 67: 280-288.

Hari R, Valta M, Uutela K. (1999). *Prolonged attentional dwell time in dyslexic adults.* Neuroscience Letters, 271: 202-204.

Hatzidaki A, Gianneli M, Petrakis E, Makaronas N, Aslanides IM. (2011). *Reading and visual processing in Greek dyslexic children: an eye-movement study.* Dyslexia, 17: 85-104.

Hawelka S, Wimmer H (2005). *Impaired visual processing of multi-element arrays is associated with increased number of eye movements in dyslexic reading.* Vision Research, 45: 855-863.

Hutzler F, Wimmer H. (2004). *Eye movements of dyslexic children when reading in a regular orthography.* Brain and Language, 89: 235-242.

Hutzler F, Kronbichler M, Jacobs AM, Wimmer H. (2006). *Perhaps correlational but not causal: no effect of dyslexic readers'magnocellular system on their eye movements during reading.* Neuropsychologia, 44: 637-648.

Hyönä J, Olson RK. (1995). *Eye Fixation patterns among dyslexic and normal readers: effect of word length and word frequency.* Journal of Experimental Psychology, Learning, Memory & Cognition, 21: 1430-1440.

Jainta S, Kapoula Z. (2011). *Dyslexic children are confronted with unstable binocular fixation while reading.* PLoS ONE, 6: 1-10.

Jones A, Stark L. (1983). *Abnormal Patterns of normal eye movements in specific dyslexia.* In: Eye Movements in Reading: Perceptual and Language Processes. Rayner Ed., Academic Press, New York.

Just MA, Carpenter PA. (1980). *A theory of reading: From eye fixations to comprehension.* Psychological Review, 87: 329-354.

Kowler E, Anton S. (1987). *Reading twisted text: implications for the role of saccades.* Vision Research, 27: 45-60.

Kowler E, Martins AJ. (1982). *Eye movements of preschool children.* Science, 215: 997-998.

Kuvač Kraljević J, Palmović M. (2011). *Spatial and temporal measurements of eye movement in children with dyslexia.* Collegium Antropologicum, 35: 191-198

Lennerstrand G, Ygge J. (1992). *Dyslexia: ophthalmological aspects 1991.* Acta Ophthalmologica, 70: 3-13.

MacKeben M, Trauzettel-Klosinski S, Reinhard J, Dürrwächter U, Adler M, Klosinski G. (2004). *Eye movement control during single-word reading in dyslexics.* Journal of Vision, 4: 388-402.

Mason A, Cornelissen P, Fowler S, Stein J. (1993). *Contrast sensitivity, ocular dominance and specific reading disability.* Clinical Vision Sciences, 8: 345-353.

Masters MC. (1988). *Orthoptic management of visual dyslexia.* British Orthoptic Journal, 45: 40-48.

McConkie GW, Kerr PW, Reddix MD, Zola D. (1988). *Eye movement control during reading: I. The location of initial eye fixations on words.* Vision Research, 28: 1107-1118.

McConkie GW, Zola D. (1989). *Some characteristics in readers' eyes movements.* In: Brain and reading. von Euler, Lundberg & Lennerstrand Eds., Macmillian Press, London.

McConkie GW, Dyre BP. (2000). *Eye fixation durations in reading: Models of frequency distributions.* In: Reading as a perceptual process, Kennedy, Radach. Heller & Pynte Eds., Elsevier, Oxford

Miall RC, Wolpert D, Stein JF. (1993). *Is the cerebellum a Smith predictor?* Journal of Motor Behaviour, 25: 203-217.

Mohler CW, Wurtz RH. (1976). *Organization of monkey superior colliculus: intermediate layer cells discharging before eye movements.* Journal of Neurophysiology, 39: 722-744.

Mosse HL, Daniels CR. (1959). *Linear dyslexia.* American Journal of Psychotherapy, 13: 826-884.

Mowforth P, Mayhew JEW, Frisby JP. (1981). *Vergence eye movements in response to spatially filtered random dot stereograms.* Perception, 10: 299-304.

Munoz DP, Wurtz RH. (1993). *Fixation cells in monkey superior colliculus. I. Characteristics of cell discharge.* Journal of Neurophysiology, 70: 559-575.

Newman SP, Wadsworth JF, Archer R, Hockley R. (1985a). *Ocular dominance, reading, and spelling ability in school children.* British Journal of Ophthalmology, 69: 228-232.

Newman SP, Karle H, Wadsworth JF, Archer R, Hockly R, Rogers P. (1985b). *Ocular dominance, reading and spelling: a reassessment of a measure associated with specific reading difficulties.* Journal of Research in Reading, 8: 127–138.

Norn MS, Rindziunski E, Skydsgaard H. (1969). *Ophthalmologic and orthoptic examinations of dyslectics.* Acta Ophthalmologica, 47: 147-160.

Oishi A, Tobimatsu S, Arakawa K, Taniwaki T, Kira J. (2005). *Ocular dominancy in conjugate eye movements at reading distance.* Neuroscience Research, 52: 263-268.

Olson RK, Kliegl R, Davidson BJ. (1983). *Dyslexic and normal readers'eye movements.* Journal of Experimental Psychology: Human Perception and Performence, 9: 816-825.

Olson RK, Conners FA, Rack JP. (1991). *Eye movements in dyslexic and normal readers.* In: Vision and visual dyslexia, Stein Ed., Houndmills, Macmillian Press, London.

O'Regan JK.(1981). *The convenient viewing hypothesis.* In: Eye movements: cognition and visual perception. Monty, Senders & Senders Eds., Erlbaum, Hillsdale, NJ.

O'Regan JK, Jacobs AM. (1992). *Optimal viewing position effect in word recognition: a challenge to current theory.* Journal of Experimental Psychology: Human Perception and Performance, 18: 185-197.

O'Regan JK, Lévy-Schoen A. (1987). *Eye movement strategy and tactics in word recognition and reading.* In Attention and Performance XII: The psychology of reading, Coltheart & Lawrence Eds., Erlbaum, N.J.

Ottes FP, Van Gisbergen JAM, Eggermont JJ. (1984). *Metrics of saccades responses to visual double stimuli: two different modes.* Vision Research, 24: 1169-1179.

Pavlidis GT. (1978). *The dyslexics' erratic eye movements : case studies.* Dyslexia Review, 1: 22-28.

Pavlidis GT. (1981a). *Do eye movements hold the key to dyslexia?* Neuropsychologia, 19: 57-64.

Pavlidis GT. (1981b). *Sequencing, eye movements and the early objective diagnosis of dyslexia.* In Dyslexia research and its application to education. Pavlidis & Miles Eds., Wiley & Sons Ltd, London.

Pavlidis GT. (1983). *The "dyslexia syndrome and its objective diagnosis by erratic eye movements".* In: Eye movements and reading, Rayner Ed., Academic Press, New York.

Pavlidis GT. (1985a). *Eye movements in dyslexia : their diagnostic significance.* Journal of Learning Disabilities, 18: 42-50.

Pavlidis GT. (1985b). *Eye movement differences between dyslexics, normal, and retarded readers while sequentially fixated digits.* American Journal of Optometry and Physiological Optics, 62: 820-832.

Pierrot-Deseilligny C,Gaymard B, Müri R, Rivaud S. (1997). Cerebral ocular motor signs. Journal of Neurology, 244: 65-70.

Pirozzolo FJ. (1979). The neuropsychology of developmental reading disorders. Praeger Ed., New York.

Pirozzolo FJ, Rayner K. (1978). *Disorders of oculomotor scanning and graphic orientation in developmental Gerstmann syndrome.* Brain & Language, 5: 119-126.

Pollatsek A. (1983). *What can eye movements tell us about dyslexia?* In: Eye movements in reading: Perceptual and language processes, Rayner Ed., Academic Press, New York.

Radach R, Inhoff A, Heller D. (2004). *Orthographic regularity gradually modulates saccade amplitudes in reading.* European Journal of Cognitive Psychology, 16: 27-51.

Rae C, Lee MA, Dixon RM, Blamire AM, Thompson CH, Styles P, Talcott J, Richardson A, Stein J. (1998). *Metabolic abnormalities in developmental dyslexia detected by 1H magnetic resonance spectroscopy.* The Lancet, 351: 1849-1852.

Rayner K. (1978). *Eye movements in reading and information processing.* Psychological Bulletin, 85: 618-660.

Rayner K. (1979). *Eye guidance in reading: fixation localization within words.* Perception, 8: 21-30.

Rayner K. (1985). *Do faulty eye movements cause dyslexia?* Developmental Neuropsychology, 1: 3–15.

Rayner K. (1986). *Eye movement and the perceptual span in beginning and skilled readers.* Journal of Experimental Child Psychology, 41: 211-236.

Rayner K, Pollatsek A. (1987). *Eye movements in reading: A tutorial review.* In: Attention and performance XII: The psychology of reading, Coltheart Ed., Erlbaum, London.

Riddell PM, Fowler MS, Stein JF. (1987a). *Poor visual direction sense in dyslexic children.* St Bartholomew's Hospital Meeting of Association of British Neurologists.

Riddell P, Fowler MS, Stein JF. (1987b). *A comparison of sighting dominance and the Dunlop Test reference eye in reading disabled children.* British Orthoptic Journal, 44: 64-69.

Riddell P, Fowler MS, Stein JF. (1988). *Vergence eye movements and dyslexia.* Dyslexia Contact, 7: 5-6.

Riddell PM, Fowler MS, Stein JF. (1990). *Spatial discrimination in children with poor vergence control.* Perception and Motor Skills, 70: 707-718.

Rubino, C.A., Minden, H. (1973). *An analysis of eye movements in children with a reading disability.* Cortex, 9: 217-220.

Sakata H, Shibutani H, Kawano K. (1980). *Spatial properties of visual fixation neurons in posterior parietal association cortex of the monkey.* Journal of Neurophysiology, 43: 1654-1672.

Schall JD. (1991). *Neuronal activity related to visually guided saccades in the frontal eye fields of rhesus monkeys: Comparison with supplementary eye fields.* Journal of Neurophysiology, 66: 559-579.

Sparks DL. (1986). *Translation of sensory signals into commands for control of saccadic eye movements. Role of primate superior colliculus.* Physiological Review, 66: 118 171.

Stanley G, Smith GA, Howell EA. (1983a). *Eye-movements and sequential tracking in dyslexic and control children.* British Journal of Psychology, 74: 181-187.

Stanley G, Smith GA, Howell EA. (1983b). *Eye-movements in dyslexic children: comments on Pavlidis reply.* British Journal of Psychology, 74: 195-197.

Stark LW, Giveen SC, Terdiman JF. (1990). *Specific dyslexia and eye movements.* In: Vision and Visual Dyslexia, Stein Ed., MacMillian Press, London:

Stein JF. (1989). *Unfixed reference, monocular occlusion, and developmental dyslexia--a critique.* British Journal of Ophthalmology, 73:319-320.

Stein JF. (1992). *The representation of egocentric space in the posterior parietal cortex.* Behavioural Brain Science, 15: 842-845.

Stein GF. (2001). The magnocellular theory of developmental dyslexia. Dyslexia, 7: 12-36.

Stein JF, Fowler S. (1982). *Diagnosis of dyslexia by means of a new indicator of eye dominance.* British Journal of Ophthalmology, 66: 332-336.

Stein JF, Fowler S. (1984). *A physiological theory of visual dyslexia.* In: Advances in Neurology. Progress in Aphasiology, Rose Ed., Raven Press, New York.

Stein JF, Fowler S. (1985). *Effect of monocular occlusion on visuomotor perception and reading in dyslexic children.* The Lancet, 2: 69-73.

Stein JF, Fowler S. (1993). *Unstable binocular control in children with specific reading retardation.* Journal of Research in Reading, 16: 30-45.

Stein JF, Riddell PM, Fowler S. (1986). *The Dunlop test and reading in primary school children.* British Journal of Ophthalmology, 70: 317-320.

Stein JF, Riddell PM, Fowler S. (1987). *Fine binocular control in dyslexic children.* Eye, 1: 433-438.

Stein JF, Riddell PM, Fowler S. (1988). *Disordered vergence eye movement control in dyslexic children.* British Journal of Ophthalmology, 72: 162-166.

Stein JF, Riddell PM, Fowler S. (1989). *Brain and Reading*, Von Euler, Lundberg & Lennerstrand Eds. Stockton, New York.

Stein JF, Talcott J. (1999). *Impaired neuronal timing in developmental dyslexia-the magnocellular hypothesis.* Dyslexia, 5: 59-77.

Stein JF, Walsh V. (1997). *To see but not to read: the magnocellular theory of dyslexia.* Trends in Neurosciences, 20: 147-152.

Tinker MA. (1958). *Recent studies of eye movements in reading.* Psychological Bulletin, 55: 215-231.

Trauzettel-Klosinski S, Koitzsch AM, Dürrwächter U, Sokolov AN, Reinhard J, Klosinski G. (2010). *Eye movements in German-speaking children with and without dyslexia when reading aloud.* Acta Ophthalmologica, 88: 681-691.

Vernet M, Kapoula Z. (2009). *Binocular motor coordination during saccades and fixations while reading: A magnitude and time analysis.* Journal of Vision, 9 (7): 1-13.

Yang SN, McConkie GW. (2001). *Eye movements during reading: a theory of saccade initiation times.* Vision Research, 41: 3567-3585.

Ygge J, Lennerstrand G, Axelsson I, Rydberg A, Wijecoon S, Pettersson BM. (1993a). *Visual functions and oculomotor functions in a Swedish population of 9-year-old dyslexics and normal readers.* Acta Ophthalmologica, 71: 1-9.

Ygge J, Lennerstrand G, Rydberg A, Wijecoon S, Pettersson BM. (1993b). *Oculomotor functions in a Swedish population of dyslexic and normally reading children.* Acta Ophthalmologica, 71: 10-21.

Zangwill OL, Blakemore C. (1972). *Dyslexia: Reversal of eye-movements during reading.* Neuropsychologia, 10: 371-373.

Zoccolotti P, De Luca M, Di Pace E, Judica A, Orlandi M, Spinelli D. (1999). *Markers of developmental surface dyslexia in a language (Italian) with a high grapheme-phoneme correspondence.* Applied Psycholinguistics, 20: 191-216.

Chapter XI

Visual Attention and Dyslexia

Although visual attention is a subject pertaining to the cognitive field, it cannot be ignored by vision scientists who deal with developmental dyslexics.

Visual attention is like a filter that enhances the recognition of a given stimulus in the visual field, helping its processing and/or inhibiting the irrelevant information from the surrounding areas [Laberge & Brown, 1989; Cave & Bichot, 1999]. More simply, visual attention is the function that promotes visual processing in a particular region of the visual space [Facoetti & Molteni, 2001]

Visual Attention and Reading

Visual attention acts in two complementary ways: the *distributed mode* and the *focused mode* [Schneider & Shriffin, 1977; Duncan, 1980; Bergen & Julesz, 1983; Jonides, 1983]. In the distributed mode, it is uniformly distributed and acts in parallel as to identify the elements of interest in a configuration without looking for a particular one: this solution is well represented by the so-called pop-out[163] visual search [McLeod et al., 1988; Duncan & Humphreys, 1992].

---

[163] Being a parallel visual search, in the pop-out task it is asked to find a target (e.g. a "C" or a vertical segment) embedded in a field of distractors (e.g. "O" or oblique segments). Serial search differs from parallel search inasmuch as it requires focused attention and considers serially every single element: In fact, differently from the latter, serial search speed depends on the number of distractors [Treisman & Gelade,1980]. In the figure below (Figure 2) it can be experienced how the identification of the target is faster in the left panel (parallel search) compared to the right (serial search).

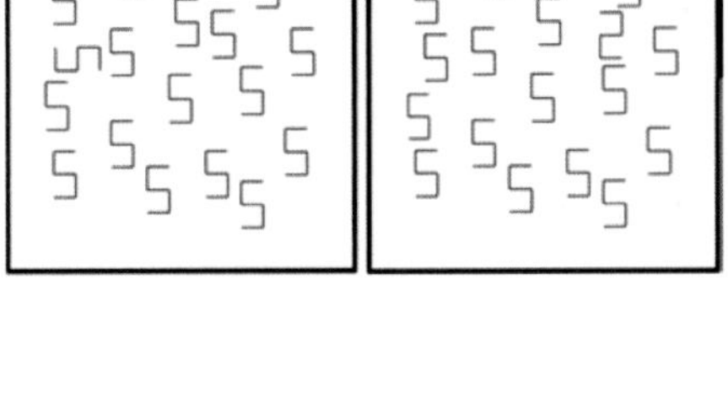

Figure 2. Parallel and serial search.

In the focused mode, the attention centers on a limited area of the visual field where the element of interest localizes[164] (Figure 1).

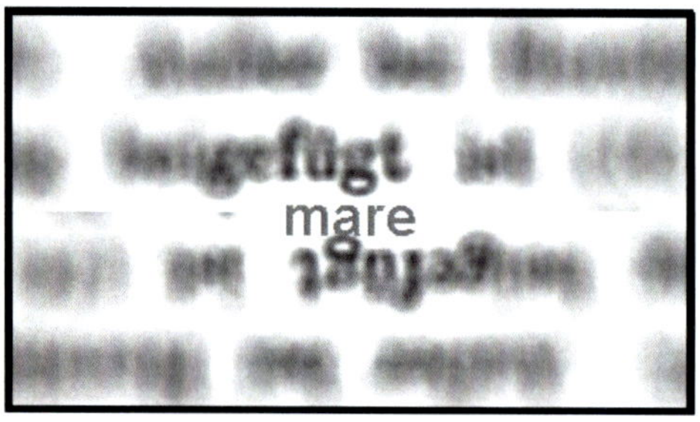

Figure 1. Focused attentional mode. Simulation.

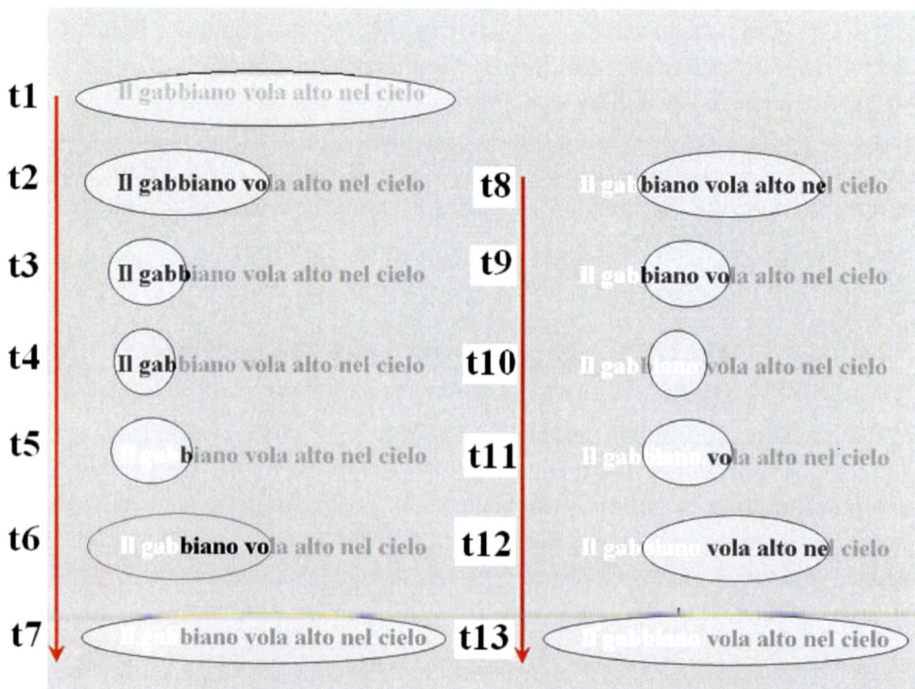

Figure 3. Visual attention during the lexical task. The attentional focus is directed on the first group of syllables (t2) and narrows (t3) until it reaches the appropriate size for their processing (t4). When the processing is complete, the focalized mode switches back to the distributed mode (t5-t7) so as to localize the second group of syllables. At this stage the distributed mode switches again into the attentional focus, which narrows and centers on the second group of syllables (t8-t10), processes them and finally returns to the distributed mode (t11-t13). Meaning of the sentence: "The seagull flies high in the sky".

---

[164] The size of the attentional focus is adjusted on the size of the stimulus so as to be as sharp as possible [Egeth, 1977; Eriksen & St. James, 1986; Castiello & Umiltà, 1990, 1992]: in fact, the sharper is the attentional focus, the faster is the acquisition of the configuration that falls within its limits because the visual function in that region turns out to be more concentrated [Egeth, 1977; Eriksen & St.James, 1986; LaBerge & Brown, 1989; Castiello & Umiltà, 1990; Benso et al., 1998; Turatto et al., 2000].

During reading, the distributed mode selects the target (for example a syllable) at the beginning of a sentence. When the target is spotted, the attentive mode switches into the focused modality, which centers on the syllable until its processing is completed. After the syllable has been processed, visual attention comes back to the distributed state in search of the next target. Thus, when reading a sentence, visual attention changes sequentially from distributed to focused condition and vice versa (Figure 3).

This view is in line with the lexical model called *DRC* (*Dual Route Cascading*, Coltheart et al., 2001]. According to the DRC model, letters are first identified in parallel through the attentional distributed mode and then processed in series via the focused mode, resulting in a sequential analysis along the lexical direction. In this paradigm, the processing of words of common use does not need the focused mode, but the parallel mode is sufficient [Kinsey et al., 2004]. Probably, the global representation of lexical configuration, i.e. the word as such, if of common use is recognized as a single entity without requiring a sequential analysis of each letter and syllable. On the contrary, in order to read correctly non-words or unfamiliar and uncommon words, sequential analysis cannot be avoided and a well-calibrated, quickly and accurately oriented attentional focus is pivotal. Therefore, the integrity of both steps of the visual attention is essential to decode both unfamiliar terms and common words: in the first case the DRC model requires both phases, while for common words often the only modality in parallel is enough.

As reported by Vidyasagar [2004], serial attention is aimed at processing both the symbol as such as well as its position with respect to the previous and the next ones.

The cerebral region in charge of the visuo-attentional processes is the right posterior parietal cortex (PPC), [Posner, 1980; Wurtz et al., 1982; Lawler & Cowey, 1987; Posner et al., 1984, 1987; Livingstone & Hubel, 1988; Arguin et al., 1993; Chelazzi, 1999; Vidyasagar, 1999; Downar et al., 2000; Corbetta & Shulman, 2002; Laberge, 2002; Bisley & Goldberg, 2003b; Costantidinis, 2006; Husain & Nachev, 2006][165]. The right PPC on the one hand provides the positional information referred to the letter; on the other hand it constantly interacts with the receptive fields of the occipital region[166], responsible for the resolution of the details of the characters [Gandhi et al., 1999; Martinez et al., 1999; Somers et al., 1999].

Indeed, such a reciprocal interaction between the parietal and the occipital cortex is at the basis of the temporal sequential processing of visual configurations and in general of the lexical function[167].

Visual Attention Impairment in Dyslexia

It is evident, now, that visual attention is an essential requisite for reading, so that its impairment can affect the lexical task[168].

165 The posterior parietal cortex (PPC) includes Brodmann areas 5, 7a and 7b and is considered as a major associative crossroads where visual, auditory and sensory inputs meet and complement each other. Together to the parietal cortex, even the lateral and inferior pulvinar [Laberge & Brown, 1989; Laberge, 1995] and the reticular nucleus of the talamus [Crick, 1984] seem be involved in the visuoattentional modulation.

166 Attentional modulatory activity has been recorded in some neurons of the area V1 of the macaque [Vidyasagar, 1998, 2001].

167 See chapter 12.

Visual attention is a function mediated by the magnocellular system [Breitmeyer & Ganz, 1976; Steinman et al., 1997; Lennie, 1993; Vidyasagar, 1999; Giaschi & Boden, 2007] and it is revealing that its anatomical site, the right posterior parietal cortex, is found to be defective in patients affected from developmental dyslexia [Kinsbourne & Warrington, 1962, Duffy et al., 1980; Wood et al., 1991; Stein, 1991, 1993, Eden et al., 1994; Stein & Walsh, 1997; Ro et al., 1998; Smania et al., 1998; Hari et al., 1999; Facoetti et al., 2001]. In confirmation of the link between visual attentional defects and reading disability, an acquired damage of this region may cause an alteration of visual attention [Kinsbourne & Warrington, 1962], which in turn leads to *secondary dyslexia* [Kinsbourne & Warrington, 1962; Shallice & Warrington, 1977; Brunn& Farah, 1991][169].

Therefore, selective attention deficits often found in dyslexics have been referred to an alteration of the right parietal cortex and of its magnocellular afferent projections [Steinman et al., 1998; Koivikko & Hari, 1999; Vidyasagar & Pammer, 1999; Facoetti & Turatto, 2000; Facoetti et al., 2001]. In addition, other areas, which cooperate with the right posterior parietal cortex in the modulation of the visuo-attentional process, such as the frontal eye fields (FEF) and especially the mediotemporal region [Posner, 1980], are shown to be functionally and morphologically inadequate in our patients. Really, in line with a previous study that reported attentional deficiencies in patients with abnormal sensitivity to dynamic configurations [Atkinson, 1991], Iles found decreased visual attention in dyslexic children with reduced motion perception and concluded that magnocellular damage in the mediotemporal area[170] can contribute to determine the attentional impairment [Iles et al., 2000]. Based on the link between the visuoattentive function and motion perception, visual attention is suggested to have a modulatory effect on the processing of dynamic stimuli [Raymond, 2000] and coherent motion perception has been adopted to study the relationship between visual attention and reading [Kinsey et al., 2004].

Apart from motion perception-related paradigms, visual attention has been investigated by using visual search paradigms. According to this approach, patients are found to be affected by a double order of attentional deficits: in the ability to *direct* the visual attention towards a target [Posner, 1980; Posner et al., 1980; Facoetti et al., 2000b], and *to focus*, i.e. to adapt the width of the attentive window to the size of the stimulus[171] [Facoetti et al., 2000b]. In fact, when the processing of a syllable is completed, for a disturbance of the attentional orientation dyslexics have difficulty in properly redirect their attentional focus towards the following cluster of letters[172] [Casco et al., 1998; Brannan & Williams, 1987; Facoetti et al., 2000b; Visser et al., 2004] and need more time to complete this operation [Jonkman et al., 1992, Hari et al., 1999; Facoetti et al., 2000b]. This latency, this slowness, suggests that the problem may be due to a developmental delay [Jonkman et al., 1992].

[168] Although attentional disorders and developmental dyslexia are two distinct conditions, 15% of dyslexics suffer from a specific attentional disorder and, in turn, 35% of patients affected by specific attentional disorders show reading problems: [Lyon, 1996; Shaywitz, 1998; Willcutt & Pennington, 2000, Pastor & Reuben, 2002].

[169] As far back as 1926, Herrmann & Pötzl coined the term *parietal dyslexia* for lesions of the parietal cortex able to determine lexical disorders like the intrusion of misspelled words into the sentence.

[170] See chapter 7.

[171] Since orientation and focusing are two independent attentive processes, they require different techniques to be investigated [Castiello & Umiltà, 1990].

[172] Reduced accuracy in processing the second of two sequential stimuli is due to the difficulty in rapidly disrupting and re-orienting the attention (*attentional blink*).

In addition, apart from its orientation, the attentional focus *per se* can be inaccurate in dyslexics [Richards et al., 1990, Sharma et al., 1991], so that after the target has been spotted, the focusing interval is too brief [Facoetti et al., 2000b]. The attentive operation is diverted too early from the syllable in fixation for the overwhelming effect of the surrounding (parafoveal) stimuli on the foveal processing. Indeed, this is the crucial point: on the one hand, the syllables in parafoveal projection promote the untimely disengagement of the attentional focus, on the other hand they directly interfere with the processing of the syllable falling on the fixation point, in both cases hindering its correct recognition [Geiger & Lettvin, 1987; Rayner et al., 1989; Morris & Rayner, 1991; Geiger et al., 1994, Old et al., 1998]. The negative influence of the parafoveal activation is therefore the main factor leading to the disruption of the normal attentional center-periphery hierarchy: the abnormal activation level of the parafoveal and peripheral (i.e. distributed) attention prevails over the focused mode centered on the fixation point, promoting its disruption and widening its radius [Williams & Bologna, 1985, Geiger & Lettvin, 1987; Facoetti et al., 2000a, b] [173]. Now, if the size of the attentional focus increases, the processing efficiency deteriorates [Egeth, 1977, Eriksen & Yeh, 1985; Eriksen & St James, 1986; Laberge, 1983].

An indirect evidence supporting this arguments is the larger number of errors made by patients when reading a line of text (whose projection extends well beyond the fixation point) compared to isolated words (and as such localized at the center) [Hill & Lovegrove, 1993].

The over sensibility to peripheral stimuli explains why dyslexics recognize more easily than normal readers a letter or a string of letters presented in the periphery of the visual field when, in the meanwhile, they are asked to identify another character projected onto the fixation point [Geiger & Lettvin, 1987]. Finally, it is revealing that the experimental narrowing of the reading field is found to improve the lexical function of many patients [Geiger et al., 1994]. In this regard, Rayner has reported the case of a professor who was dyslexic since he was a boy. The researcher noticed in the patient a specific attentional defect characterized by an exuberant effect of the peripheral attention compared to the visual attention directed onto the fixation point: the result was the difficult processing of letters and syllables in foveal projection for the abnormal interference of the parafoveal ones.

In this case, a moving window aimed at masking the more eccentric regions of the string (especially on the right) so as to help focusing on the syllable under fixation, led to an improvement of the lexical performance [Rayner et al., 1989] [174]. The progressive narrowing

[173] The stronger parafoveal influence in dyslexics would therefore make the pre-processing of the syllable on the right able to interfere with the current processing of the fixated syllable [Geiger & Lettvin, 1987]. This perspective, confirmed by Perry [Perry et al., 1989], fits well with the wider extent of visual attention on the right of the fixation point as shown by the *form resolving field* of dyslexics (see below).

[174] The model of the *moving window* [McConkie & Rayner, 1975; Rayner & Bertera, 1979] allows to measure the size of the so-called "actual visual field during the reading" [Rayneret al., 1995] that could match the so-called *visual span*, i.e. the extension of visual space that can be processed at each fixation (see chapter 13). The paradigm of the moving window presents a sentence made up of a central readable part of a given length; at the left and right side of the central part, the letters of the sentence are replaced by random characters or"xs". The fixation is monitored by a tracking system and interfaced with the computer program so that the window moves sequentially along the sentence at the same pace of the subject's fixations. This way, the change in reading rate as a function of the size of the window can be measured. It is observed that in normal subjects reading rate increases proportionally with the widening of window until the function reaches a "ceiling". The decrease of the number of fixations and especially the reduction of their duration are responsible for this lexical improvement [Underwood & Zola, 1986, Rayner et al., 1989]. In fact, as explained by Rayner, the larger is the window, the longer is the part of the sentence projected on the left and on the right of the fixation point, i.e. on the parafovea. So, provided the window is wide enough, the parafovea is able to pre-process the

of the moving window till to an optimum extension enabled this patient to reach his maximum reading rate.

To underline the importance that a visuoattentive defect may have in preventing from fluent reading, Valdois described the case of a 10 years old dyslexic girl whose disability was ascribed to a visual attentive defect and defined her type of dyslexia as *visuo-attentional dyslexia* or *selective attentional dyslexia*. [Valdois et al., 1995].

The Form Resolving Field (FRF)

The distribution of the visual attention across the visual field can be described as a gradient that slopes from both sides of the fixation point (the "core" of the attentional focus).

This double gradient, called *Form Resolving Field* (FRF) [Geiger & Lettvin 1987, 1989, Perry et al., 1989, Geiger et al., 1992], has been assessed by measuring the reaction time or the accuracy in recognizing a target (such as a letter) displayed at different eccentricities across the visual field when another stimulus is projected onto the fixation point [Laberge & Brown, 1989; Geiger et al., 1992; Geiger et al., 1994; Smania et al., 1998; Facoetti et al., 2000a, Lorusso et al., 2004].

In normal subjects, the two gradients of the FRF are steep, since the recognition speed or accuracy drops more and more as the distance of the target from the fixation point increases[175] [Laberge & Brown, 1989; Smania et al., 1998; Facoetti et al., 2000a]. In occidental readers, the FRF is found slightly narrower on the right side, i.e. in the direction of reading in western languages[176] [Geiger et al., 1992, 1994, Zegarra-Moran & Geiger, 1993].

On the contrary, both in children [Geiger et al., 1994; Lorusso, et al., 2004, 2005] and adult dyslexics [Geiger & Lettvin, 1987[177], 1989, 2000; Perry et al., 1989; Geiger et al., 1992], the slight and physiological asymmetry of the FRF tends to disappear, since the widening of the attentional focus causes an enlargement compared to controls with a smoother gradient in the right hemifield [Lorusso et al., 2004, 2005][178].

The difference is significant at 7.5, 9, 10 and 12.5 degrees of eccentricity on the right side of the fixation point [Geiger et al., 1994; Lorusso et al., 2004] (Figure 4). The normal asymmetry of the FRF is reduced also in poor readers (*poor readers*, not dyslexics), but the difference is significant only for the most eccentric values (10 and 12.5 deg) and not for the more proximal ones (7.5 deg) [Lorusso et al., 2004].

---

part of the text projected on each side of the fixation point, and this ability improves as the size of the window gets wider. The lexical improvement is due to the fact that very short words or high frequency words (i.e. of common use) do not need to be fixated but may be processed simply via parafoveal pre-processing: evidently, the paroveal pre-processing enables a consistent save of time during reading [Blanchard et al., 1989].

175 Aubert-Foerster law [Aubert &Foerster, 1857].

176 On the contrary, in Hebrew readers the profile of the FRF is reversed, in agreement with the opposite direction of lexical processing (from right to left: Geiger et al., 1992].

177 In this study, the FRF was estimated only on the right side.

178 Yet, in other investigations the FRF of normal and dyslexic readers turned out to be approximately the same [Goolkasian & King, 1990; Klein et al., 1990; Bjaalid et al., 1993]. According to Geiger, such a difference in the experimental results would depend on the device used to generate the stimuli: in fact, cathode ray tubes (CRT) tend to make the letters jagged; on the contrary, with the slide projector employed by Geiger the stroke of the characters resulted regular. The jagged appearance of the letters generated by the CRT would bias the FRF of dyslexics, making it similar to that of normal readers.

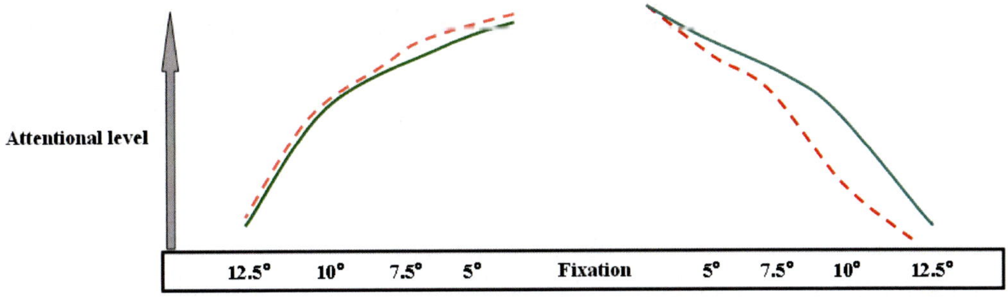

Figure 4. The FRF in normal readers (dashed line) and in dyslexics (solid line). Note the different slope in the right hemifield (*Modified reprint from: Vision Research, Vol. 44, Issue 20, Lorusso ML, Facoetti A, Pesenti S, Cattaneo C, Molteni M, Geiger G, Wider recognition in peripheral vision common to different subtypes of dyslexia, pages 2413-2424, 2004, with permission from Elsevier).*

In summary, compared to normal readers, in patients the visual attention on the right side of the fixation point drops more gradually than expected, whereas on the left side it does not show significant differences: it is arguable, therefore, that the abnormally high attentive level for the parafoveal letters on the right side of the fixation point ends up to interfere with the foveal syllable processing.

According to some authors, the attentional imbalance in dyslexics is not limited to the increased interference of peripheral visual attention on the right side of the FRF but is associated with reduced attentional activity in the left hemifield [Koivikko & Hari, 1999; Facoetti & Turatto, 2000; Facoetti & Molteni, 2001][179]. According to this solution, in the right hemifield the distributed mode, predominant, tends to overcome the focused mode [Geiger & Lettvin, 1987; Geiger et al., 1994; Facoetti et al., 2000a]: as a result, a peripheral over-distractibility makes the patients unable to appropriately center his visual attention on the target. In contrast, the reduced interference of the letters projected on the left side predisposes the left characters to be ignored, that is to say to left hemi-attention. These two conditions (increased interference of visual attention in the right hemifield associated with a reduced interference in the left hemifield) have been called *right over-distractibility* and *left inattention*, respectively [Facoetti & Turatto, 2000; Facoetti & Molteni, 2001].

Now, is it possible to consider the reduced gradient on the right side of the FRF a marker for developmental dyslexia?

An index called "criterion 2" (C2) has been computed from the right and left side of the FRF [Lorusso et al., 2004]. Criterion 2 is the ratio between the percentage of correctly recognized letters for the stimuli presented at 2.5 degrees of eccentricity and the sum of the percentages at 10 and 12.5 degrees. Therefore, a reduced C2 means higher frequency of

[179] According to Hari, the crucial point is not the right over-distractibility but the left inattention so that dyslexics would suffer from a left *mini-hemineglect* [Koivikko & Hari, 1999, Hari et al., 2001], a possibility previously advanced by Stein [1993]. In hemineglect, visual inattention is limited to one hemifield (right or left). However, the authors underlined that this asymmetry, frequently reported in patients suffering from right cerebral hemisphere lesions [Husain et al., 1997], is modest in dyslexics. Yet, Jaśkowski & Rusiak [2005] remarked that subjects with left hemineglect tend to make reading mistakes that do not match the typical errors of dyslexics, since the reversal of characters, confusion of syllables and confusion of mirror letters in the former are missing. Moreover, a slight hemineglect can be observed not only in disabled readers, but even in the normal population [Polikoff et al., 1995].

recognition in the periphery, that is to say the lower is C2, the higher is the peripheral visual attention.

In accordance with the reduced rate of decrease of the FRF on the right side, in the right hemifield of dyslexic patients C2 is lower compared to normal readers (C2: 1.77 vs. 4.11, respectively), whereas on the left side no significant differences have been observed (C2 = 1.44 vs. 1.53). It has been computed that a C2 cutoff referred to the right hemifield = 2 enables to identify patients in 91% of cases and normal readers in 78% of cases.

Although the evidence for visual attention impairment in developmental dyslexia is consistent, the relationship between attentional and impaired reading requires further investigation and the possible cause/effect relationship must be ascertained.

An Italian study compared the lexical behavior of children with a selective attention defect with the reading performance of a group of normal subjects [Casco et al., 1998]. The experiment is interesting, since it starts from the attentional problem to evaluate its impact on the lexical function and not *vice versa* (i.e., it investigates the reading function in patients with attentional problems rather than the attentional deficits in disabled readers). In this research, the lexical performance of the inattentive group was worse compared to normal children. As a conclusion, the occurrence of lexical problems in children with visuo-attentional deficit together with the previously reported finding of attentional disorders in dyslexics support a cause-effect relationship between the two clinical conditions. Indeed, based on this result, visual attention impairment could be a marker of lexical disability. Moreover, as visual attention can be investigated since the preschool age, it may allow the early diagnosis of dyslexia.

Interestingly, the FRF of dyslexic children is broader and less asymmetric compared to adult patients. This FRF difference suggests the existence of a plastic phase during the visuo-attentional development: with a timely diagnosis and an early specific training, it could be possible to modulate the maturation of the form resolving field, narrowing its right slope. Therefore, under this perspective a solution based on the visual rehabilitation training can be considered[180] [Geiger et al., 1994; Rettenbach & Sireteanu, 1995, Geiger & Lettvin, 2000].

Asymmetry of Attentional Orientation

In addition to the balancing between peripheral and central attention and between distributed and focused attentional mode, an adequate capacity to orient the visual attention across the written page is required to achieve the normal lexical function [Inhoff et al., 1989; Facoetti et al., 2000b].

Normally, the orientation of the visual attention toward a hemifield promotes the attentional process in the same hemifield and, at the same time, inhibits the attentional process in the contralateral hemifield [Posner & Rafal, 1987; Cohen et al., 1994]. A target presented in the left hemifield drives the visual attention orientation to divert on the left, activating the right cerebral hemisphere, which in turn inhibits the left one via interemispheric connections. It follows that when visual attention is diverted toward the left hemifield, the attention in the contralateral hemifield is inhibited. The same happens when visual attention is

[180] See chapter 15.

diverted toward the right hemifield, so that in normal readers visuo-attentional orientation turns out to be symmetric (Figure 5).

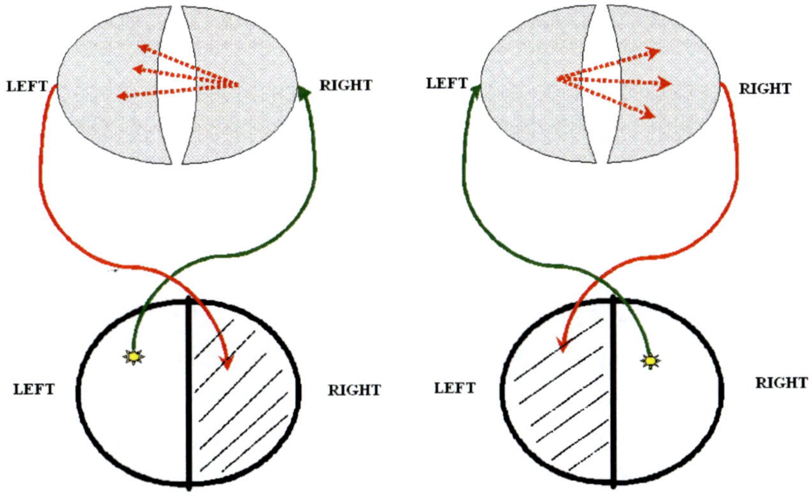

Figure 5. Orientation of the visual attention in a normal reader. In green is the excitatory impulse, in red the inhibitory one. The dashed hemifield is inhibited. The red dotted arrows refer to the direction of the interemispheric inhibition.

In dyslexics, the situation is different and depends on the side: when the target is presented on the left hemifield, the activation of the right cerebral emisphere fails to inhibit adequately the left hemisphere: this event would account for the lack of suppression of the attentional process in the right hemifield (right over-distractibility).

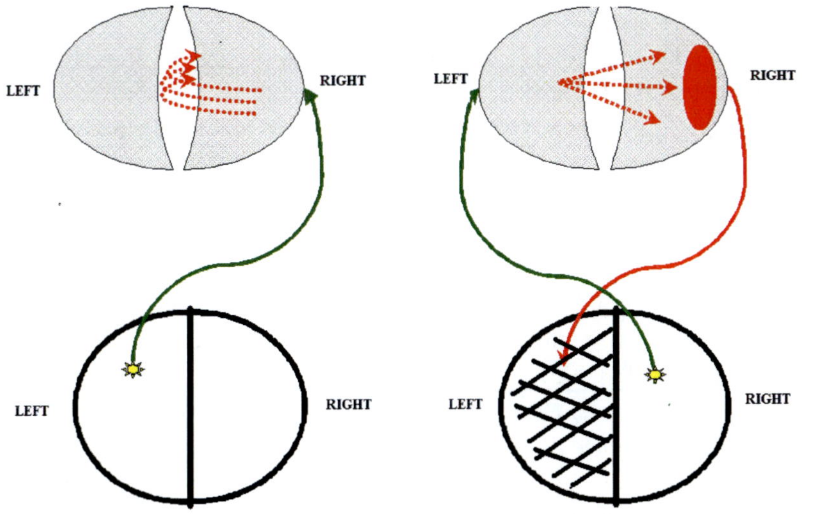

Figure 6. Orientation of visual attention in a dyslexic subject. As in the previous figure, in green is the excitatory impulse, in red the inhibitory one and the dotted arrows indicate interemispheric inhibition. The red spot refers to excessive hemispheric inhibition. The filled hemifield is over inhibited.

On the contrary, a stimulus presented on the right side activates the left cerebral emisphere, which in turn inhibits the contralateral hemisphere more strongly than in normal readers: the result is an excessive inhibition of the visual attention in the left hemifield (left inattention: Facoetti et al., 2001) (figure 6).

Therefore, unlike normal readers, the orientation of visual attention in dyslexics is asymmetric. The origin of this unbalancing lies in the malfunctioning of the right posterior parietal cortex [Ro et al., 1998; Smania et al., 1998; Facoetti et al., 2001], that on the one hand suffers from defective interemispheric communication[181], on the other hand would be affected by a dysfunction of the large ganglion cells.

Visual Attention, M System and Ocular Movements

Actually, since visual attention is a magnocellular function, in dyslexics the anatomical substrate of the attentional impairment would lie once more in a magnocellular anomaly [Lorusso et al., 2004].

A damage of the M-system is supposed to act by disrupting the relationship between focused and distributed attentional mode, hampering the former and favoring the maintenance of the latter.

Since visual attention has a modulatory effect on the triggering of saccadic movements [Shepherd et al., 1986; Inhoff et al., 1989; Henderson & Ferreira, 1990; Johnson, 1994] and that both functions are driven by the magnocellular system, such a disruption would affect the oculomotor pattern [Morris & Rayner, 1991, Eden et al., 1994]. In addition, the right temporal parietal cortex is found to be involved not only in visuo-attentional processes but even in the modulation of saccades and fixations [Andersen, 1989; Corbetta et al., 1998; Anderson et al., 1994; Bisley & Goldberg, 2003a, b]. More specifically, the regions in charge of the oculomotor control are the Parietal Eye Field (PEF), the mediotemporal area (MT), and the medial superotemporal area (MST) [Pierrot-Deseilligny et al., 1997]. So, malfunctioning of these regions can lead both to abnormal saccadic pattern and attentional deficit: the difficulty in orienting and focusing the attention would have a negative impact respectively on the saccades programming and on the fixation stability during reading [Facoetti et al., 2000b]. Indeed, since PEF is responsible for saccadic latency and precision [Pierrot-Deseilligny et al., 1991a, b] and MT/MST modulate the slow eye movements[182] [Pierrot-Deseilligny et al., 1997], such an impairment would cause increased saccadic latency and reduced precision, together to an alteration of the SEMs.

Effective attentional focusing and its correct orientation are not yet enough to ensure the normal lexical process: the peculiarity of reading, in fact, is *sequential analysis* [Vidyasagar, 1999; 2004]. A correct sequential analysis requires the serial visual search to be effective: Vidyasagar stated that the only reliable visual tests able to identify dyslexics are those based on serial visual search [Vidyasagar, 2004] and claimed that the reading rate depends on the

[181] This finding is confirmed by the analysis of the cerebral electrical activity (Event-Related Potentials: ERP) referred to the attentional orientation. In fact, ERP supports an abormal development of the interemispheric asymmetry [Wijers et al., 2005].

[182] SEM, see chapter 10.

visual search rate. The possibility to train visual search and to make it able to work in a sequential manner is therefore the main condition to learn to read correctly. Indeed, sequential analysis makes reading a demanding task, more difficult to acquire than the serial search: serial search is the basis for the sequential analysis, but it is not enough *per se* to enable the sequential analysis of a configuration.

It has been suggested that a general attentional problem, causing difficulties in performing the psychophysical exams, would bias the results obtained in the dyslexics, simulating a magnocellular impairment [Peli & Garcia-Pérez, 1997; Roach & Hogben, 2004]. Therefore, since the attentional defect is generalized, such a poor performance is expected to involve even the parvocellular pathway: and yet, the P-function in patients is not impaired compared to normal readers[183].

Moreover, the reduced steepness of the right side of the FRF in patients has been advanced to depend on the increased strength of the lateral masking[184] [Geiger & Lettvin, 1987, 1989; Geiger et al., 1992]. Indeed, this relation would account for many of the signs and symptoms typical of dyslexics [Geiger & Lettvin, 1999]. Still, lateral masking acts on a local level, being ineffective when the distance between adjoining letters in the more central region of the visual field is wider than few tenths of degree. Thereby, it is unlikely that lateral masking, acting across so short a spatial interval, is the fundament of visual attention, which on the contrary encompasses a far wider range.

Nonetheless, like visual attention, lateral masking is perhaps the most promising line of investigation under a visual perspective.

References

Andersen RA. (1989). *Visual and eye movement functions of the posterior parietal cortex.* Annual Review of Neuroscience, 12: 377-403.

Anderson TJ, Jenkins IH, Brooks DJ, Hawken MB, Frackowiak RSJ, Kennard C. (1994). *Cortical control of saccades and fixation in man. A PET study.* Brain, 117: 1073-1084.

Arguin M, Joanette Y, Cavanagh P. (1993). *Visual search for feature and conjunction targets with an attentional deficit.* Journal of Cognitive Neuroscience, 5: 436-452.

Atkinson J. (1991). *Review of human visual development: crowding and dyslexia.* In: Vision and visual dyslexia, Stein Ed., MacMillian Press, Houndmills, London.

Aubert H, Foerster A. (1857). *Beitraege zur Kenntniss des indirecten Sehen.* Graefes Archives of Ophthalmology, 3: 1−37.

Bergen JR, Julesz B. (1983). *Parallel versus serial processing in rapid pattern discrimination.* Nature, 28: 241-248.

Bisley JW, Goldberg ME. (2003a). *The role of the parietal cortex in the neural processing of saccadic eye movements.* Advances in Neurology, 93: 141-157.

Bisley JW, Goldberg ME. (2003b). *Neuronal activity in the lateral intraparietal area and spatial attention.* Science, 299: 81-86.

[183] Consider for example contrast sensibility at high spatial frequencies and low temporal frequencies [Lovegrove et al., 1980; Mason et al., 1993]

[184] See chapter 13.

Bjaalid IK, Høien T, Lundberg I. (1993). *Letter identification and lateral masking in dyslexics and normal readers.* Scandinavian Journal of Educational Research, 37: 151-161.

Blanchard HE, Pollatsek A, Rayner K. (1989). *Parafoveal processing during eye fixation in reading.* Perception & Psychophysics, 46: 85-94.

Benso F, Turatto M, Mascetti GG, Umiltà C. (1998). *The time course of atentional focusing.* European Journal of Cognitive Psychology, 10: 373-388.

Boden C, Giaschi D. (2007). *M-stream deficits and reading-related visual processes in developmental dyslexia.* Psychological Bulletin, 133: 346-366.

Brannan J, Williams M. (1987). *Allocation of visual attention in good and poor readers.* Perception & Psychophysics, 41: 23-28.

Breitmeyer BG, Ganz L. (1976). *Implications of sustained and transient channels for theories of visual pattern masking, saccadic suppression, and information processing.* Psychological Review, 83: 1-36.

Brunn JL, Farah MJ. (1991). *The relation between spatial attention and reading: evidence for the neglect syndrome.* Cognitive Neuropsychology, 8: 59-75.

Casco C, Tressoldi P, Dellantonio A. (1998). *Visual selective attention and reading efficiency are related in children.* Cortex, 34: 531-546.

Castiello U, Umiltà C. (1990). *Size of the attentional focus and efficiency of processing.* Acta Psychologica, 73: 195-209.

Castiello U, Umiltà C. (1992). *Splitting focal attention.* Journal of Experimental Psychology: Human Perception and Performance, 18: 837-848.

Cave KR, Bichot NP. (1999). *Visuospatial attention: beyond a spotlight model.* Psychonomic Bulletin and Review, 6: 204-223

Chelazzi L. (1999). *Serial attention mechanisms in visual search: a critical look at the evidence.* Psychological Research, 62: 195-219.

Cohen JD, Romero RD, Servan-Schreiber D, Farah MJ. (1994). *Mechanisms of spatial attention: the relation of macrostructure to microstructure in parietal neglect.* Journal of Cognitive Neuroscience, 6: 377-387.

Coltheart M, Rastle K, Perry C, Langdon R, Ziegler J. (2001). *DRC: a dual route cascaded model of visual word recognition and reading aloud.* Psychological Review, 108: 204-256.

Corbetta M, Shulman GL. (2002). *Control of goal-directed and stimulus driven attention in the brain.* Nat Reviews Neuroscience, 3: 201-215.

Corbetta M, Akbudak E, Conturo TE, Snyder AZ, Ollinger JM, Drury HA, Linenweber MR, Petersen SE, Raichle ME, Van Essen DC, Shulman GL. (1998). *A Common Network of Functional Areas for Attention and Eye Movements.* Neuron, 21: 761-773.

Costantinidis C. (2006). *Posterior parietal mechanisms of visual attention.* Reviews in the Neurosciences, 17: 415-427.

Crick F. (1984). *Function of the talamic reticular complex : The searchlight hypothesis.* Proceedings of the National Academy of Sciences of the United States of America, 81: 4586-4590.

Downar J, Crawley DJ, Mikulis DJ, Davis KD. (2000). *A multimodal cortical network for the detection of changes in the sensory environment.* Nature Neuroscience, 3: 277-283.

Duffy FH, Denckla MB, Bartels PH, Sandini B. (1980). *Dyslexia: regional differences in brain electrical activity by topographical mapping.* Annals of Neurology, 7: 412-420.

Duncan J. (1980). *The locus of interference in the perception of simultaneous stimuli.* Psychological Review, 87: 272-300.

Duncan J, Humphreys G. (1992). *Beyond the search surface: visual search and attentional engagement.* Journal of Experimental Psychology: Human Perception and Performance, 18: 578-588.

Eden GF, Stein JF, Wood MH, Wood FB. (1994). *Differences in eye movements and reading problems in dyslexics and normal children.* Vision Research, 34: 1345-1358.

Egeth H. (1977). *Attention and preattention.* In: The psychology of Learning and Motivation, Bower Ed., Academic Press, New York.

Eriksen CW, St. James JD. (1986). *Visual attention within and around the field of focal attention: A zoom lens model.* Perception & Psychophysics, 40: 225-240.

Eriksen CW, Yeh Y. (1985). *Allocation of attention in the visual field.* Journal of Experimental Psychology: Human Perception and Performance, 5: 583-595.

Facoetti A, Turatto M. (2000). *Asymmetrical visual field distribution of visual attention in dyslexic children: a neuropsychological study.* Neuroscience Letters, 290: 216-218.

Facoetti A, Paganoni P, Lorusso ML. (2000a). *The spatial distribution of visual attention in developmental dyslexia.* Experimental Brain Research, 132: 531-538.

Facoetti A, Paganoni P, Turatto M, Marzola V, Mascetti GG. (2000b). *Visual-spatial attention in developmental dyslexia.* Cortex, 36: 109-123.

Facoetti A, Molteni M. (2001). *The gradient of visual attention in developmental dyslexia.* Neuropsychologia, 39: 352-357.

Facoetti A, Turatto M, Lorusso ML, Mascetti GG. (2001). *Orienting of visual attention in dyslexia: evidence for asymmetric hemispheric control of attention.* Experimental Brain Research, 138: 46-53.

Gandhi SP, Heeger DJ, Boynton GM. (1999). *Spatial attention affects brain activity in human primary visual cortex.* Proceedings of the National Academy of Sciences of the United States of America, 96: 3314-3319.

Geiger G, Lettvin JY. (1987). *Peripheral vision in persons with dyslexia.* New England Journal of Medicine, 316: 1238-1243.

Geiger G, Lettvin JY. (1989). *Dyslexia and reading as examples of alternative visual strategies.* In: Brain and reading, Von Euler, Lundberg & Lennerstrand Eds., Macmillian Press, New York.

Geiger G, Lettvin JY. (1999). *How dyslexics see and learn to read well.* In: Reading and Dyslexia: Visual and Attentional Processes in Reading and Dyslexia, Everatt Ed., Routledge: London, New York.

Geiger G, Lettvin JY. (2000). *Developmental dyslexia: A different perceptual strategy and how to learn a new strategy for learning.* Saggi, 26: 73-89.

Geiger G, Lettvin JY, Zegarra-Moran O. (1992). *Task-determined strategies of visual process.* Cognitive Brain Research, 1: 39-52.

Geiger G, Lettvin JY, Fahle M. (1994). *Dyslexic children learn a new visual strategy for reading: a controlled experiment.* Vision Research, 34: 1223-1233.

Goolkasian P, King J. (1990*). Letter identification and lateral masking in dyslexic and average readers*. American Journal of Psychology, 103: 519-538.

Hari R, Koivikko H. (1999). *Left side mini-neglect and attentional sluggishness in dyslexic adults* [Abstract]. Society for Neuroscience, 25: 1634.

Hari R, Valta M, Uutela K. (1999). *Prolonged attentional dwell time in dyslexic adults.* Neuroscience Letters, 271: 202-204.

Hari R, Renvall H, Tanskanen T. (2001). *Left minineglect in dyslexic adults.* Brain, 124: 1373-1380.

Henderson JM, Ferreira F. (1990). *Effects of foveal processing difficulty on the perceptual span in reading: implications for attention and eye movement control.* Journal of Experimental Psychology, Learning, Memory & Cognition, 16: 417-429.

Herrmann GP, Pötzl O. (1926). *Über die Agraphie.* Karger, Berlin.

Hill R, Lovegrove WJ. (1993). *One word at a time: A solution to the visual deficits in SRDs?* In: Facets of dyslexia and its remediation, Wright, Groner & Kauffman-Hayoz Eds., Elsevier, Amsterdam.

Husain M, Shapiro K, Martin J, Kennard C. (1997). *Abnormal temporal dynamics of visual attention in spatial neglect patients.* Nature, 385: 154-156.

Iles J, Walsh V, Richardson A. (2000). *Visual search performance in dyslexia.* Dyslexia, 6: 163-177.

Inhoff AW, Pollatsek A, Posner MI, Rayner K. (1989). *Covert attention and eye movements during reading.* Quaterly Journal of Exprimental Psychology, 41: 63-89.

Jaśkowski P, Rusiak P. (2005). *Posterior parietal cortex and developmental dyslexia.* Acta Neurobiologiae Experimentalis, 65: 79-94.

Johnson, J. (1994). *Visual attention and the control of eye movements in early infancy.* In: Attention and performance, Umiltà & Moscovitch Eds., MIT Press, Cambridge.

Jonides J. (1983). *Further toward a model of the mind's eye's 'movement.* Bulletin of the Psychonomic Society, 21: 247-250.

Jonkman I, Licht R, Bakker DJ, Van den Broek-Sandmann TM. (1992). *Shifting of attention in subtyped dyslexic children: An event-related potential study.* Developmental Neuropsychology, 8: 243-259.

Kinsbourne M, Warrington EK. (1962). *A variety of reading disability associated with right hemisphere lesions.* Journal of Neurology, Neurosurgery & Psychiatry, 25: 339-344.

Kinsey K, Rose M, Hansen P, Richardson A, Stein J. (2004). *Magnocellular-mediated visual-spatial attention and reading ability.* NeuroReport, 15: 1-5.

Klein R, Berry G, Briand K, D'Entremont B, Farmer M. (1990). *Letter identification declines with increasing retinal eccentricity at the same rate for normal and dyslexic readers.* Perception & Psychophysics, 47: 601-606.

Laberge D. (1983). *Spatial extent of attention to letters and words.* Journal of Experimental Psychology: Human Perception and Performance, 9: 371-379.

Laberge D. (2002). *Attentional control: Brief and prolong.* Psychological Research, 66: 230-233.

Laberge D, Brown V. (1989). *Theory of attentional operations in shape identification.* Psychological Review, 96: 101-124.

Laberge D. (1995). *Computational and anatomical models of selective attention in object identification.* In: The cognitive neurosciences, Gazzaniga Ed., MIT Press, Cambridge.

Lawler KA, Kowey A. (1987). *On the role of posterior parietal and prefrontal cortex in visuo-spatial perception and attention.* Experimental Brain Research, 65: 695-698.

Lennie P. (1993). *Roles of M and P pathways.* In, Contrast sensitivity. Proceeding on the retina research foundation symposia. Vol 5, Shapley & Man-Kit-Lam Eds., MIT Press, Cambridge.

Livingstone M, Hubel D. (1988). *Segregation of form, color movement, and dept: anatomy, physiology, and perception.* Science, 240: 740-749.

Lorusso ML, Facoetti A, Pesenti S, Cattaneo C, Molini m, Geiger G. (2004). *Wider recognition in peripheral vision common to different subtypes of dyslexia.* Vision Research, 44: 2413-2424.

Lorusso ML, Facoetti A, Toraldo A, Molteni M. (2005). *Tachistoscopic treatment of dyslexia changes the distribution of visual-spatial attention.* Brain and Cognition, 57: 135-142.

Lovegrove WJ, Bowling A, Badcock D, Blackwood M. (1980). *Specific reading difficulty: Differences in contrast sensitivity as a function of spatial frequency.* Science, 210: 439-440.

Lyon GR. (1996). *Learning disabilities*. Future Child, 6: 54-76.

Martinez A, Anllo-Vento L, Sereno MI, Frank LR, Buxton RB, Dubowitz DJ, Wong EC, Hinrichs H, Heinze HJ, Hillyard SA. (1999). *Involvement of striate and extrastriate visual cortical areas in spatial attention*. Nature Neuroscience, 2: 364-369.

Mason A, Cornelissen P, Fowler MS, Stein JF. (1993). *Contrast sensitivity, ocular dominance and reading disability*. Clinical Visual Science, 8: 345-353.

McConkie GW, Rayner K. (1975). *The span of the effective stimulus during a fixation in reading,* Perception & Psychophysics, 17: 578–586.

McLeod P, Driver J, Crisp J. (1988). *Visual search for a conjunction of movement and form is parallel*. Nature, 332: 154-155.

Morris RK, Rayner K. (1991). *Vision and Visual Dyslexia*, Stein Ed., MacMillian Press, London.

Nachev P, Husain M. (2006). *Disorders of visual attention and the posterior parietal cortex.* Cortex, 42: 375-425.

Pastor PN, Reuben CA. (2002). *Attention deficit disorder and learning disability: United States 1997-98*. Vital and Health Statistics, 10: 206, 1-12.

Peli E, Garcia-Pèrez MA. (1997). *Contrast sensitivity in dyslexia: deficit or artefact?* Optometry & Vision Science, 74: 986-988.

Perry AR, Dember WN, Warm JS, Sacks JG. (1989). *Letter identification in normal and dyslexic readers: A verification.* Bulletin of the Psychonomic Society, 27: 445-448.

Pierrot-Deseilligny C, Rivaud S, Gaymard B, Agyd Y. (1991a). *Cortical control of reflexive visually guided saccades in man,* Brain, 114: 1473-1485.

Pierrot-Deseilligny C, Rivaud S, Gaymard B, Agyd Y. (1991b). *Cortical control of memory-guided saccades*. Annals of Neurology, 37: 557-567.

Pierrot-Deseilligny C, Gaymard B, Müri R, Rivaud S. (1997). *Cerebral ocular motor signs.* Journal of Neurology, 244: 65-70.

Polikoff BR, Evans BJ, Legg CR. (1995). *Is there a visual deficit in dyslexia resulting from a lesion of the right posterior parietal lobe?* Ophthalmic and Physiological Optics, 15: 513-517.

Posner MI. (1980). *Orienting of attention*. Quarterly Journal of Experimental Psychology, 32: 3-25.

Posner MI, Snyder CRR, Davidson BJ. (1980). *Attention and the detection of signals.* Journal of Experimental Psychology: General, 109: 160-174.

Posner MI, Rafal RD. (1987). *Cognitive theories of attention and the rehabilitation of attentional defects.* In: Neuropsychological rehabilitation, Meier & Benton Eds., Guilford Press, New York.

Posner MI, Walker JA, Friedrich FJ, Rafal RD. (1984). *Effects of parietal injury on covert orienting of attention.* The Journal of Neuroscience, 4: 1863-1874.

Posner MI, Walker JA, Friedrich FJ, Rafal RD. (1987). *How do the parietal lobes direct covert attention?* Neuropsychologia, 25: 135-145.

Raymond JE (2000). *Attentional modulation of visual motion perception.* Trends in Cognitive Sciences, 2: 42-50.

Rayner K, Bertera JH. (1979). *Reading without a fovea.* Science, 206: 468-470.

Rayner K, Murphy LA, Henderson JM, Pollastek A. (1989). *Selective attentional dyslexia.* Cognitive Neuropshychology, 6: 357-378.

Rayner K, Pollatsek A, Bilsky AB. (1995). *Can a temporal processing deficit account for dyslexia?* Psychonomic Bulletin Review, 2: 501-507.

Richards GP, Samuels SJ, Turnure JE, Ysseldyke JE. (1990). *Sustained and selective attention in children with learning disabilities.* Journal of Learning Disabilities, 23: 129-136.

Ro T, Cohen A, Ivry RB, Rafal RD. (1988). *Response channel activation and the temporoparietal junction.* Brain Cognition, 37: 461-476.

Roach NW, Hogben JH. (2004). *Attentional modulation of visual processing in adult dyslexia: a spatial-cuing defect.* Psychological Science, 15: 650-654.

Schneider W, Shiffrin RM. (1977). *Controlled and automatic human information processing; I: detection, search and attention.* Psychological Review, 84: 1-66.

Shallice T, Warrington EK. (1977). *The possible role of selective attention in acquired dyslexia.* Neuropsychologia, 15: 31-41.

Sharma V, Halperin JH, Newcorn JN, Wolf NE. (1991). *The dimension of focussed attention: relationship to behaviour and cognitive functioning in children.* Perceptual and Motor Skills, 72: 787-793.

Shaywitz SA. (1998). *Dyslexia.* New England Journal of Medicine, 338: 307-312.

Shepherd M, Findlay JM, Hockey RJ. (1986). *The relationship between eye movements and spatial attention.* The Quarterly Journal of Experimental Psychology, 38: 475-491.

Sireteanu R, Rettenbach R. (1995). *Perceptual learning in visual search: Fast, enduring but not specific.* Vision Research, 35: 2037-2043.

Smania N, Martini MC, Gambina G, Tomelleri G, Palmara A, Natale E, Marzi CA. (1998). *The spatial distribution of visual attention in hemineglect and extinction patients.* Brain, 121: 1759-1770.

Somers DC, Dale AM, Seiffert AE, Tootell RB. (1999). *Functional MRI reveals spatially specific attentional modulation in human primary visual cortex.* Proceedings of the National Academy of Sciences of the United States of America, 96: 1663-1668.

Stein JF. (1991). *Visuospatial sense, hemispheric asymmetry and dyslexia. Vision and Visual dysfunction.* In: Vision and Visual Dyslexia, vol 13, Stein Ed., CRC Press, Boca Raton, FL.

Stein JF. (1993). *Visuospatial perception in disabled readers.* In: Visual Processes in Reading and Reading Disabilities Willows, Kruk & Corcos Eds., Lawrence Erlbaum Associates, Inc., Hillsdale, NJ.

Stein JF, Walsh V. (1997). *To see but not to read: the magnocellular theory of dyslexia.* Trends in Neurosciences, 20: 147-152.

Steinman BA, Steinman SB, Lehmkuhle S. (1997). *Transient visual attention is dominated by the magnocellular stream.* Vision Research, 37: 17-23.

Steinman SB, Steinman BA, Garzia RP. (1998). *Vision and attention. II. Is visual attention a mechanism through which a deficient magnocellular pathway might cause reading disability?* Optometry & Vision Science, 75: 674-781.

Treisman A, Gelade G. (1980). *A feature integration theory of attention.* Cognitive Psychology, 12: 97-136.

Underwood NR, Zola D. (1986). *The span of letter recognition of good and poor readers.* Reading Research Quaterly, 21: 6-19.

Turatto M, Benso F, Facoetti A, Galfano G, Mascetti GG, Umiltà C. (2000). *Automatic and voluntary focusing of attention.* Perception & Psychophysics, 62: 935-952.

Valdois S, Gérard C, Vanault P, Dugas M. (1995). *Peripheral developmental dyslexia: a visual attentional account?* Cognitive Neuropsychology, 12: 31-67.

Vidyasagar TR. (1998). *Gating of neuronal responses in macaque primary visual cortex by an attentional spotlight.* NeuroReport, 9: 1947-1952.

Vidyasagar TR. (1999). *A neural model of attentional spotlight: parietal guiding the temporal.* Brain Research Review, 30: 66-76.

Vidyasagar TR. (2001). *From attentional gating in macaque primary visual cortex to dyslexia in humans.* Progress in Brain Research, 134: 297-312.

Vidyasagar TR. (2004). *Neural underpinnings of dyslexia as a disorder of visuo-spatial attention.* Clinical and Experimental Optometry, 87: 4-10.

Vidyasagar TR, Pammer K. (1999). *Impaired visual search in dyslexia relates to the role of the magnocellular pathway in attention.* NeuroReport, 10:1283-1287.

Visser T, Boden C, Giaschi D. (2004). *Children with dyslexia: evidence for visual attention deficits in perception of rapid sequences of objects.* Vision Research, 44: 2521-2535.

Wijers AA, Been PH, Romkes KS. (2005). *Dyslexics show a deviant lateralization of attentional control: a brain potential study.* Neuroscience Letters, 374: 87-91.

Willcutt EG, Pennington BF. (2000). *Psychiatric comorbidity in children and adolescents with reading disability.* Journal of Child Psychology and Psychiatry, 41: 1039-1048.

Williams MC, Bologna NB. (1985). *Perceptual gouping in good and poor readers.* Perception & Psychophysics, 38: 367-374.

Wood F, Felton R, Flowers L, Naylor C. (1991). *Neurobehavioural definition of dyslexia.* In: The reading brain, Dwayne & Grey Eds., Parkton Press. New York.

Wurtz RH, Goldberg ME, Robinson DL. (1982). *Brain mechanisms of attention.* Scientific American, 246: 124-135.

Zegarra-Moran O, Geiger G. (1993). *Visual recognition in the peripheral field: letters versus symbols and adults versus children.* Perception, 22: 77-90.

Chapter XII

The Theory of the Deficit of the Temporal Rate Processing

Although developmental dyslexia is a condition intimately related to the phonological environment [Liberman & Shankweiler, 1985; Vellutino, 1987; Bishop & Snowling, 2004; Vellutino et al.,2004], due to the growing interest for the visual perspective aspect (supported by a great amount of evidence collected over more than a century), its aetiopathogenesis has to be dialectically re-theorized.

In the light of the experimental findings, the new speculative trend makes the phonological and the visuoperceptual aspect not as two opposite points of view, but related to a common supramodal anomaly (Stein & Walsh, 1997], stemming from a generalized[185] defect of the magnocellular pathway.

Many researchers have argued that the heterogeneous results found in dyslexics are ascribable to an impairment of the so-called *temporal rate processing (TRP)*, which is to say to an alteration in processing rapid sequences of stimuli (auditory, visual or tactile) [Bakker, 1970; Tallal & Piercy, 1973; Tallal, 1980, Livingstone et al.,1991,Tallal et al.,1993; Farmer & Klein, 1995; Hari & Kiesilä, 1996; Stein & Walsh, 1997; Helenius et al., 1999; Walker et al., 2006]. Therefore, defective temporal rate processing would be the common denominator accounting for the heterogeneity of the defects found in the different sensorial modalities [Tallal, 1984; Tallal & Curtiss, 1990].

In their thorough review, Farmer & Klein [1995] gathered the results supporting a defect of this function in the dyslexic population and considered the TRP as a valuable tool to justify the inhomogeneity of their clinical manifestations.

More in detail, the TRP is the response to two or more rapid sequential stimuli, whatever they be (for example visual, auditory or tactile) and consists of 4 stages [Farmer & Klein, 1995] (Figure 1):

1. *Detection and recognition*: the first step is the detection and the recognition of the stimulus: in case of composed stimuli, their recognition occurs when all their features are correctly detected and integrated.

[185] It is noteworthy that CAT 301, an antibody selective for the magnocells, localizes not only in the visual and auditory cortical areas but even in the somatosensory and motor cerebral regions [McGuire et al., 1989].

2. *Stimulus individuation*: the second stage is the ability to distinguish two stimuli as separated by a very short interval of time (*interstimulus interval*, ISI). Therefore, the stimulus individuation requires the detection of a temporal discontinuity between the two targets. The stimulus individuation can be studied as *fusion task*, as *gap detection task* or as *integration task*.

In the first case, the aim is to measure the minimum ISI required to perceive two sequential stimuli as separated.

The gap detection task measures the minimum ISI required to detect the disruption of a quasi-continuous stimulation. Hence, unlike the fusion task, the gap detection task is not aimed at assessing whether a single or double stimulation is presented, but if a non-stimulation (time interval) occurs within a single configuration.

The integration task measures the ISI threshold needed to recognize two tachistoscopic stimuli (for example the vertical and horizontal bar of a cross) as such (two bars) and not merged into a single configuration (a cross).

3. *Temporal order judgment*: the third stage is the evaluation of the temporal order between two different targets: in other words, given two sequential presentations the aim is to judge which stimulus appears first.
4. *Sequence discrimination*: the fourth and last stage is the discrimination of the ordering of a temporal sequence of stimuli.

In such a hierarchical order, the superior function to be effective requires the normality of the inferior one, so that a temporal sequence of stimuli (fourth level) cannot be adequately recognized if the temporal order judgment between two stimuli (third level) is impaired. In turn, this judgment requires that the involved stimuli are perceived as separated (second level) after their detection or recognition (first level) has occurred.

No difference was found between dyslexic and normal readers in the first stage of the TRP for visual (letters: Mason, 1980; Blackwell et al., 1983; Klein et al., 1990)[186] or auditory (composed tones: Tallal, 1980) configurations. Instead, temporal separation threshold for the identification of two stimuli is higher when measured as gap detection task[187] and as integration task[188].

Also the temporal order judgment is defective in dyslexics, regardless of the presentation mode [Tallal et al., 1981; Brannan & Williams, 1988][189], so that the discrimination of visual [Zurif & Carson, 1970; Farmer & Bryson, 1989 as reported by Farmer & Klein, 1995] and auditory sequences turns out to be inaccurate[190] [Zurif & Carson, 1970; Bryden, 1972; McGivern et al., 1991; McAnally & Stein, 1996; Stein & McAnally, 1996]. In the auditory domain, a correlation is found between the lexical ability and both the temporal order

186 But see Gross-Glenn & Rothenberg [1984] for a counter evidence.
187 To be perceived as separate, in normal subjects the ISI for visual stimuli must be as long as 20 msec [Hirsh & Sherrick, 1961]. This interval in dyslexics is higher both in the visual domain [Stanley & Hall, 1973; Lovegrove et al., 1980; Badcock & Lovegrove, 1981; Di Lollo et al., 1983; Slaghuis & Lovegrove, 1985] and in the auditory domain [Haggerty & Stamm, 1978; McCroskey & Kidder, 1980].
188 As found in adult dyslexics aged 18-37 years [Winters et al., 1989].
189 Not only in children but even in adults [Kinsbourne et al., 1991].
190 The same impairment has been observed in dysphasics [Tallal & Piercy, 1973, 1974, 1975], but see Bryden [1972] for a counter evidence.

judgment [Tallal et al., 1981] and the sequence discrimination [Zurif & Carson, 1970; Bryden, 1972].

In summary, dyslexics are found to suffer from a multimodal alteration of the temporal rate processing and would be unable to analyze accurately both visual and auditory sequential stimuli [Witton et al. 1998, Helenius et al. 1999, De Martino et al., 2001; Van Ingelghem et al., 2001]. In confirmation of such a close auditory-visual link, the discrimination threshold for auditory transients correlates with motion perception, and both auditory transients and motion perception correlate with the reading performance of non-words [Witton et al., 1998][191].

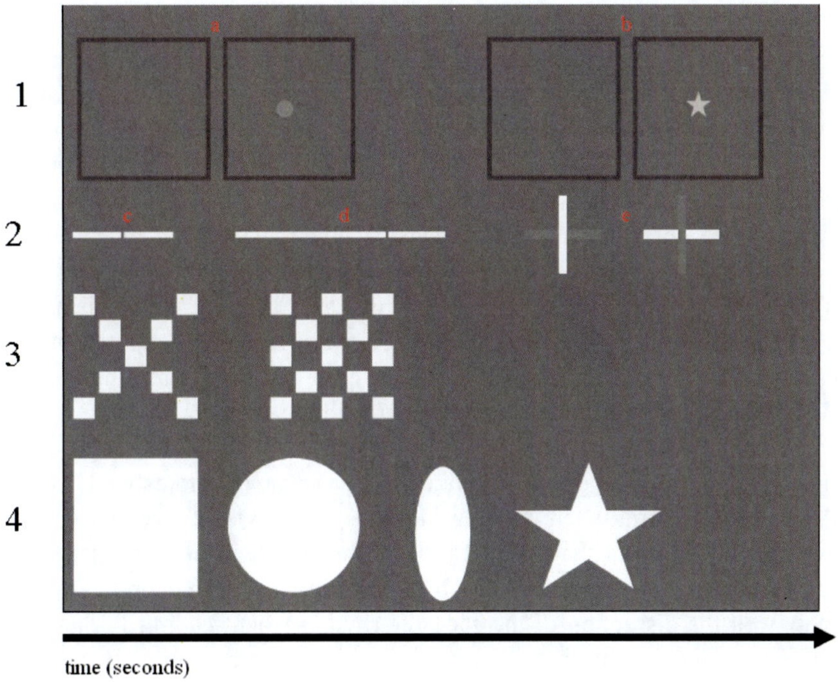

Figure 1. Representation of the hierarchical organization of the TRP. The first level is the detection of a simple stimulus (a) or its recognition (b). The second is the identification of the stimulus as *fusion task* (c) for which two sequential stimuli are perceived as separate, as *gap detection task* (d) for which the subject has to be aware of a very brief interruption during the presentation of the stimulus, or as *integration task* (e). The third level is the *temporal order judgment* between two subsequent configurations: in this case the pattern "X" would appear first, then the checkerboard. Finally, the fourth level is the *sequence discrimination*, i.e. the discrimination of the order of a sequence of stimuli.

The magnocellular system is believed to be the responsible for the defective sequential *timing* [Williams et al., 1989; Eden et al., 1995]. Indeed, the M-system is in charge of transient processing not only in the visual domain, but even in the auditory and in the motor ones [Tallal et al., 1993; Trussell, 1998]. The neurons sensitive to changes in amplitude and frequency of the sounds that form the phonemes, in fact, are arranged along the magnocellular pathway that projects onto the auditory cortex [Trussell, 1998] and a reduction in their

[191] In dyslexic and in normal readers.

number and in their size has been documented in the medial geniculate body [Galaburda et al., 1994][192]

Probably, this supramodal characteristic of the *transient* system is responsible for the association of phonological and visual signs [Tallal, 1976; Breitmeyer, 1993], like the reduced ability to process the modulated sounds sequences in the spoken language [McAnally & Stein, 1996, Stein & McAnally, 1996] and the difficulty to recognize the spatial sequence of printed letters in the written texts, respectively.

In this perspective, it remains unclear whether the defective temporal rate processing in a given domain affects the temporal rate processing in another domain: actually, some evidence supports this position [Kinsbourne et al., 1991] whereas other researchers are skeptical [Reed, 1989].

However in dyslexics the TRP alteration, far from being limited to the sensorial domain (including tactile sensibility: Grant et al., 1999; Stoodley et al., 2000)[193], is found to extend even to the motor control [Fawcett & Nicolson, 1992, 1994; Nicolson & Fawcett 1993, 1994, 1995; Rae et al., 1998; Nicolson et al., 1999]: as a matter of fact, sequential motor tasks that require coordination (such as tapping the fingers of the right hand and of the left hand asynchronously) are defective in many dyslexic children [Wolff et al., 1990], as well as mirror movements [Gladstone et al., 1989; Moore et al., 1995]. Therefore, patients show problems when performing simultaneous tasks involving different automatisms and different domains: on the one hand the visual recognition of two strings of letters presented at the same time is problematic [Sangosse-Lassus et al., 2008], on the other hand the motor balance is reduced if patient is asked to count down when walking on a beam [Nicolson & Fawcett, 1990].

Such an impaired motor balance may affect the saccadic pattern as well. Thereby, even if abnormal saccadic pattern when reading depends on a visuoperceptive imbalance, this perspective does not rule out that an alteration of the temporal rate processing on the motor (or better *oculomotor*) side may act as an aggravating factor. Theoretically, indeed, it is striking how well the disruption of the saccadic rhythm when reading fits the hypothesis of the deficit of the temporal rate processing, so that the saccadic anomalies may be regarded also as the manifestation of an impaired oculomotor TRP on the oculomotor plan [Pavlidis 1981a, b, 1985].

Still, the motor problems stemming from a defective TRP do not involve the whole dyslexic population, but are mainly referred to patients affected by the so-called ADHD (*attention-deficit hyperactivity disorder*) [Denckla et al., 1985; Yap & van der Leij, 1994]. This finding suggests that in order to avoid methodological errors when studying the relationship between temporal rate processing and lexical disability, it is crucial to adopt classification criteria.

However, even after the patients have been divided into different subgroups, assessing the damage of the TRP is still difficult, since its features may change with the development of the child: in particular the *stimulus individuation* and *sequence discrimination* tasks have a developmental trend both in the auditory and in the visual domain[194].

[192] Especially the left one. The medial geniculate body is an intermediate station along the auditory pathway.

[193] The skin of dyslexics is less sensitive to mechanical vibration according to Stoodley, to tactile sensitivity according to Grant.

[194] See Farmer & Klein [1995] for further considerations on this subject and references.

In addition, whether the development rate of the TRP is the same or changes according to its stage (*stimulus individuation, temporal order judgment* and *sequence discrimination*), what is the anatomical region underlying the alteration of the TRP and what is the relationship between TRP and the visuoperceptive anomalies described thus far, remain all open questions.

Regarding the first issue, the cerebral structures potentially in charge of the temporal rate processing are the thalamus and the cerebellum. The thalamus may play a role for its modulatory effect in both the auditory and visual domain [Farmer & Klein, 1995]. Modulation takes place in the reticular thalamic nucleus where axons carrying the visual and auditory input (as well as the somatosensory information) are interconnected and their discharge frequency is adjusted via a reciprocal GABA-mediated inhibitory interaction [Berne & Levy, 1988]. The final goal is to fine-tune the discrimination of the stimuli so that a sequence of configurations can be recognized and categorized quickly and with a high degree of accuracy: in other words, the final goal is to promote the temporal rate processing.

Another cerebral structure that deserves consideration is the cerebellum [Nicolson et al., 1995, 1999, 2001][195]. As mentioned, many dyslexics suffer from postural impairment and posture is a cerebellar function. In a French experiment, 60 patients[196] showed a postural deficiency syndrome [Quercia et al., 2005]. It was observed that patients were less stable than normal readers when they were asked to stand on one leg and this ability was correlated with their lexical performance (r =0.52) [Stoodley et al., 2005]. Dyslexics, therefore, would be impaired in tasks requiring the cerebellar activation [Fawcett et al., 1996][197]. Even in this case such alterations would depend on the magnocellular *pool*: since a substantial number of magnocellular inputs coming from different sensory and motor centers project to the cerebellum, this anatomical structure has been considered as the most important station of the magnocellular quota in charge of the temporal sequential processing [Laycock & Crewther, 2008]. Its aforementioned role in modulating the saccadic movements and in maintaining stable fixation[198] should be considered also in this respect [Miall et al., 1993]. Even if some dyslexics manage to read by means of compensatory strategies, patients are unable to reach the lexical fluency typical of the normal readers [Shaywitzet al., 1999; Wolf et al., 2000]: in fact, for this cerebellar and/or thalamic dysfunction, they fail to achieve the oculomotor automatism which characterizes the normal TRP.

Indeed, the reduced performance for tasks involving visual attention in subjects with a cerebellar damage got a considerable interest [Townsend et al., 1999], since in these patients the visuo-attentional defect would end up disrupting the delicate dynamics of the TRP. Now, as previously reported[199], also in dyslexics an abnormal cerebellar function may lead to visuo-attentional alterations [Hari et al., 1999, 2001]. The posterior parietal cortex is another region involved in the visuo-attentional process. This area is particularly interesting as it is a crossroads for the integration of the auditory and visuoperceptive[200] afferent inputs [Farah et

[195] According to Nicolson et al. [2001] a cerebellar deficit alone would be able to explain the signs and symptoms of developmental dyslexia.

[196] Mean age: 11 years.

[197] The cerebellar impairment refers in particular to the right side, as shown by PET [Nicolson et al., 1999] and magnetic resonance spectroscopy [Rae et at, 1998; Eckert et al., 2003] investigations.

[198] See chapter 10.

[199] Chapter 11.

[200] The posterior parietal cortex is responsible for the control of gaze aimed at locating objects in the visual space [Galletti et al., 1991] and for the perceptual constancy of the visual space surrounding a target when the

al., 1989; Vidyasagar, 1999; Downar et al., 2000]. Therefore, as for the temporal rate processing, the cerebellar and parietal deficits may be two faces of the same coin: the visual attention [Jaśkowsi & Rusiak, 2005].

Defective temporal rate processing is argued to be the consequence of a more generalized attentional deficit [Segalowitz et al., 1992], not restricted to the visuoperceptive sphere but involving also the auditory [Asbjørnsen & Bryden, 1998; Vidyasagar, 1999; Hari & Renvall, 2001; Renvall & Hari, 2002; Facoetti et al., 2003; Facoetti et al.,2005] and tactile domain [Grant et al.,1999].

Still, the normal performance for many tasks requiring normal attentional levels in dyslexics does not support a cause/effect relationship [Farmer & Klein, 1995] and if the TRP alteration were simply the result of an attentional deficit, the performance would be defective irrespective of the type of task. On the contrary, in some experimental conditions TRP of patients is normal as well as in normal readers affected by attentional deficit [Ludlow et al., 1983]. So, in dyslexic children it is unlikely that the TRP defect depends on a mere attentive disturbance.

To understand better the relationship between TRP and other sensorial (including visuoperceptive) anomalies, researchers have tried to assess whether impaired auditory, phonological, visual and the cerebellar motor automatisms could affect the same patients.

In an English survey, the phonological, auditory, visual and cerebellar functions have been evaluated in a group of 17 adult dyslexics with a set of specific tests [Ramus et al., 2003]. To assess the visuoperceptive function, M- and P-mediated contrast sensitivity by means of sinusoidal gratings[201] as well as motion perception were estimated. The phonological and auditory function turned out to be affected in 44-62% of cases, while the cerebellar performance was found to be impaired in 25% of the recruited sample. Only 12.5% of the patients showed a magnocellular visuoperceptive defect. Therefore, in most dyslexics the main problem is auditory and phonological, whereas the visuoperceptive impairment involves just one tenths of the disabled readers. Apart from these different functional involvements, the results demonstrate the importance of classifying patients rather than treating developmental dyslexia as a single entity.

In conclusion, the basic assumptions, the speculative structure and the experimental evidence make the temporal rate processing deficit an important element in the aetiopathogenetical *panorama* of developmental dyslexia; it shows a dialectical agility that makes it worthy of consideration.

In line with Habib [Habib, 2000], it is plausible that dyslexics have difficulties in integrating rapidly changing stimuli, both in the phonological domain and in the visuospatial arrangement of letters and words.

Above all, the theory of the deficit of the temporal rate processing has pinpointed the multimodal involvement typical of developmental dyslexia, thereby moving the academic world toward an interdisciplinary approach.

---

position of the observer moves. If the observer moves to or from the target, the relationship between target and surrounding area changes, so that after the movement the same target may be mistaken for a new target. The perceptual constancy ensures a tolerance, so that after the observer's displacement the target is correctly recognized as the same [Motter & Mountcastle, 1981].

201 M- and P-related contrast sensitivity was estimated by displaying sinusoidal gratings. For the M-system, gratings of 0.5 cycles/deg with temporal frequency of 15 Hz were presented in scotopic conditions; to asses the P-function, stationary gratings of spatial frequency of 8 cycles/degree were displayed in photopic conditions.

References

Asbjornsen AE, Bryden MP. (1998). *Auditory attention shifts in reading disabled students: Quantification of attentional effectiveness by the attentional shift index.* Neuropsychologia, 36: 143-148.

Badcock DR, Lovergrove WJ. (1981). *The effect of contrast, stimulus duration and spatial frequency on visible persistence in normal and specifically disabled readers.* Journal of Experimental Psychology: Human Perception and Performance, 7: 495-505.

Bakker DJ. (1970). *Temporal order perception and reading retardation.* In: specific reading disability, advances in theory and method, Bakker & Satz Eds., Rotterdam University Press, Rotterdam.

Berne RM, Levy MN. (1988). *Physiology*, Berne & Levi Eds., St Louis, MO: Mosby Inc, Academic Press, Orlando.

Bishop DV & Snowling MJ. (2004). *Developmental dyslexia and specific language impairment: same or different?* Psychological Bulletin, 130: 858-866.

Blackwell SL, McIntyre CW, Murray ME. (1983). *Information processed from brief visual displays by learning-disabled boys.* Child Development, 54: 927-940.

Brannan J, Williams M. (1988). *Developmental versus sensory deficit effects on perceptual processing in the reading disabled.* Perception & Psychophysics, 44: 437-444.

Breitmeyer, BG. (1993). *The roles of sustained and transient channels in reading and reading disabilities.* In: Facets of dyslexia and its Remediation, Wright & Groner Eds., Elsevier, Amsterdam.

Bryden MP. (1972). *Auditory-visual and sequential-spatial matching in relation to reading ability.* Child Development, 43: 824-832.

Castles A, Coltheart M. (1993). *Varieties of developmental dyslexia.* Cognition, 47: 149-180.

De Martino S, Espesser R, Rey V, Habib M. (2001). *The "temporal processing deficit" hypothesis in dyslexia: New experimental evidence.* Brain Cognition, 46: 104-108.

Denckla MB, Rudel RG, Chapman C, Krieger J. (1985). *Motor proficiency in dyslexic children with and without attentional disorders.* Archives of Neurology, 42: 228-231.

Di Lollo V, Arnett JL, Kruk RV. (1982). *Age-related changes in rate of visual information processing. Journal of Experimental Psychology: Human Perception & Performance,* 8: 225-237.

Di Lollo V, Hanson D, McIntyre JS. (1983). *Initial stages of visual information processing in dyslexia.* Journal of Experimental Psychology, 9: 923-935.

Downar J, Crawley AP, Mikulis DJ, Davis KD. (2000). *A multimodal cortical network for the detection of changes in the sensory environment.* Nature Neuroscience, 3: 277-283.

Eckert MA, Leonard CM, Richards TL, Aylward EH, Thomson J, Berninger VW. (2003). *Anatomical correlates of dyslexia: frontal and cerebellar findings.* Brain, 126: 482-494.

Eden GF, Stein JF, Wood HM, Wood FB. (1995). *Temporal and spatial processing in reading disabled and normal children.* Cortex, 31: 451-468.

Facoetti A, Lorusso ML, Paganoni P, Cattaneo C, Galli R, Umiltà C, Mascetti GG. (2003). *Auditory and visual automatic attention deficits in developmental dyslexia.* Cognitive Brain Research 2003, 16: 185-191.

Facoetti A, Lorusso ML, Cattaneo C, Galli R, Molteni M. (2005). *Visual and auditory attentional capture are both sluggish in children with developmental dyslexia.* Acta Neurobiologiae Experimentalis, 65: 61-72.

Farah MJ, Wong AB, Wong MA, Monheit MA, Morrow LA. (1989). *Parietal lobe mechanisms of spatial attention: Modality-specific or supramodal?* Neuropsychologia, 27: 461-470.

Farmer ME, Bryson SE. (1989). *Reproduction of simultaneously or sequentially presented letter sets by dyslexic and normal readers.* Manoscritto non pubblicato, Dalhousie University, Halifax, Canada.

Farmer ME, Klein RM. (1995). *The evidence for a temporal processing deficit linked to dyslexia.* Psychonomic Bulletin Review, 2: 460-493.

Fawcett AJ, Nicolson RI. (1992). *Automatisation deficits in balance for dyslexic children.* Perceptual & Motor Skills, 75: 507-529.

Fawcett AJ, Nicolson RI. (1994). *Naming speed in children with dyslexia.* Journal of Learning Disabilities, 27: 641-646.

Fawcett AJ, Nicolson RI, Dean P. (1996). *Impaired performance of children with dyslexia on a range of cerebellar tasks.* Annals of Dyslexia, 46: 259-283.

Galaburda AM, Menard MT, Rosen GD. (1994). *Evidence for aberrant auditory anatomy in developmental dyslexia.* Proceedings of the National Academy of Sciences of the United States of America, 91: 8010-8013.

Galletti C, Battaglini P, Fattori P. (1991). *Functional properties of neurons in the anterior bank of the parieto-occipital sulcus of the macaque monkey.* European Journal of Neuroscience, 3: 452-461.

Gladstone M, Best CT, Davidson RJ. (1989). *Anomalous bimanual coordination among dyslexic boys.* Developmental Psychology, 25: 236-246.

Grant AC, Zangaladze A, Thiagarajah MC, Sathian K. (1999). *Tactile perception in developmental dyslexia: a psychophysical study using gratings,* Neuropsychologia, 37: 1201-1211.

Gross-Glenn K, Rothenberg S. (1984). *Evidence for deficit in interhemispheric transfer of information in dyslexic boys.* The International Journal of Neuroscience, 24: 23-35.

Habib M. (2000). *The neurological basis of developmental dyslexia. An overview and working hypothesis.* Brain, 123: 2373-2399.

Haggerty R, Stamm JS. (1978). *Dichotic auditory fusion levels in children with learning disabilities.* Neuropsychologia, 16: 349-360.

Hari R, Kiesilä P. (1996). *Deficit of temporal auditory processing in dyslexic adults.* Neuroscience Letters, 205: 138-140.

Hari R, Renvall H. (2001). *Impaired processing of rapid stimulus sequences in dyslexia.* Trends in Cognitive Sciences, 5: 525-532.

Hari R, Valta M, Uutela K. (1999). *Prolonged attentional dwell time in dyslexic adults.* Neuroscience Letters, 271: 202-204.

Hari R, Renvall H, Tanskanen T. (2001). *Left minineglect in dyslexic adults.* Brain, 124: 1373-1380.

Helenius P, Uutela K, Hari R. (1999). Auditory stream segregation in dyslexic adults. Brain, 122: 907-913.

Hirsh IJ, Sherrick CE Jr. (1961). *Perceived order in different sense modalities.* Journal of Experimental Psychology, 62: 423-432.

Jaśkowski P, Rusiak P. (2005). *Posterior parietal cortex and developmental dyslexia.* Acta Neurobiologiae Experimentalis, 65: 79-94.

Kinsbourne M, Rufo DT, Gamzu E, Palmer RL, Berliner AK. (1991). *Neuropsychological deficits in adults with dyslexia.* Developmental Medicine & Child Neurology, 33: 763-775.

Klein R, Berry G, Briand K, D'Entremont B, Farmer M. (1990). *Letter identification declines with increasing retinal eccentricity at the same rate for normal and dyslexic readers.* Perception & Psychophysics, 47: 601-606.

Lassus-Sangosse D, N'guyen-Morel M, Valdois S. (2008). *Sequential or simultaneous visual processing deficit in developmental dyslexia?* Vision Research, 48: 979-988.

Laycock R, Crewther SG. (2008). *Towards an understanding of the role of the 'magnocellular advantage' in fluent reading.* Neuroscience and Biobehavioral Reviews, 32: 1494-1506.

Liberman IY, Shankweiler D. (1985). *Phonology and the problems of learning to read and write.* Remedial & Special Education, 6: 8-17.

Livingstone MS, Rosen GD, Drislane FW, Galaburda AM. (1991). *Physiological and anatomical evidence for a magnocellular defect in developmental dyslexia.* Proceedings of the National Academy of Sciences of the United States of America, 88: 7943-7947.

Lovergrove WJ, Heddle M, Slaghuis W. (1980). *Reading disability: spatial frequency specific deficits in visual information store.* Neuropsychologia, 18: 111-115.

Ludlow C, Cudahy EA, Bassich C, Brown GL. (1983). *Auditory processing skills of hyperactive, language-impaired and reading-disabled boys.* In: Central auditory processing disorders, Lasky & Katz Eds., University Park Press, Baltimore.

Mason A. (1980). *Reading ability and the encoding of item and location information.* Journal of Experimental Psychology: Human Perception and Performance, 6: 89-98.

Mc Anally KI, Stein JF. (1996). *Auditory temporal coding in dyslexia.* Proceedings of the National Academy of Sciences of the United States, 263: 961- 965.

McCroskey RL, Kidder HC. (1980). *Auditory fusion among learning disabled, reading disabled, and normal children.* Journal of Learning Disabilities, 13: 18-25.

McGivern RF, Berka C, Languis ML, Chapman S. (1991). *Detection of deficts in temporal pattern discrimination using the Seashore Rhythm test in young children with reading impairments.* Journal of Learning Disabilities, 24: 58-62.

McGuire PK, Hockfield S, Goldman-Rakic PS. (1989). *Distribution of Cat-301 immunoreactivity in the frontal and parietal lobes of the macaque monkey.* The Journal of Comparative Neurology, 288: 280-296.

Miall RC, Wolpert D, Stein JF. (1993). *Is the cerebellum a Smith predictor?* Journal of Motor Behaviour, 25: 203-217.

Moore LH, Brown WS, Markee TE, Theberge DC, Zvi JC. (1995). *Bimanual coordination in dyslexic adults.* Neuropsycologia, 33: 781-793.

Motter BC, Mountcastle VB. (1981). *The functional properties of the light-sensitive neurons of the posterior parietal cortex studied in waking monkeys: foveal sparing and opponent vector organization.* Journal of Neuroscience, 1: 3-26.

Nicolson RI, Fawcett AJ. (1990). *Automaticity: a new framework for dyslexia research?* Cognition, 35: 159-182.

Nicolson RI, Fawcett AJ. (1993). *Children with dyslexia automatize temporal skills more slowly.* Annals of the New York Academy of Sciences, 682: 390-392.

Nicolson RI, Fawcett AJ. (1994). *Reaction times and dyslexia.* The Quarterly Journal of Experimental Psychology [A], 47: 29-48.

Nicolson RI, Fawcett AJ. (1995). *Dyslexia is more than a phonological deficit.* Dyslexia, 1: 19-36.

Nicolson RI, Fawcett AJ, Dean P. (1995). *Time estimation deficits in developmental dyslexia: evidence of cerebellar involvement.* Proceedings: Biological Sciences, 259: 43-47.

Nicolson RI, Fawcett AJ, Berry EL, Jenkins IH, Dean P, Brooks DJ. (1999). *Association of abnormal cerebellar activation with motor learning difficulties in dyslexic adults.* The Lancet, 353: 1662-1667.

Nicolson RI, Fawcett AJ, Dean P. (2001). *Developmental dyslexia: the cerebellar deficit hypothesis.* Trends in Neurosciences, 24: 508-511.

Pavlidis GT. (1981a). *Do eye movements hold the key to dyslexia?* Neuropsychologia, 19: 57-64.

Pavlidis GT. (1981b). *Sequencing, eye movements and the early objective diagnosis of dyslexia.* In: Dyslexia research and its application to education, Pavlidis & Miles Eds., Wiley & Sons Ltd, London.

Pavlidis GT. (1985). *Eye movement differences between dyslexics, normal, and retarded readers while sequentially fixated digits.* American Journal of Optometry and Physiological Optics, 62: 820-832.

Quercia P, Seigneuric A, Chariot S, Vernet P, Pozzo T, Bron A, Creuzot-Garcher C, Robichon F. (2005). *Ocular proprioception and developmental dyslexia. Sixty clinical observations.* Journal Français d Ophtalmologie, 28 : 713-723.

Rae C, Lee MA, Dixon RM, Blamire AM, Thompson CH, Styles P, Talcott J, Richardson A, Stein J. (1998). *Metabolic abnormalities in developmental dyslexia detected by 1H magnetic resonance spectroscopy.* The Lancet, 351: 1849-1852.

Ramus F, Rosen S, Dakin SC, Day BL, Castellote JM, White S, Frith U. (2003). *Theories of developmental dyslexia: insights from a multiple case study of dyslexic adults.* Brain, 126: 841-865.

Reed MA. (1989). *Speech perception and the discrimination of brief auditory cues in reading disabled children.* Journal of Experimental Child Psychology, 48: 270-292.

Renvall A, Hari R. (2002). *Auditory cortical responses to speech-like stimuli in dyslexic adults.* Journal of Cognitive Neuroscience, 14: 757-768.

Segalowitz S, Wagner WJ, Menna R. (1992). *Lateral versus frontal ERP predictors of reading skill.* Brain & Language, 20: 85-103.

Shaywitz SE, Fletcher JM, Holahan JM, Shneiden AE, Marchione KE, Stuebing KK, Francis DJ, Pugh, KR, Shaywitz BA. (1999). *Persistence of dyslexia: the Connecticut Longitudinal Study at adolescence.* Pediatrics, 104: 1351-1359.

Slaghuis WL, Lovergrove WJ. (1985). *Spatial-frequency-dependent visible persistence and specific reading disability.* Brain and Cognition, 4: 219-240.

Stanley G, Hall R. (1973). *A comparison of dyslexics and normals in recalling letter arrays after brief presentation.* British Journal of Education Psychology, 43: 301-304.

Stein JF, McAnally KI. (1996). *Impaired auditory temporal processing in dyslexics.* Irish Journal of Psychology, 16: 220-228.

Stein JF, Walsh V. (1997). *To see but not to read: the magnocellular theory of dyslexia.* Trends in Neurosciences, 20: 147-152.

Stoodley CJ, Talcott JB, Carter EL, Witton C, Stein CF. (2000). *Selective deficits of vibrotactile sensitivity in dyslexic readers*. Neuroscience Letters, 295: 13-16.

Stoodley CJ, Fawcett AJ, Nicolson RI, Stein JF. (2005). *Impaired balancing ability in dyslexic children.* Experimental Brain Research, 167: 370-380.

Tallal P. (1976). *Auditory perceptual factors in language and learning disabilities*. In: The Neuropsychology of Reading Disorders, Knights &.Bakker Eds, University Park Press, Baltimore.

Tallal P. (1980). *Auditory temporal perception, phonics, and reading disability in children.* Brain & Language, 9: 182-198.

Tallal P. (1984). *Temporal or phonetic processing deficit in dyslexia? That is the question.* Applied Psycholinguistics, 5: 167-169.

Tallal P, Curtiss S. (1990). *Neurological basis of developmental language disorders*. In: Brain and Behavior in child psychiatry, Rothenberg Ed., Springer-Verlag, New York.

Tallal P, Piercy M. (1973). *Defects of non-verbal auditory perception in children with developmental aphasia.* Nature, 241: 468-469.

Tallal P, Piercy M. (1974). *Developmental aphasia: rate of auditory processing and selective impairment of consonant perception.* Neuropsychologia, 12: 83-93.

Tallal P, Piercy M. (1975). *Developmental aphasia: the perception of brief vowels and extended stop consonants*. Neuropsychologia, 13: 69-74.

Tallal P, Galaburda AM, Llinas RR, Von Euler C. (1993). *Temporal information processing in the nervous system: Special reference to dyslexia and dysphasia.* Annals of the New York Academy of Sciences, 682: 27-47.

Tallal P, Stark R, Kallman C, Mellits D. (1981). *A re-examination of some nonverbal perceptual abilities of language-impaired and normal children as a function of age and sensory modality*. Journal of Speech & Hearing Research, 24: 351-357.

Townsend JT, Courchesne E, Covington J, Westerfield M, Singer Harris N, Lynden P, Lowry TP, Press GA. (1999). *Spatial attention deficits in patients with acquired or developmental cerebellar abnormality*. The Journal of Neuroscience, 19: 5632-5643.

Trussell LO. (1998). *Cellular mechanisms for preservation of timing in central auditory pathways.* Current Opinion in Neurobiology, 7: 487-492.

Van Ingelghem M, van Wieringen A, Wouters J, Vandenbussche E, Onghena P, Gesquière P. (2001). *Psychophysical evidence for a general temporal processing deficit in children with dyslexia.* Neuroreport, 12: 3603-3607.

Vellutino FR. (1987). *Dyslexia.* Scientific American, 256: 34-41.

Vellutino FR, Fletcher JM, Snowling MJ, Scanlon DM. (2004). *Specific reading disability (dyslexia): what have we learned in the past four decades?* Journal of Child Psychology and Psychiatry, 45: 2-40.

Vidyasagar TR. (1999). *A neural model of attentional spotlight: parietal guiding the temporal.* Brain Research Review, 30: 66-76.

Walker KM, Hall SE, Klein RM, Phillips DP. (2006). *Development of perceptual correlates of reading performance.* Brain Research, 1124: 126-141.

Werner LA, Marean GC, Halpin CF, Spetner NB, Gillenwater JM. (1992). *Infant auditory temporal acuity: Gap detection.* Child Development, 63: 260-272.

Williams MC, Molinet K, LeKluyse K. (1989). *Visual masking as a measure of temporal processing in normal and disabled readers*. Clinical Vision Science, 4: 137-1444.

Winters RL, Patterson R, Shontz W. (1989). *Visual persistence and adult dyslexia*. Journal of Learning Disabilities, 22: 641-645.

Witton C, Talcott JB, Hansen PC, Richardson AJ, Griffiths TD, Rees A, Stein JF, Greef GGR. (1998). *Sensitivity to dynamic auditory and visual stimuli predicts nonword reading ability in both dyslexic and normal readers*. Current Biology, 8: 791-797.

Wolf M, Bowers PG, Biddle K. (2000). *Naming-sped processes, timing and reading: a conceptual view*. Journal of Learning Disabilities, 33: 387-407.

Wolff PH, Michel GF, Ovrut M, Drake C. (1990). *Rate and timing precision of motor coordination in developmental dyslexia*. Developmental Psychology, 26: 349-359.

Yap RL, van der Leij A. (1994). *Testing the automatization deficit hypothesis of dyslexia via a dual-task paradigm*. Journal of Learning Disabilities, 27: 660-665.

Zurif EG, Carson G. (1970). *Dyslexia in relation to cerebral dominance and temporal analysis*. Neuropsychologia, 8: 351-361.

Chapter XIII

Dyslexia and Crowding

The perception of a visual configuration is made of two steps: the first is the recognition of its individual constituents (or *features*), the second is their integration.

Each receptive field along the visual pathway is responsible for the processing of the elementary constituents of a stimulus, for example the three horizontal bars and the vertical bar making the letter “E”. However, in order to recognize the configuration, the identification of the single features (*first-rate analysis* or *feature detection*) is not enough: they must be properly integrated with each other. This integration process is defined *second-rate analysis* or *feature binding integration* [Selfridge, 1959; Campbell & Robson, 1968; Thomas et al.. 1969; Treisman & Gelade, 1980; Sagi & Julesz, 1984; Olzak & Thomas, 1986; Chubb et al., 2001]. Feature binding integration depends strictly on feature detection. This is proven by the fact that the recognition efficiency of a configuration (a word) gets worse as the amount of its features (namely its complexity: the letters) increases [Pelli et al.. 2003].

A defective recognition of a configuration may depend on the first phase of the process, i.e. on the defective detection of its elementary features, or can be confined to the second phase, that is to say to the failure of their integration.

Masking phenomena, namely the interference of another stimulus on the target, may account for both cases: the *ordinary masking* is responsible for the first eventuality, *the lateral masking*

[Townsend et al., 1971], also defined *contour interaction* [Flom et al., 1963], but better known in clinical neurophtalmological field as *crowding effect* (or simply *crowding*), is responsible for the second[202].

In ordinary masking, the masking stimulus (or *distractor*) acts on the same receptive field engaged by the target. This occurs when a grating configuration [Legge & Foley, 1980; Levi et al., 2002a] or a background noise [Pelli & Farell, 1999] overlaps or is located so close to the target as to be processed by the same detector [Legge & Foley, 1980; Foley & Chen, 1990]. In this case, the signal deteriorates till to disappear and the higher is the resemblance

[202] As pointed out by Strasburger [2005], the term *lateral masking* belongs to the vocabulary of experimental psychology. The term crowding has been introduced by the Scandinavian ophthalmologist Ehlers in 1936. If it is defined as the result of the interaction among contiguous stimuli, to a certain extent in the peripheral visual field it is a normal physiological process [Levi, 2008]. If it refers to an excessive integration between close configurations, the term takes on a pathological meaning.

between the properties of the mask (spatial frequency, orientation, position) and the properties of the target, the stronger is the effect [Legge & Foley, 1980; Levi et al., 2002a]. Therefore, the loss of visibility of the signal depends on the failure of its detection and, consequently, effective second-rate analysis is not possible.

On the contrary, in lateral masking distractors do not act on the same receptive field engaged by the target but on the neighboring detectors: the activation of the neighboring detectors ends up perturbing the processing of the target. Unlike the previous case, its elementary constituents remain detectable (since there is no spatial overlapping), and yet the configuration is no longer recognizable because it seems to incorporate also the features of the mask.

As shown in figure 1a, the signal (in this case the word) becomes almost unrecognizable when a mask acts on the same receptive fields. In fact, the detestability of the elementary constituents (the letters) of the target (the word) is reduced so that the subsequent feature binding integration is prevented.

In figure 1b, when the observer looks steadily at the asterisk, although he is aware of the presence of three letters on the right side, these letters are not recognizable. In this case the masking does not act via direct suppression of the signal but produces a confusing and unstable perception: the features of each character seem to influence each other, failing to combine in the respective configurations. When two of the three symbols are covered with a finger, crowding ceases and the features of the remaining configuration can finally be integrated, making the letter identifiable.

Since the lateral masking is not effective on the stimulus detection but on the subsequent integration mechanism, it applies only to compounds stimuli (e.g. characters) and not to their constituents (the features of the character).

In conclusion, the ordinary masking prevents the detection of the target, the lateral masking its resolution.

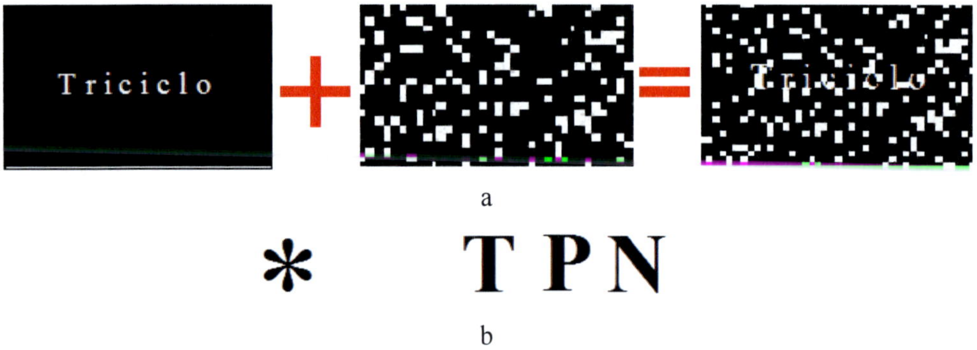

Figure 1. Ordinary masking and lateral masking. In ordinary masking (a) a background noise is superimposed on the stimulus and, acting on the same detectors, hinders its recognition. On the contrary, in lateral masking (b) the effect of the distractors (the flanked letters) takes place on the neighboring detectors rather than on the same receptive field activated by the target (the central letter). Therefore, since the masking stimuli do not overlap the target, the features of the target remain visible: and yet the target is no more recognizable, as its features perceptually *merge* with the features of the adjoining configurations (the distractors). Indeed, when looking steadily at the asterisk it is difficult to name the letters, but covering the two lateral ones with the fingers, the crowding effect disappears and the central character eventually becomes recognizable.

Crowding occurs for a great variety of tasks: not only for visual acuity but also for vernier acuity[203] [Westhermer & Hauske, 1975; Levi et al., 1985a], orientation discrimination [Andriessen & Boume, 1976; Westheimer et al., 1976], stereoacuity [Butler & Westheimer, 1978], motion perception [Bex et al., 2003, Bex & Dakin, 2005], and even faces recognition (*holistic crowding*: Louie et al., 2007). However, given the possible implication of crowding on the lexical function, we will focalize on the alphabetic symbols.

By progressively reducing the distance between three adjoining letters (whose the central one represents the target and the others the distractors) placed outside of the fixation point, below a given interval the target is no more recognizable. This interval is defined *critical spacing* and represents the spatial extent of crowding.

Therefore, when studying crowding, the critical spacing is taken as a measure of the lateral masking. The critical spacing can be assessed by measuring contrast threshold for alphanumeric symbols (letters) as a function of their separation. As the distance between the characters widens, the threshold remains constant up to a certain extent, beyond which it drops abruptly and then levels off: the critical spacing is referred to this extent (Figure 2).

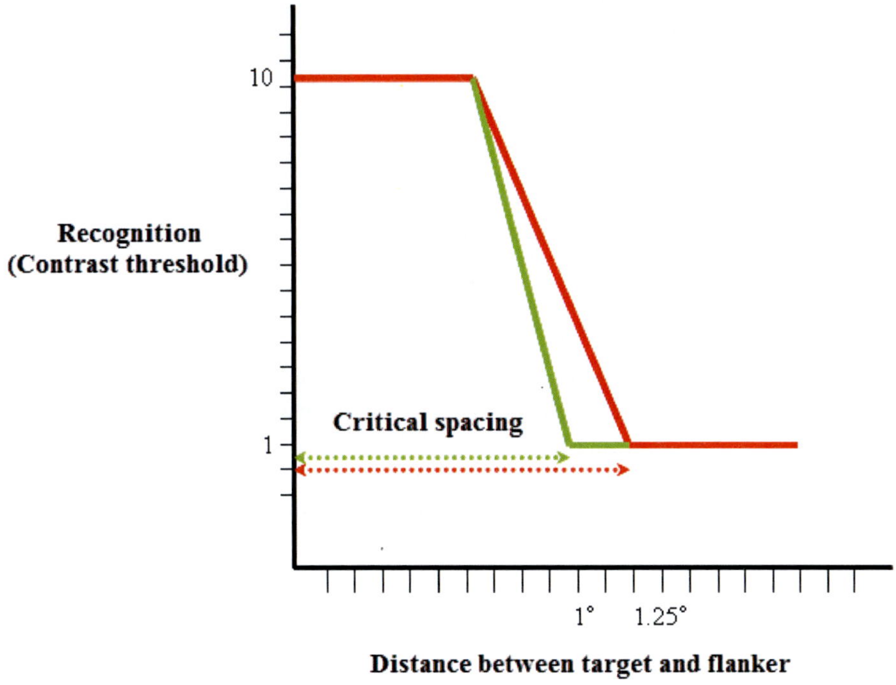

Figure 2. The critical spacing. Recognition threshold at 4 degrees of eccentricity in presence of a distractor on the right (red line) and on the left (green line) of the target. The contrast threshold remains constant up to a separation of 1.25 deg on the right and 1 deg on the left of the target and then it decreases abruptly. (*Modified reprint from: Journal of Vision, Vol. 4, Issue 12, Pelli DG, Palomares M, Majaj, Crowding is unlike ordinary masking: distinguishing feature integration from detection, pages 1136-1169, 2004, with permission from The American Research for Vision and Ophthalmology).*

[203] Vernier acuity deals with the ability to detect the misalignment of the two parts of a broken line slightly displaced along the vertical axis. Visual acuity, is an hyperacuity, because its resolution threshold is lower than the resolution threshold of visual acuity.

The width of the critical spacing does not depend on the size of the target or of the distractors [Pelli et al., 2004; Martelli et al., 2009], does not narrow when increasing the presentation time [Townsend et al., 1971] and does not depend on the complexity of the type character [Pelli et al., 2004].

Crowding is effective if the contrast level of the distractors is equal or greater than the contrast of the target [Chung et al., 2001; Pelli et al., 2004], and is made stronger by the resemblance of the distractors with the target [Banks et al., 1979; Chastain, 1981, 1983; Baylis & Driver, 1992; Nazir, 1992] as for shape, size, orientation [Andriessen & Bouma, 1976, Levi et al., 2002b], color [Bouma, 1969], and polarity [Kooi et al., 1994]. Finally, the strength of the lateral masking depends on the number of the distractors [Strasburger et al., 1991; Felisberti et al., 2005; Pöder & Wagemans 2007][204].

However, the crucial variable is the position of the stimuli in the visual field, since crowding increases with eccentricity: indeed, given a triplet of letters, the critical spacing widens as they depart from the center of fixation[205].

The widening of the critical spacing with the eccentricity of the target is a linear function known as the *Bouma's law*. According to the Bouma's law, the critical spacing on the right and on the left of the target is about half its eccentricity[206] and its extent depends upon a constant which in the case of letters[207] is 0.4-0.5[208] [Bouma, 1970; Toet & Levi, 1992; Kooi et al., 1994] (figure 3).

$$CS=K\varphi$$

CS is the critical spacing, K is the constant computed by Bouma (0.4-0.5) and φ is the eccentricity in degrees.

It follows that on the foveal region lateral masking is at its minimum (or absent) and the recognition of stimuli placed so close as to activate the same detector can be affected only by ordinary masking. Actually, it is estimated that at the foveal level the critical spacing matches approximately the size of the target (0.4 degrees for a letter of 0.32 degrees: Pelli et al., 2004) but it is advanced to be even smaller, not wider than 4-6 minarc [Flom et al., 1963; Bouma 1970; Toet & Levi, 1992; Liu & Arditi, 2000; Danilova & Bondarko, 2007].

On the contrary, at 4 degrees from the fixation point the effect of the lateral masking is evident and the critical spacing extends up to about 1 degree to the left and to the right of the character [Leathers et al., 2004][209] irrespective of the increase of the size of the letters.

---

[204] The "ceiling" effect is reached for four-five [Strasburger et al., 1991; Felisberti et al., 2005] or seven [Pöder & Wagemans, 2007] distractors.

[205] Instead, increasing the size of the central character is ineffective in improving its recognition: this is a key feature that makes lateral masking different from ordinary masking.

[206] Both critical spacing and eccentricity are computed in angular values (degrees).

[207] The same value applies to numbers [Strasburger et al., 1991], to "T" [Tripathy & Cavanagh, 2002], to triplets of bars [Latham & Whitaker, 1996], to the spatial frequency or contrast of gratings [Wilkinson et al., 1997], as well as to the orientation task for lines [Andriessen & Bouma, 1976].

[208] The critical spacing calculated by Bouma is based on the blank area between the characters, while in the current literature it refers to the center- to-center distance between two adjacent letters. In this case the original value (0.4-0.5) must be increased to about 0.6.

[209] Indeed, the finding satisfies the Bouma's law: 2°/4°=0.5.

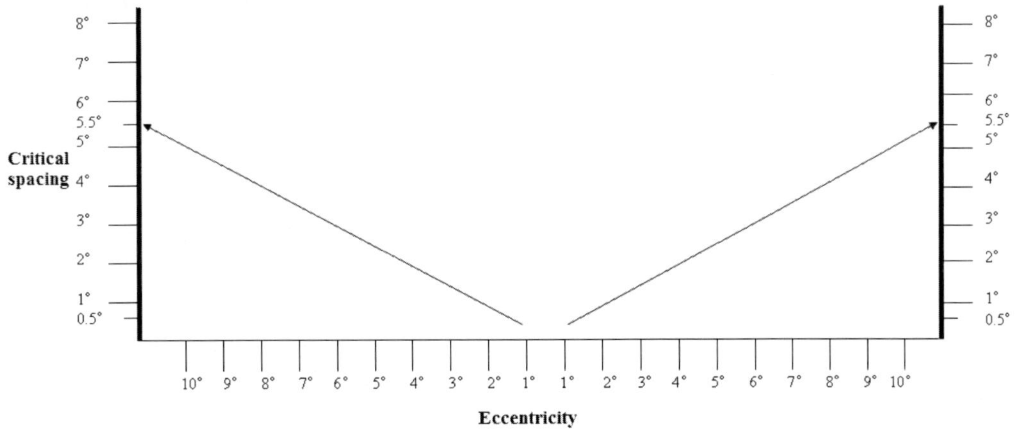

Figure 3. The critical spacing as a function of the eccentricity of the target. According to the Bouma's law, the critical spacing is about half its eccentricity. The figure does not take into account the outward-inward anisotropy (see further on in the text).

Therefore, in the extrafoveal region the reading rate increases as the character size enlarges up to a certain value, beyond which crowding hinders a further improvement. This is the reason why in normal readers peripheral reading cannot match the level registered at the foveal level [Chung et al., 1998].

Asymmetry and Anisotropy of Crowding

Crowding is an anisotropic phenomenon[210]. The anisotropy referred to lateral masking is of three types: inside/outside anisotropy, radial/tangential anisotropy and horizontal/vertical anisotropy.

Due to the inside/outside anisotropy, originally described by Bouma [1970, 1973] and later confirmed in other studies [Townsend et al., 1971; Krumhansl & Thomas, 1977; Banks et al., 1979; Chastain & Lawson, 1979; Wolford & Shum, 1980; Chastain, 1982; Toet & Levi, 1992], critical spacing depends on the side of the target. In fact, it is larger on the peripheral side and smaller towards the fixation point. At 4 degrees of eccentricity, for example, given a reference target, the critical spacing is 1.25 degrees wide toward the periphery and 1 degree wide in the direction of the fixation point [Pelli et al., 2004]. This perceptive arrangement makes the masking effect of a distractor placed on the external (peripheral) side of the target (distal flanker) stronger than an identical and equidistant one, placed between the target and the fovea (proximal flanker). It follows that the final (peripheral) letters of a word are less confusing than the initial (proximal) characters[211]. In fact, on the right of the fixation point the masking effect on the final letter is provided by the character on its left, which acts as proximal flanker, whereas the initial letter is masked by the character on its right that acts as

[210] In visual psychophysics, a perceptual phenomenon is anisotropic if it shows different characteristics depending on the direction or orientation (for example vertical/horizontal/oblique).

[211] The inside/outside anisotropy is not typical of the alphabetical symbols but affects also Gabor patches (i.e. distributions of luminance with sinusoidal modulation) of different orientation [Petrov & Popple, 2007].

distal flanker. Since the proximal distractors are weaker than the distal ones, the last character of a word is less subjected to crowding than the initial one (figure 4). This is the reason why in the studies of Bouma the outer letters were less often confused than the inner characters[212].

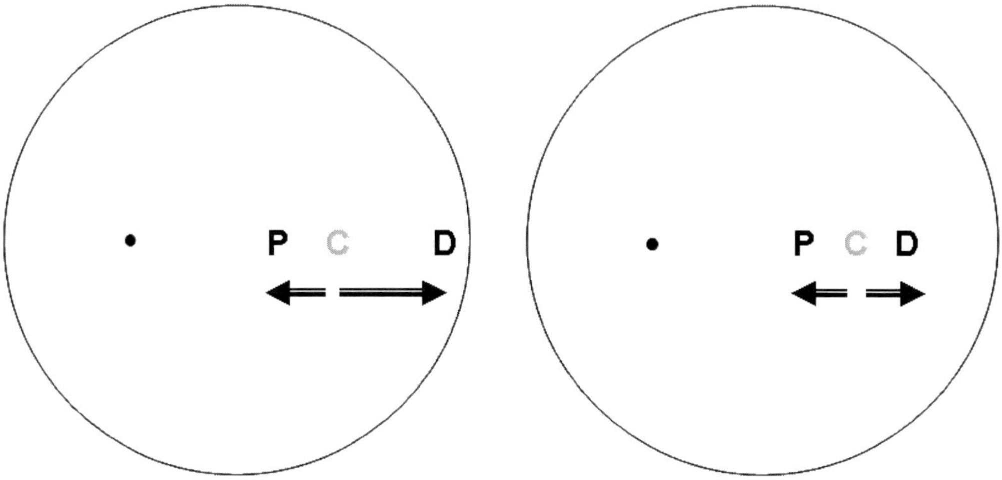

Figure 4. Inside/outside anisotropy. Given an eccentric target C and two distractors, P proximal and D distal, the critical spacing is wider towards the periphery and smaller towards the fixation point. On the left it is shown the separation PC+CD between target and distractors required to allow the recognition of C. To be noted that the distance between the target and P (the weaker flanker) is smaller than the distance between the target and D (the stronger flanker). Looking steadily at the dot, C should be barely recognizable despite the two flankers. On the right the separation between target and distractors is made symmetrical so that PC = CD. Staring steadily at the dot, the recognition of C should become more difficult. In summary, the inside/outside anisotropy makes the distal flanker stronger compared to the proximal one, so that the masking effect turns out to be higher from the peripheral side of the target. In the lexical task, when reading a word (made of characters equally spaced) projected on the right side of the foveal region, the last letter of the string turns out to be less crowded than the first character, since the last letter suffers from the weaker masking effect of the proximal flankers while the first letter is more strongly affected by the adjoining (distal with respect to the fixation point) characters on its right.

The radial/tangential anisotropy makes critical spacing different according to the radial or tangential arrangement of the stimuli, taking as a reference the fixation point. Toet & Levi [1992] mapped the *spatial interaction zones* along the vertical and the horizontal meridian: given a target and two distractors, the spatial interaction zone is the bidimensional spatial extent where the probability to recognize the target is 75%. Therefore, the spatial interaction zones correspond to the critical spacing along the *x-, y*-axis.

The critical spacing is wider for radial configurations, so that along the vertical axis[213] characters arranged in column (radial disposition) require wider separations to be recognized compared to the side by side alignment (tangential disposition), while the contrary is observed along the horizontal coordinate[214] [Chambers & Wolford, 1983; Toet & Levi, 1992].

---

[212] The anatomical basis of the phenomenon lies in the anisotropic mapping of the visual space on the striate cortex. Given two distractors (external and internal) equidistant from the target, the cortical representation makes the distal distractor closer to the target compared to the proximal one, making the former more masking than the latter [Motter & Simoni, 2007].

[213] Below and presumably above the fixation point.

[214] Nasally and presumably temporally to the fixation point.

For this discrepancy the spatial interaction zones, circular in shape in the foveal region, turn elliptical in the peripheral field, with the focal axis facing the fixation point (Figure 5). Furthermore, their size rises in the eccentric regions, according to the Bouma's law: so, at the foveal level the spatial interaction zones are 3.6 minarc wide, whereas at 0.4 degrees of eccentricity along the horizontal meridian their radial length (side by side stimuli) increases fourfold and its tangential length (stimuli in column) doubles [Toet & Levi, 1992]. Likewise, along the vertical meridian the recognition threshold increase is steeper the radial direction (stimuli in column) compared to the tangential one (side by side stimuli). In summary, along the radial axis the critical spacing is about 0.5φ wide while along the tangential meridian it is just 0.1φ [Toet & Levi, 1992].

The third type of anisotropy can be observed in the four quadrants of the visual field along the horizontal and the vertical axis. The asymmetry makes lateral masking stronger for the horizontal alignments compared to the vertical ones[215]. Therefore, in the four quadrants of the visual field recognition threshold is lower for vertically aligned configurations and higher for stimuli arranged horizontally, suggesting a greater integration (that is a stronger crowding effect) along the horizontal coordinate[216] (Figure 6).

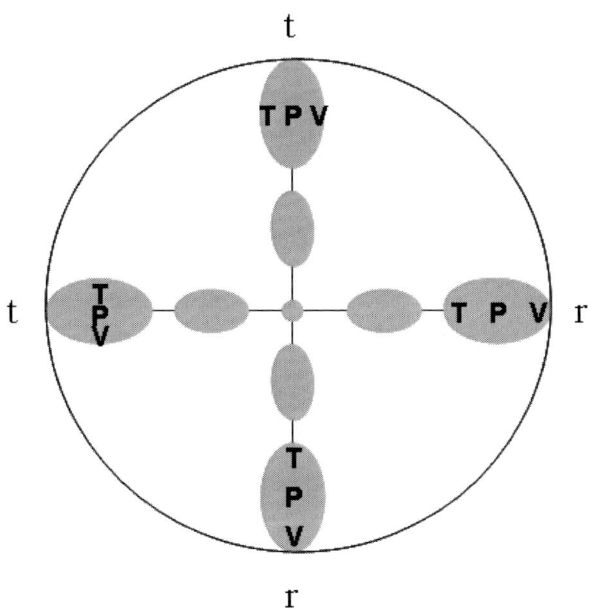

Figure 5. Radial/tangential anisotropy. In grey are represented the spatial interaction zones (not to scale) along the vertical and horizontal meridian. The critical spacing is wider for radially arranged configurations (r) and smaller for tangentially arranged configurations (t). Consequently, the spatial interaction zones in the periphery of the visual field are elliptical with the focal axis facing the fixation point. Note the circular shape and the small size of the spatial interaction zone at the center of the visual field (the fixation point, corresponding to the foveal region of the retina).

---

215 This perceptual phenomenon has been investigated with triplets of "T" or "C" [Feng et al., 2007].

216 The result is in agreement with the radial /tangential asimmetry for stimuli arranged along the horizontal meridian but not along the vertical axis. The source of this discrepancy may lie on a stronger effect of the radial/tangential anisotropy compared to the horizontal /vertical asimmetry, so that along the vertical coordinate the first prevails on the second. In addition, the discrepancy can be due to methodological differences in the experimental designs (see Feng et al., 2007 for details).

Lower processing threshold along the vertical axis from now on will be defined *vertical anisotropy*.

Vertical anisotropy does not depend on alphabetical configurations, since similar results have been obtained also with non-alphabetical stimuli[217]. Still, it could simply depend on higher spatial resolution acuity along the vertical axis and not on the predominant effect of the lateral masking along the horizontal coordinate. And yet, the lack of vertical anisotropy for acuity tasks as Vernier acuity and in particular bisection acuity[218] [Feng et al., 2007] rules out this eventuality.

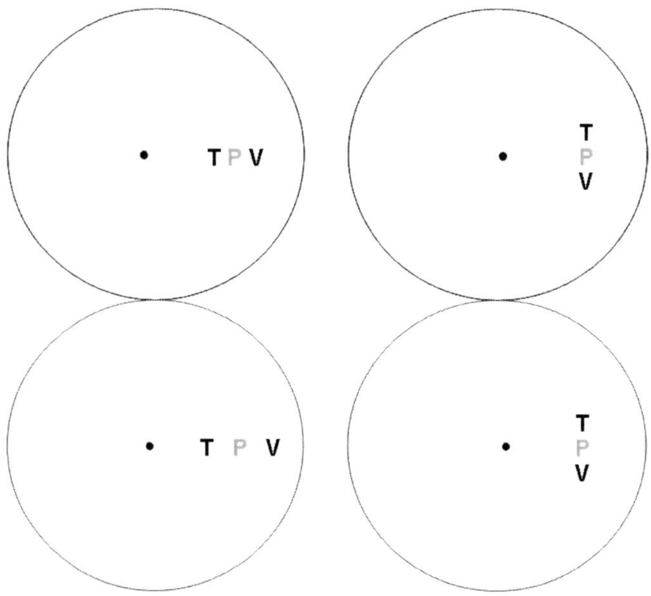

Figure 6. Horizontal/vertical anisotropy. The lateral masking, i.e. the critical spacing, is greater for horizontal alignments so that the spatial interval that enables the recognition of letters in column (upper right) is not wide enough to allow the recognition of the same characters aligned along the horizontal axis (upper left). The recognition of the central character of the horizontal triplet, therefore, requires a greater interletter distance among the three characters (bottom left) compared to the vertical triplet (bottom right).

Modeling of Crowding

It is still unclear the way crowding affects the recognition threshold: whether via lateral inhibition of the distractors on the target [Estes, 1972, 1974, Bjork & Murray, 1977] or improper spatial grouping of the elementary constituents of the stimulus when distractors are added (*perception pooling* theory: Wolford, 1975; Krumhansl & Thomas, 1977, Wilkinson et al., 1997; Parkes et al., 2001; Levi et al., 2002a, b; Pelli et al., 2004).

The first solution implies that features belonging to adjacent letters inhibit each other. According to this model, called the *interactive channels model* [Estes, 1972, 1974, 1982] (figure 7a), the recognition of a character among other characters is reduced as a function of

[217] For example pairs of segments [Feng et al., 2007].

[218] The bisection acuity can be assesed estimating the coaxial misalignment in a series of stimuli: for example the lateral displacement of the central of three aligned dots.

their similarity. So, letters that share some features, such as "E" and "F", if close enough interact and their elementary constituents compete to engage the channels responsible for their processing. The correspondent detector, when activated by the "winner" feature of a character, inhibits the contiguous receptive field aimed at processing the same feature belonging to the adjoining letter.

Hence, according to the interactive channels model, resembling symbols are expected to be particularly susceptible to competitive inhibition because many of their elementary constituents are identical and as such engage the same detector[219].

Correctly, based on this paradigm, increased interletter distance is expected to lower the probability of features competition whereas a progressive reduction of the interactive channels in the peripheral visual field would favor the competitive interaction, that is to say lateral masking. This way, the model accounts for two crucial characteristics of crowding: its disappearance beyond the critical spacing and its stronger effect as a function of the eccentricity.

As an alternative solution, the elementary constituents belonging to close configurations would tend to be pooled and mixed, resulting in visual confusion. In this *feature perturbation model* [Wolford, 1975] (figure 7b), the interactive inhibition between contiguous channels is replaced by a disturbing effect affecting the positional coding of the features making up the characters.

Therefore, the perturbation effect removes some features of a letter (for example the upper and middle horizontal bar of an 'E') and transposes them on the adjoining letter (for example an 'I'). As a result, the two characters are perceptually transformed into different letters (first letter: E → L, adjoining letter: I → F).

Unlike the *interactive channels model*, since the pooling of elementary constituents of letters which share similar features is expected to alter their shape to a less extent [Krumhansl & Thomas, 1977], resemblance between characters would minimize the effect of the perturbation.

Instead (in agreement to the interactive channels model) increased interletter spacing is expected to reduce the feature perturbation, as the wider is the distance between two characters, the less likely is the migration of their features.

Finally, since the perceptual pooling paradigm relies on the spatial integration zones and the spatial integration zones increase in size as a function of the eccentricity, the same is expected to occur for the perturbation effect. As a result, feature perturbation increases with the eccentricity of the characters, as predicted by the Bouma's law.

In summary, according to the interactive channels model are the elementary constituents to get lost, according to the feature perturbation model is their positional coding to be defective.

---

[219] According to this solution, lateral masking is expected to be stronger for stimuli that share common characteristics. Yet, in a recent investigation crowding is found to be weaker (or even absent) for triplets of Gabor patches with the same orientation and stronger when the orientation was different [Petrov & Popple, 2007].

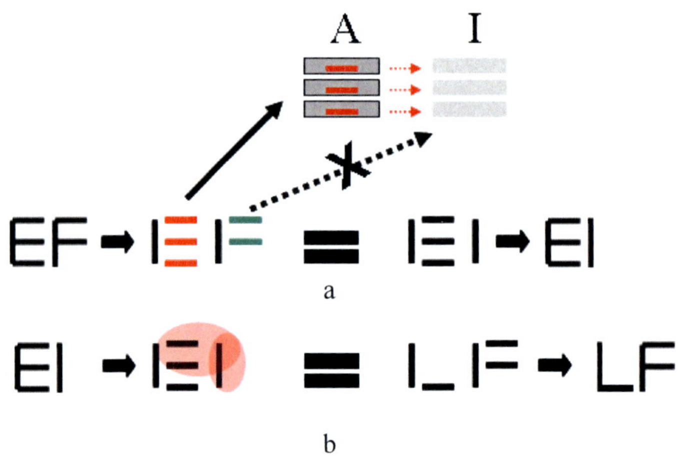

Figure 7. The interactive channels model (a) and the feature perturbation model (b).
In a) it is shown a pair of letters whose features compete for activating the detectors responsible for their processing. In this case the three horizontal bars of the 'E' win the competition on the corresponding two horizontal bars of the nearby letter, the 'F', and engage the respective detectors. The detectors, when activated by the "winner" features of the 'E', inhibit the contiguous receptive fields aimed at processing the same feature belonging to the adjoining letter (the 'F'). Therefore, the 'F' is perceived as 'I'. A: activated detectors, I: inhibited detectors; dotted red arrows: inhibitory effect of the activated detectors on the adjacent detectors. In b) the perturbing effect removes from the letter 'E' some of its features (the upper and middle horizontal bars), turning the 'E' into 'L'. The two elementary constituents involved in the perturbation are shift on the contiguous character, an 'I', which in turn becomes an 'F'. The oval spots represent the spatial integration areas, made asymmetric for clarity so as to cover the second character and two features of the first letter.

The two paradigms may be complementary, so that in some cases the interactive channels model accounts well for the experimental results, in others the feature perturbation model is more reliable. Therefore, a third solution that encompasses the previous two has been developed [Krumhansl & Thomas, 1977]. In this new paradigm, on the one hand identical features belonging to two adjacent letters can lead to reciprocal lateral inhibition, according to the interactive channels model; on the other hand, one or more features belonging to a character can shift, merging with the adjacent letter, in agreement with the feature perturbation model.

In this operation, however, the result of the pooling is not a simple overlapping of the features, but a selective integration of the features of the distractors that differ from the elementary constituents of the target (*anisotropic feature contrast model,* Petrov & Popple, 2007).

The way crowding leads to visual confusion has been investigated by estimating the percentage of errors when asked to recognize strings made up of 5 letters [Liu & Arditi, 2001]. By reducing the interletter spacing from a value equivalent to the size of the characters up to one tenth, the lexical performance worsens by 25-46% and the most frequent errors are found to affect the central letters; on the contrary, the characters at the ends of the string tend to be less involved. In this survey, the inhibition of the elementary constituents of the characters together to their wrong pooling within the final configuration has been postulated.

The Anatomofunctional Basis of Crowding

There is no doubt that crowding stems from the cortex and not from the retina, since it occurs even when the target is directed to one eye and the distractors to the other[Flom et al., 1963; Taylor & Brown, 1972; Levi et al., 1985a; Tripathy & Levi, 1994]. In particular, its anatomical source would be the long range connections of the cortical horizontal cells, since a correlation between their length and the critical spacing has been documented [Gilbert et al., 2000][220]. Indeed, once the detection and recognition of the elementary constituents of a visual configuration have been processed, specific cortical modules defined *integration fields* account for their integration [Toet & Levi, 1992; Pelli et al., 2004]. Therefore, the goal of the integration fields is to arrange the local configurations within a more global pattern (for example to arrange the features of a letter in the letter and the letters in a word).

In the visual field, the size of the integrative fields increases with the eccentricity [Pelli et al., 2004]. In the foveal region the size is small[221], so that in the fixation point the visual integration takes place on a reduced scale, allowing the composition of the elementary constituents of a target (like a letter or a syllable) and at the same time neutralizing possible interferences from the surrounding regions. On the contrary, in the peripheral visual field the dimension of the integration fields may exceed the size of the target, involving a neighboring region of visual space. It follows that some features of the surrounding stimuli may fall within the boundaries of the integration field aimed at the target: as a result, the surrounding features are perceptually integrated within the target, thereby preventing the proper recognition of its global configuration.

On the cortex, the rate of change of the integration field size as a function of eccentricity is about 0.4-0.5φ, in full accordance with the Bouma's law. Thereby, the relation critical spacing/eccentricity described by Bouma would stem from the gradient of the visual space representation on the cerebral cortex, where the size of the integration fields depends on their distance from the foveal representation. Since the progressive widening of the critical spacing toward the periphery depends on the progressive increase of the integration span of the features making up a visual configuration, the visual space turns out to be perceptually more and more "shrunk", "compressed"[222] towards the periphery. This anisotropic trend is undoubtedly of the utmost importance for the hypothesis we are presenting in the second part of this treatise.

To date, the cortical region in charge of the lateral masking is unknown. V1 could be involved, since in V1 the binocular columns integrate the input coming from each of the two eyes and lateral masking occurs also in dichoptic conditions (as stated above). Yet, functional magnetic resonance studies have shown a metabolic response to crowding not in V1 but as from V2 [Arman et al., 2006]. The proportionality factor that relates the eccentricity with the size of the cortical receptive fields tends to increase from V1 to V2-V4: the coefficient is just 0.1 in V1, 0.2 in V2 and 0.5 in V4 [Motter, 2002]: therefore, in V4 the factor matches the coefficient of the Bouma's law. According to this finding, the region responsible for the

---

[220] But see Levi [2008].

[221] The width of the integration fields in the foveal region is about 4 minarc, in accordance with the extent of the critical spacing in the fixation point (about 4-6 minarc: Flom et al., 1963; Bouma 1970; Toet & Levi, 1992 ;Liu & Arditi, 2000; Bondarko & Danilova, 2007).

[222] Indeed, to integrate means to minimize the separations, i.e. to compress.

crowding effect could be V4. In addition, V4 shows anisotropic functional characteristics[223] similar to those described for the critical spacing [Toet and Levi, 1992] and, as aforementioned, seems to be involved in the attentional process[224]. Eventually, crowding is shown to affect even the recognition of faces [Louie et al., 2007] and the recognition of faces does not involve V1 but the temporal cortex [Desimone, 1991; Allison et al., 1994][225].

Crowding and Lexical Function

In clinical field, crowding has been studied paying particular attention to the reading task.

Lateral masking hinders the recognition of letters or words, making the integration of their elementary constituents strong enough to make the processing of the lexical material simultaneous rather than sequential: the result is visual confusion or perceptive annihilation. When reading, lateral masking gives rise to localization errors, both locally in the positional coding of the features that make up the characters and at a more global level, in the arrangement of the letters within the string [Huckauf & Heller, 2002]. Therefore, a defective positional coding at the local level (characters) generates errors in letters recognition, while at the global level (words) it determines letters/syllables exchanges and inversions. The increase of the localization errors at the more eccentric positions is in line with the *pooling hypothesis* and with the enlargement of the spatial interaction zones toward the periphery.

The lateral masking hampers the reading task because the widening of the critical spacing *shrinks* the so-called *visual uncrowded span* [Law et al., 2001].

The *visual span* must be distinguished from the *perceptual span* [O'Regan, 1990]: the *visual span* is the number of characters readable[226] at each fixation in an extra lexical context, therefore when the cognitive component is ruled out. On the contrary, the *perceptual span* refers to letters arranged in words. Since the perceptual span benefits from a cognitive linguistic anticipatory component, it turns out to be wider compared to the visual span. The perceptive span encompasses up to 11-15 characters (approximately 2.5° -3°) on the right of the fixation point [McConkie & Rayner, 1975][227] and no more than 3-4 on the left [Rayner et al., 1980, 1982][228]. The visual span is made of 6 letters on the right and 4 letters on the left of the fixation point in occidental readers [Legge et al., 2001][2]. The perceptual and visual span can be assessed presenting respectively words and meaningless strings of characters (non-words). However, from now on, the terms *perceptual span* and *visual span* will be put together under the global term of (generic) *visual span*.

As shown in figure 8, the visual span depends on the critical spacing[229] because if the critical spacing is wider, the number of characters of the string recognizable at each fixation decreases and more fixations are needed to read the whole sentence [Leathers et al., 2007].

---

[223] Anisotropy about 2:1 [Pinon et al., 1998].

[224] Yet, in the macaque, attentional modulation is found even in neurons of the area V1 [Vidyasagar, 1998, 2001].

[225] Reduced crowding has been reported in patients suffering from ischemia of the posterior thalamus [Michael & Desmedt, 2004], suggesting a possible involvement of the pulvinar, as well.

[226] Because not crowded.

[227] In high school students.

[228] In western languages.

[229] According to an fMRI study, the anatomical substrate of the visual span is advanced to be the left superior parietal lobe, found impaired in a group of 12 dyslexic children [Peyrin et al., 2011].

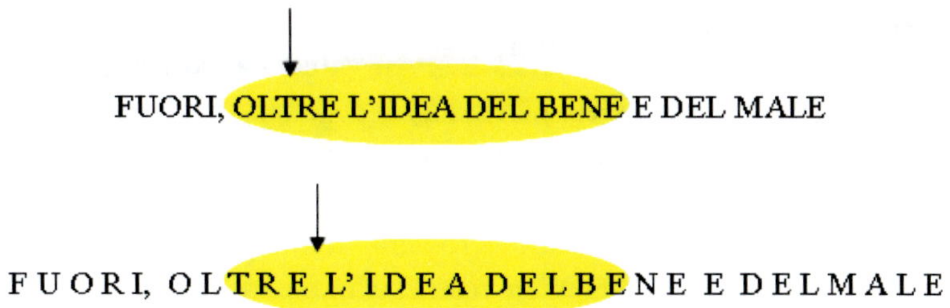

Figure 8. Visual span and critical spacing. The oval area represents the visual span, i.e. the number of characters processed at every single fixation. A single fixation enables the reader to process the sentence within the boundaries of the oval region but not beyond, since beyond the visual span the letters are crowded. If the critical spacing widens, a greater interletter distance is needed to allow their recognition: it follows that the number of letters within the window of processing, that is to say the visual span, is reduced.
The arrow shows the position of the fixation. The meaning of the sentence is "outside, beyond the idea of the good and the evil". The representation is not to scale.

It is well known that reading rate depends on the visual span [Sperling, 1960; Levi et al., 2007; Kwon et al., 2007].

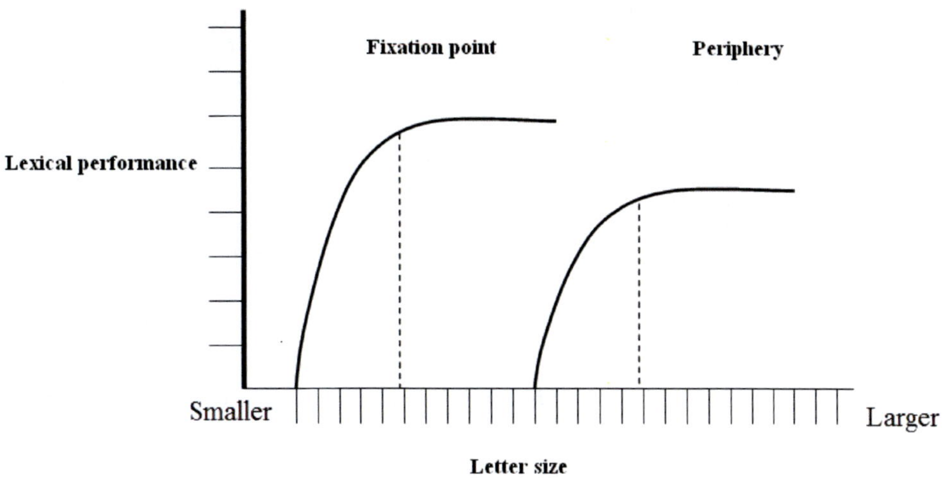

Figure 9. The asymptotic function that relates reading rate and character size (simulation). In the fixation point, the reading rate rapidly increases with the size of the characters up to a level represented by the dashed segment (*critical print size*). From this point, the gradient tends to stabilize and the lexical performance depends only on the visual span. In the extrafoveal region the curve is shifted to the right: in fact, the characters size has to be larger because in the peripheral visual field the visual acuity is reduced compared to the foveal region. Therefore, the critical print size is larger but the shape of the function is the same: rapid rise till the character size has reached the CPS (whose value depends on the eccentricity), then the "ceiling". Yet, the ceiling" in the extrafoveal region is located to a lower level compared to the fixation point, since the critical spacing outside of the fixation point, that is wider, makes the visual span shorter: thereby, the highest level of performance of the extrafoveal region would never match the foveal one.

Thus, if the critical spacing is wider than the interletter distance of the ordinary print size, the more peripheral characters of the visual span are masked because they happen to localize beyond its boundary, and as such can no longer be processed. It follows that the visual span is reduced and reading rate and accuracy decrease [Levi et al., 2007; Pelli et al., 2007]. Instead, the size of the character affects reading only when it is smaller than a given value. Therefore, the function that relates reading rate and print size shows a steep gradient that tends to stabilize when the size of the letters exceeds a given value, called *critical print size* (CPS) (Figure 9). From this point on, the lexical performance depends only on the visual span. In the extrafoveal region the curve is similar but is shifted to the right: in fact since the peripheral acuity is lower, letters have to be larger to be recognized. Besides, the "ceiling" is placed to a lower reading rate level because the increased crowding in the peripheral visual field shortens the visual span [Law et al., 2001]. This is the reason why the maximum level of performance in the peripheral visual field, irrespective of the size of the characters, cannot be the same as at the fixation point [Chung et al., 1998].

Therefore, lateral masking shortens the visual span and the visual span in turn correlates with the lexical function, so that its enlargement increases the reading rate whereas its contraction worsens the lexical function [Legge et al., 2007a, b, Kwon et al., 2007].

The size of the visual span would account for up to 52% of the variance of the reading rate of normal children [Kwon et al., 2007]. As a matter of fact, a wider visual span implies more characters to be processed at each fixation, allowing thereby longer saccades. It follows that the number of fixations required to complete the sentence is reduced, so that the oculomotor pattern is optimized and, eventually, the reading rate increases.

Once assessed that the visual span extent depends on crowding [Legge et al., 2007a, b], it is worthwhile wondering whether the compensation of the reinforced lateral masking via widening of the interletter spacing may help to improve the lexical function. Yet, even if this compensation may enhance the processing of words [Latham & Whitaker, 1996], it does not necessarily increase the reading rate [Chung, 2002; Berger et al., 2003; Yu et al., 2007]. Indeed, the enlargement of the interletter distance to a value greater than the critical spacing improves the recognition of the individual characters, but the visual span (rather than widening) narrows, and for this reason the lexical speed does not increase as expected [Yu et al., 2007].

Two rehabilitative investigations may help to illuminate on such a relationship between crowding and visual span.

In the first [Chung et al., 2004], normal adult readers were trained to recognize sequences of three letters presented in the periphery of the visual field. In this case subjects were asked to identify all the letters of the trigram, without focusing on the central one. At the end of the training, reading rate improved by 41% as a result of the widening of the visual span.

In the second study, normal readers were trained using the same method and the same number of sessions[230] [Chung, 2007]. However, unlike the previous case, subjects were required not to recognize all the letters of the trigram but only the central one. At the end of the training program, the lateral masking reduction was revealed by the increase of the proportion of correct answers from 34% to 64%.

Interestingly, the results obtained at a given interletter spacing transferred to other interletter distances[231]. This improvement led to a reduction of the critical spacing by 38%. In turn, the narrowing of the critical spacing allowed a reduction of the critical print size by 0.14 degrees[232].

[230] One hour a day for six days. The presentation time was 150 msec, short enough to rule out the trigger of saccadic movements.
[231] In this work the interletter distances ranged from 0.8 to2 times the horizontal extent of the character.
[232] From 1.28 to 1.14 degrees.

Still, despite the decline of crowding, after the training the reading rate improved only by 7.2%[233]. Therefore, the training was effective only on the reduction the critical print size: in other words trainees after the practice were able to read at their maximum reading rate (which remained unchanged) texts printed with a smaller size. As suggested by the researchers, in the first experiment (the observer was trained to recognize all the letters of the trigram) the practice had led to the widening of the visual span, while in the second investigation (the efforts of the subject were directed only to the central character) the result was only the reduction of the lateral masking.

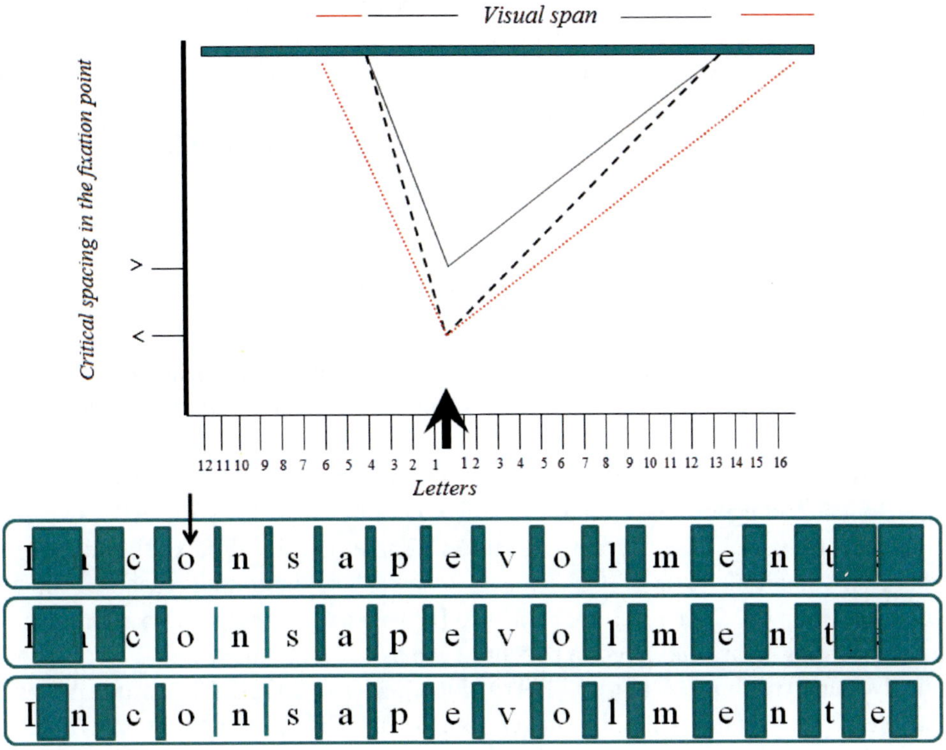

Figure 10. Visual span (perceptual span) and lateral masking in normal readers. Solid line: normal lateral masking around the fixation point. Crowding increases with the eccentricity in accordance with the Bouma's law until the critical spacing matches and then exceeds the interletter distance. This equivalence takes place after about 11-15 characters on the right of the fixation point and 3-4 characters on the left and limits the visual span. Broken line: lateral masking after a training (one session of one hour a day for six days) aimed at identifying the central letter in trigrams. Around the fixation point the critical spacing is shrunken but the width of the visual span remains unchanged. Thin dotted line: lateral masking after a training (one session of one hour a day for six days) aimed at identifying all the letters making up the trigrams. Around the fixation point the critical spacing is shrunken and the width of the visual span increases. The three lower panels show the relationship between crowding and visual span. Top panel: simulation of the normal distribution of the critical spacing across the string. Middle panel: distribution of the critical spacing after the first type of training. Crowding is reduced around the fixation point but the width of the visual span remains unchanged. Lower panel: distribution of the critical spacing after the second type of training. Crowding is reduced not only around the fixation point but along the whole string, resulting in an enlargement of the visual span: it follows that more peripheral characters become recognizable at each fixation. The arrow shows the position of the fixation. The interletter distance is not to scale.

[233] Not statistically significant.

According to a personal interpretation, in the latter study the visual span did not widen because the contraction of the critical spacing occurred only in the fixation point, while in the first experiment the reduction involved the whole reading line (figure 10).

In ordinary conditions peripheral crowding is not deleterious but is necessary to avoid that the eccentric lexical information interferes with the central processing. The incremental gradient of the critical spacing towards the periphery has its *raison d'être* in such a selective exclusion of the more eccentric lexical stimuli, which act as distractors in respect to the central ones: so, the more peripheral letters (i.e. those outside the boundary of the visual span) are neutralized by crowding, allowing an undisturbed analysis of the foveal and parafoveal characters.

In conclusion, the physiological peripheral crowding enhances the attentional focusing, so that it can be regarded as a pre-attentive process that tends to isolate the spatial region of interest from the potentially disturbing neighboring information (see below) [Pelli et al., 2004].

Crowding in Dyslexics

Since increased lateral masking prevents the lexical task via a reduction of the visual span, it has to be ascertained whether this factor is involved in the pathogenesis of developmental dyslexia[234].

It is well known that patients read better single letters rather than letters arranged in words [Bouma & Legein, 1977] and single words rather than lines of text [Lovegrove & MacFarlane, 1990; Hill & Lovegrove, 1993]. Therefore, in dyslexics the recognition threshold for stimuli made up of 4-6 elements is higher than in normal readers[235], whereas it is equivalent when just 2 elements are presented [Hawelka & Wimmer, 2005]. This difference suggests crowding to be reinforced in patients, such as to hinder the recognition of words and eventually fluent reading [Atkinson, 1991; Spinelli et al., 2002]. The argument has been investigated by presenting stimuli in foveal projection [Geiger & Lettvin, 1987; Atkinson, 1991, 1993, Spinelli et al., 2002] or letters displayed in the neighboring (parafoveal) regions [Bouma & Legein, 1977]. These studies showed that in patients interletter spacing outside of the fixation point[236] must be about one and a half wider compared to normal readers[237], in order to match their level of reading efficiency [Martelli et al., 2009].

It follows that the gradient of the function critical spacing/eccentricity in dyslexics is greater than the value predicted by the Bouma's law, i.e. steeper compared to normal subjects ($k = 0.95$, vs. 0.62) [Martelli et al., 2009]: in other words, lateral masking increases at a faster rate than expected when the stimulus is shifted towards the periphery.

---

[234] On the contrary, ordinary masking is excluded: when noise is added to lexical stimuli, contrast sensitivity threshold raises by 0.7 log units without significant differences between dyslexics and normal readers and whatever the length of the string be [Martelli et al., 2009]. This finding confirms once more that the impairment does not lie on the identification of individual stimuli (*first rate analysis*) but on the integration between sequential letters (*second rate analysis*).

[235] Not in the whole sample, but only in half of the subjects.

[236] At 4, 8, 10, 12 degrees from the fovea.

[237] The widening does not involve the whole dyslexic sample. In addition, even in a proportion of normal readers the strenght of the lateral masking is comparable to that observed in patients [Atkinson, 1991, 1993].

Apart from the reinforcement of crowding, even its distribution in the visual field is found to be abnormal in dyslexics. Usually, lateral inhibition is weaker around the fixation point and increases with the eccentricity: as a result, the recognition of the stimuli in the fixation point is enhanced because the surrounding visual information, masked, is unable to interfere. Farther from the fixation point, stronger lateral masking helps visual attention to shift along the reading direction, preventing any peripheral stimulation that can mislead its orientation.

On the contrary, in dyslexics crowding is stronger in the central regions [Atkinson, 1991, 1993] and especially around the fixation point[238] [Bouma & Legein, 1977; Geiger & Lettvin, 1987; Atkinson, 1991; Geiger et al., 1992] and tends to decrease in the direction of reading[239]. In patients, the critical spacing is found to be wider at 4 degrees of eccentricity compared to the more peripheral regions [Martelli et al., 2009].

Therefore, letters surrounded by distractors presented parafoveally[240] are less recognizable by dyslexics compared to normal readers [Bouma & Legein, 1977].

In conclusion, the distribution of crowding in dyslexics shows a double anomaly: first, increased lateral masking in paracentral area (acting especially in the proximal direction) that prevents from processing the syllable projected onto the fixation point; second, reduced peripheral crowding, that allows the more distal portions of the string to interfere on the proximal lexical processing. The final outcome is that in dyslexics the peripheral information tends to prevent the central processing [Geiger & Lettvin, 1987; Rayner et al., 1989; Geiger et al., 1992; Geiger et al., 1994, Facoetti et al., 2000], forcing to analyze shorter fragments of the string. Therefore, especially for long words, the sequential integration requires more saccades and more fixations[241] [De Luca et al., 1999; De Luca et al., 2002; Hutzler & Wimmer, 2004].

Investigation on Lateral Masking in Dyslexics with Compensatory Approaches

It is worthwhile to assess whether the wider critical spacing in dyslexics can be balanced by suitably manipulating the reading material, so as to increase the distance between the letters: doing so, the enlargement of the visual span and eventually the improvement of the lexical performance is expected.

Reading rate as a function of the print size [O'Brien et al., 2005] has been evaluated in a group of 22 dyslexic children[242] and a sample of 12 age-matched normal readers. A similar

---

238 Reinforced lateral masking is a tipical feature of amblyopia. Indeed, the distribution of crowding across the visual field is one aspect that makes amblyopia different from developmental dyslexia. In fact, although both conditions suffer from a widening of the critical spacing due to a reinforcement of the lateral masking, in amblyopes this anomaly involves the fixation point while in dyslexics it is observed especially in the parafoveal region. Even the reading rate of amblyopes is slower than expected, but it can be normalized by increasing the interletter distance [Levi et al., 2007].

239 From left to right in western patients, from right to left in Hebrew dyslexics [Geiger & Lettvin, 1987; Geiger et al., 1992].

240 And tachistoscopically.

241 Dyslexics need to make up to 4 fixations to read a word of 6-8 letters, while in normal readers 2 fixations are enough.

242 Age: 6.3-10.4 years.

experiment would be conducted a few years later on a sample of older dyslexics[243] [Martelli et al., 2009].

Critical spacing and critical print size are closed linked: in both cases, in fact, the ability to recognize groups of letters rises with a linear trend, up to stabilize. Indeed, increasing the print size does not involve just the size of the characters, but even the interval between them. In agreement with previous studies [Chung et al., 1998; Law et al., 2001], both in patients and in controls reading rate is found to increase up to the CPS, then the function levels.

The CPS is higher in dyslexics (0.34 deg vs. 0.21 deg in controls: Martelli et al., 2009), so that even after the print size is increased, reading rate in patients remains lower than in controls by a factor 2. These results confirm that dyslexics suffer from a stronger lateral masking, thereby from wider critical spacing: and yet, trying to correct this parameter is not enough to solve their problem.

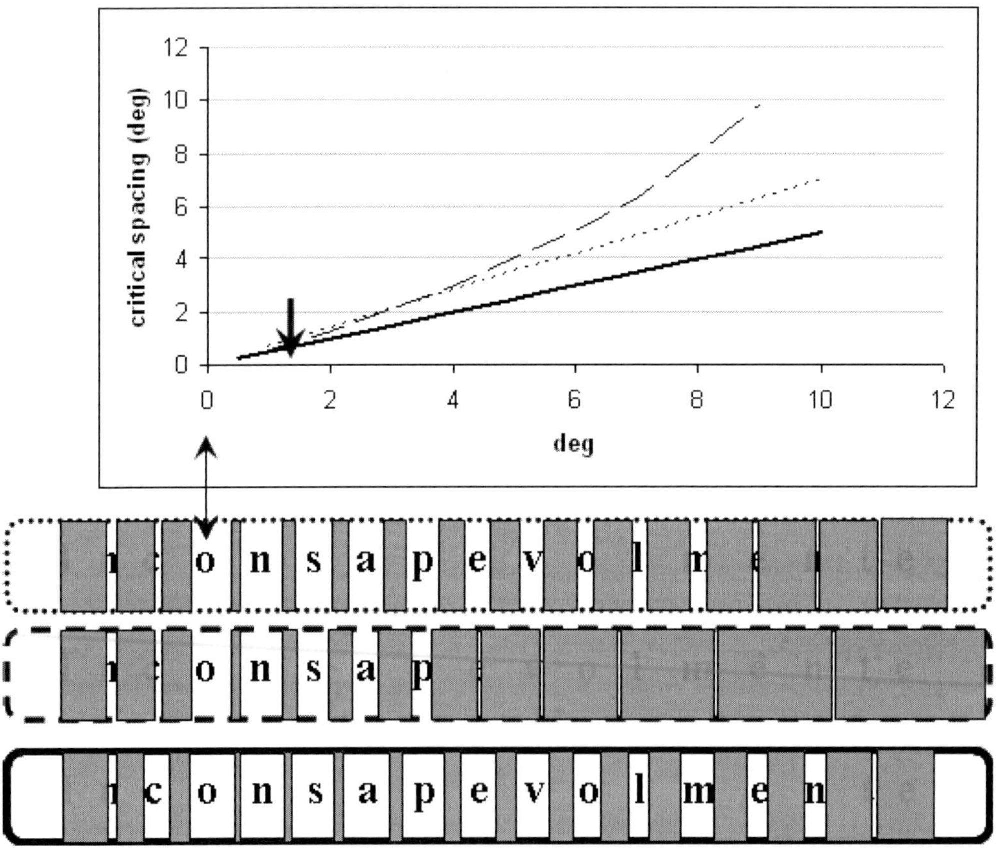

Figure 11. Critical spacing and visual span. The solid line describes the critical spacing as a function of the eccentricity in a normal reader. Bouma coefficient k=0.5. The effect on the text is simulated in the bottom panel. The thin dotted line refers to the critical spacing for k=0.7: the critical spacing widens at a faster but constant rate. The effect on the text is simulated in the upper panel. The thick dashed line represents the critical spacing for a coefficient varying from 0.5 →1.2: the critical spacing increases according to a non-linear trend. The effect on the text is reported in the central panel. The arrow refers to the fixation.

[243] Mean age: 11.7 years. In this investigation, words 6-9 letters long were presented individually.

As for normal readers, in patients the effect of crowding on the lexical function acts via a reduction of the visual span according to one of the following *scenarios* (figure 11):

- the critical spacing is larger at all the eccentricities by a proportionality factor higher than the Bouma's coefficient (0.5-0.6), but remains constant along the horizontal meridian.
- the critical spacing increases towards the periphery according to a factor that is not constant but shows an incremental gradient.

Whatever be the solution, the outcome is clear: the visual span is reduced, as recently confirmed by Hatzidaki et al. [2011].

However, the analysis of the individual data reveals a considerable variability, so that only 35% of dyslexics show a significantly steeper increase of the critical spacing as a function of eccentricity compared to controls [Martelli et al., 2009]. Indeed, taking as a *cutoff* the mean critical spacing found in normal subjects +1 DS, the results found in the two groups overlap, so that on the one hand only a part of dyslexics is set above this limit [Spinelli et al., 2002], on the other hand the effect of crowding seems to be abnormal even in a part of normal readers [Atkinson 1991, 1993]. In patients, the frequent inconsistence of the relationship between critical spacing and reading rate is demonstrated by the fact that the statistical significance of the correlation between the latter and the critical print size is borderline ($p = 0.06$)[244] [O'Brien et al., 2005].

A possible explanation for such a weak correlation is that the prevailing effect of an additional phonological-linguistic factor contributes to hinder the lexical process irrespective of the visuoperceptive impairment. As a matter of fact, even if the widening of the critical spacing were compensated by a proportional increase of the print size (thereby of the interletter spacing), the reading rate in patients would not normalize but would remain lower by approximately 30% [O'Brien, et al., 2005].

In conclusion, reinforced crowding is not the only factor responsible for the reading disability in developmental dyslexia. In fact, it accounts for about 48% or 60% of the reading impairment (Spinelli et al., 2002 and Martelli et al., 2009, respectively) in transparent orthographies so that other (linguistic) factors are expected to be responsible for the remaining quota [Martelli et al., 2009].

The similarities between visual attention, which selects the visual space containing the stimulus, and lateral masking, which aims at neutralizing the surrounding lexical configurations to enhance the processing of the target, have led to believe that lateral masking stems from the spatial attention [Strasburger et al., 1991; Strasburger & Rentschler, 1995; He et al., 1996; Strasburger, 2005]. Some authors suggested that crowding is the limit of the so-called *attentional resolution*, that is to say the limit of the ability to select the target among other visual configurations [Intriligator & Cavanagh, 2001].

The relationship between visual attention and lateral masking is supported by the finding that the visual attention enhancement provided by an attentional cue (as a circle presented in the locus where the target is expected to be displayed a few moments later) reduces the effect of crowding.

---

[244] Whereas it is significant in normal readers ($p = 0.001$).

Moreover, the attentional focus (*attentional spotlight*) has been identified with the aforementioned spatial interaction zones delimiting the influence of the lateral masking [Strasburger, 2005]: indeed, the attentional focus and the spatial interaction zones share common characteristics such as the radial/tangential anisotropy [He et al., 1996; Intriligator & Cavanagh, 2001].

Yet, a body of evidence does not identify crowding with the attentional resolution but rather assigns to it a preattentive local role [Nazir, 1992; Wilkinson et al., 1997; Pelli et al., 2004]. As a matter of fact, crowding acts across short separation angles whereas the attentional gradient is wider[245]. Therefore, the lateral masking is a local phenomenon, while the attentional gradient would encompass the overall central visual field.

In addition, the attentional gradient has been defined as the reduction of the cognitive resolution of the background [Geiger et al., 1992] maybe referring to the activation of superior, associative cerebral modules [Geiger & Lettvin, 2000]. On the contrary, crowding depends on lower (non-cognitive) cortical mechanisms [Kooi et al., 1994] and as such it is located at a prelinguistic level, being the effect similar for lexical and non-lexical symbols. Finally, the anatomical site of visual attention and crowding are probably different: (visual attention: parietal cortex; crowding: V2 or V4).

Thereby, crowding is unlikely to be merely the expression of the attentional focus.

Effect of Visual Training on Crowding

As previously reported, visual training is found to be effective in improving crowding in normal readers [Chung et al., 2004; Chung, 2007].

The reduction of the lateral masking in normal readers after visual training has been confirmed by another investigation [Huckauf & Nazir, 2007][246]. Interestingly, this study aimed at estimating the effect of training on trigrams made of words and non-words as well. At the end of the session, the recognition rate improved by 25.4% for words and only by 16.2% for non-words. The result was found to last for at least the first 24 hours and after prolonged practice with words the improvement extended also to trigrams not presented during the training session.

Therefore, visual training can reduce crowding in normal readers and if the practice is long enough, the effect extends to other locations in the visual field, to different interletter spacings and especially to lexical configurations other from those trained.

Evidently, these findings suggest that a rehabilitative treatment centered on reducing the abnormal lateral masking so as to increase dyslexics' reading rate is theoretically possible.

As argued, in order to improve the reading skills in dyslexics the rehabilitation must aim at widening the visual span: as a matter of fact, successful shrinking of the critical spacing in correspondence of the fixation point is not enough but (as previously discussed) the

[245] See chapter 11.

[246] Normal readers were asked to recognize the central character of trigrams presented tachistoscopically at two different eccentricities (separation between characters: 1 degree, presentation time: 50 msec, eccentricity: 4 and 7 degrees). The ameliorative effect was measured as the percentage of correct answers. After the training, an increase of correct answers by 12% was observed.

improvement of crowding must occur along the whole extension of the string to obtain the widening of the visual span.

As far as we know, to date studies on this topic in dyslexics are scarce. However, the ameliorative effect of visual training on lateral masking, visual span and reading rate observed in normal readers could apply even in patients, provided the treatment is administered during the lexical developmental phase. This last consideration is supported by the fact that in beginner normal readers the lexical practice is crucial for the development of visual span in the scholar period from the third to the seventh grade. Indeed, this is a confirmation that the visual span develops at the same rate with the lexical experience of the child [Kwon et al., 2007][247].

All this aspects are worth being considered, since disclose the possibility to modulate by a suitable visual training the extent of the visual span in dyslexic children.

References

Allison T, Ginter H, McCarthy G, Nobre AC, Puce A, Luby M, Spencer DD. (1994). *Face recognition in human extrastriate cortex.* Journal of Neurophysiology, 71: 821-825.

Andriessen JJ, Bouma H. (1976). *Eccentric vision: Adverse interactions between line segments.* Vision Research, 16: 71-78.

Arman AC, Chung STL, Tjan BS. (2006). *Neural correlates of letter crowding in the periphery* [Abstract]. Journal of Vision, 6: 804.

Atkinson J. (1991). *Review of human visual development: crowding and dyslexia.* In: Vision and visual dyslexia, Stein Ed., MacMillian Press, Houndmills, London.

Atkinson J. (1993). *Vision in dyslexics: letter recognition acuity, visual crowding, contrast sensitivity, accommodation, convergence and sight reading music.* In: Facets of dyslexia and its remediation, Studies in Visual Information Processing, Wright and Groner Eds., Elsevier, Amsterdam.

Banks WP, Larson DW, Prinzmetal W. (1979). *Asymmetry of visual interference.* Perception & Psychophysics, 25: 447-456.

Baylis GC, Driver J. (1992). *Visual parsing and response competition: The effect of grouping factors.* Perception & Psychophysics, 51: 145-162.

Berger TD, Martelli M, Su M, Aguayo M, Pelli DG. *Reading quickly in the periphery.* (2003). [Abstract]. Journal of Vision, 3(9): 806a.

Bex PJ, Dakin SC. (2005). *Spatial interference among moving targets.* Vision Research, 45: 1385-1398.

Bex PJ, Dakin SC, Simmers AJ. (2003). *The shape and size of crowding for moving targets.* Vision Research, 43: 2895-2904.

Bjork EL, Murray JT. (1977). *On the nature of input channels in visual processing.* Psychological Review, 84: 472-484.

Bouma H. (1969). *Visual isolation in eccentric form vision, the role of colour.* IPO Annual Progress Report, 4: 95-99.

Bouma H. (1970). *Interaction effects in parafoveal letter recognition.* Nature, 226: 177–178.

[247] See part II, appendix B.

Bouma H. (1973). *Visual interference in the parafoveal recognition of initial and final letters of words.* Vision Research, 13: 767-782.

Bouma H, Legein CHP. (1977). *Foveal and parafoveal recognition of letters and words by dyslexics and by average readers.* Neuropsychologia, 15: 69-80.

Butler TW, Westheimer G. (1978). *Interference with stereoscopic acuity: Spatial, temporal, and disparity tuning.* Vision Research, 18: 1387-1392.

Campbell FW, Robson JG. (1968). *Application of Fourier analysis to the visibility of gratings.* Journal of Physiology, 197: 551-566.

Chambers L, Wolford G. (1983). *Lateral masking vertically and horizontally.* Bulletin of the Psychonomic Society, 21: 459-461.

Chastain G. (1981). *Inhibition of feature extraction with multiple instances of the target feature in different orientations.* Psychological Research, 43: 45-56.

Chastain G. (1982). *Confusability and interference between members of parafoveal letter pairs.* Perception & Psychophysics, 32: 576-580.

Chastain G. (1983). *Task and contrast effects on performance with parafoveal stimulus pairs.* Psychological Research, 45: 147-156.

Chastain G, Lawson L. (1979). *Identification asymmetry of parafoveal stimulus pairs.* Perception & Psychophysics, 26: 363-368.

Chubb C, Olzak L, Derrington A. (2001). *Second-order processes in vision: Introduction.* Journal of the Optical Society of America A, 18: 2175-2178.

Chung STL (2002). *The effect of letter spacing in central and peripheral vision.* Investigative Ophthalmology & Visual Science, 43: 1270-1276.

Chung STL, Legge GE, Cheung SH. (2004). *Letter recognition and reading speed in peripheral vision benefit from perceptual learning.* Vision Research, 44: 695-709.

Chung STL. (2007). *Learning to identify crowded letters: does it improve reading speed?* Vision Research, 47: 3150-3159.

Chung STL, Mansfield JS, Legge GE. (1998). *Psychophysics of reading. XVIII. The effect of print size on reading speed in normal peripheral vision.* Vision Research, 38: 2949–2962.

Chung STL, Levi DM, Legge GE. (2001). *Spatial-frequency and contrast properties of crowding.* Vision Research, 41: 1833-1850.

Danilova MV, Bondarko VM. (2007). *Foveal contour interactions and crowding effects at the resolution limit of the visual system.* Journal of Vision, 7 (25): 1-18.

De Luca M, Di Pace E, Judica A, Spinelli D, Zoccolotti P. (1999). *Eye movements patterns in linguistic and non-linguistic tasks in developmental surface dyslexia.* Neuropsychologia, 37: 1407-1420.

De Luca M, Borrelli, Judica A, Spinelli D, Zoccoletti P. (2002). *Reading words and pseudo-words: an eye movement study of developmental dyslexia.* Brain and Language, 80: 617-626.

Desimone R. (1991). *Face-Selective Cells in the Temporal Cortex of Monkeys.* Journal of Cognitive Neuroscience, 3: 1-8.

Estes WK. (1972). *Interactions of signal and background variables in visual processing.* Perception & Psychopshysics, 12: 278-286.

Estes WK. (1974). *Redudancy of noise elements and signals in visual detection of letters.* Perception & Psychophysics, 16: 53-60.

Estes WK. (1982). *Similarity-related channel interactions in visual processing.* Journal of Experimental Psychology: Human Perception & Performance, 8: 353-382.

Facoetti A, Paganoni P, Lorusso ML. (2000). *The spatial distribution of visual attention in developmental dyslexia.* Experimental Brain Research, 132: 531-538.

Felisberti FM, Solomon JA, Morgan MJ. (2005). *The role of target salience in crowding.* Perception, 34: 823-833.

Feng C, Jiang Y, He S. (2007). *Horizontal and vertical asymmetry in visual spatial crowding effects.* Journal of Vision, 7 (2), 13: 1-10.

Flom MC. (1991). *Contour interaction and the crowding effect.* Problems in Optometry 1991; 3:237-257.

Flom MC, Heath GG, Takahashi E. (1963). *Contour interaction and visual resolution: Contralateral effect.* Science, 142: 979-980.

Foley JM, Chen CC. (1999). *Pattern detection in the presence of maskers that differ in spatial phase and temporal offset: Threshold measurements and a model.* Vision Research, 39: 3855-3872.

Geiger G, Lettvin JY. (1987). *Peripheral vision in persons with dyslexia.* New England Journal of Medicine, 316: 1238-1243.

Geiger G, Lettvin JY, Zegarra-Moran O. (1992). *Task-determined strategies of visual process.* Cognitive Brain Research, 1: 39-52.

Geiger G, Lettvin JY, Fahle M. (1994). *Dyslexic children learn a new visual strategy for reading: a* controlled experiment. Vision Research, 34: 1223-1233.

Geiger G, Lettvin JY. (2000). *Developmental dyslexia: A different perceptual strategy and how to learn a new strategy for learning.* Saggi, 26: 73-89.

Gilbert C, Ito M, Kapadia M, Westheimer G. (2000). *Interactions between attention, context and learning in primary visual cortex.* Vision Research, 40: 1217-1226.

Hatzidaki A, Gianneli M, Petrakis E, Makaronas N, Aslanides IM. (2011). *Reading and visual processing in Greek dyslexic children: an eye-movement study.* Dyslexia, 17: 85-104.

Hawelka S, Wimmer H. (2005). *Impaired visual processing of multi-element arrays is associated with increased number of eye movements in dyslexic reading.* Vision Research, 45: 855-863.

He S, Cavanagh P, Intriligator J. (1996). *Attentional resolution and the locus of visual awareness.* Nature, 383: 334-337.

Hill R, Lovegrove WJ. (1993). *One word at a time: A solution to the visual deficits in SRDs?* In: Facets of dyslexia and its remediation, Wright, Groner & Kauffman-Hayoz Eds., Elsevier, Amsterdam.

Huckauf A, Heller D. (2002). *What various kinds of errors tell us about lateral masking effects.* Visual Cognition, 9: 889-910.

Huckauf A, Nazir TA. (2007) *How odgcrnwi becomes crowding: Stimulus-specific learning reduces crowding.* Journal of Vision, 7: 1-12.

Hutzler F, Wimmer H. (2004). *Eye movements of dyslexic children when reading in a regular ortography* Brain and Language, 89: 235-242.

Intriligator J, Cavanagh P. (2001). *The spatial resolution of visual attention.* Cognitive Psychology, 43: 171-216.

Kooi FL, Toet A, Tripathy SP, Levi, D. M. (1994). *The effect of similarity and duration on spatial interaction in peripheral vision.* Spatial Vision, 8: 255-279.

Korte W. (1923). *Uber die Gestaltauffassung im indirekten Sehen.* Zeitschrift für Psychologie, 93: 17-82.

Krumhansl CL, Thomas EA. (1977). *Effect of level of confusability on reporting letters from briefly presented visual displays.* Perception & Psychophysics, 21: 269-279.

Kwon M, Legge GE, Dubbels BR. (2007). *Developmental changes in the visual span for reading.* Vision Research, 47: 2889-2900.

Latham K, Whitaker D. (1996). *A comparison of word recognition and reading performance in foveal and peripheral vision.* Vision Research, 36: 2665-2674.

Legge GE, Foley JM. (1980). *Contrast masking in human vision.* Journal of the Optical Society of America, 70: 1458-1471.

Legge GE, Mansfield JS, Chung ST. (2001). *Psychophysics of reading. XX. Linking letter recognition to reading speed in central and peripheral vision.* Vision Research, 41: 725–743.

Legge GE, Cheung SH, Yu d, Chung STL, Lee HW, Owens DP. (2007a). *The case for the visual span as a sensory bottlenech in reading.* Journal of Vision, 7(2), 9: 1-15.

Legge GE, Lee HW, Owens D, Cheung SH, Chung STL. (2007b). *Visual span: a sensory bottleneck on reading speed.* Journal of Vision, 2 (7): 279.

Levi DM. (2008). *Crowding-An essential bottleneck for object recognition: A mini-review.* Vision Research, 48: 635-654.

Levi DM. Klein SA, Aitsebaomo AP. (1985a). *Vernier acuity, crowding and cortical magnification.* Vision Research, 25: 963-977.

Levi DM, Klein SA. (1985b). *Vernier acuity, crowding and amblyopia.* Vision Research, 25: 979-991.

Levi DM, Klein SA, Hariharan S. (2002a). *Suppressive and facilitatory spatial interactions in foveal vision: Foveal crowding is simple contrast masking.* Journal of Vision, 2: 140-166.

Levi DM, Hariharan S, Klein SA. (2002b). *Suppressive and facilitatory spatial interactions in peripheral vision: Peripheral crowding is neither size invariant nor simple contrast masking.* Journal of Vision, 7 (2), 3: 167-177.

Levi DM, Song S, Pelli DG. (2007). *Amblyopic reading is crowded.* Journal of Vision 7 (2), 21: 1-17.

Liu L, Arditi A. (2000). *Apparent string shortening concomitant with letter crowding.* Vision Research, 40: 1059–1067.

Liu L, Arditi A. (2001). *How crowding affects letter confusion.* Optometry and Vision Science, 78: 50-55.

Louie EG, Bressler DW, Whitney D. (2007). *Holistic crowding: Selective interference between configural representations of faces in crowded scenes.* Journal of Vision, 7 (2), 24: 1-11.

Lovergrove WJ, MacFarlane T. (1990). *The effect of text presentation on reading in dyslexic and normal readers.* Perception, 19: 386.

Martelli M, Di Filippo G, Spinelli D, Zoccolotti P. (2009). *Crowding, reading, and developmental dyslexia.* Journal of Vision, 9 (4), 14: 1-18.

McConkie GW, Rayner K. (1975). *The span of the effective stimulus during a fixation in reading,* Perception & Psychophysics, 17: 578–586.

Michael GA, Desmedt S. (2004). *The human pulvinar and attentional processing of visual distractors.* Neuroscience Letters, 362: 176-181.

Morris RK, Rayner K. (1991). *Vision and Visual Dyslexia.* Stein Ed., MacMillian Press, London,

Motter, B. C. (2002). *Crowding and object integration within the receptive field of V4 neurons* [Abstract]. Journal of Vision, 2(7): 274a.

Motter BC, Simoni DA. (2007). *The roles of cortical image separation and size in active visual search performance.* Journal of Vision, 7 (2), 6: 1-15.

Nazir TA. (1992). Effects of lateral masking and spatial precueing on gap-resolution in central and peripheral vision. Vision Research, 32: 771-777.

O'Brien BA, Mansfield JS, Legge GE. (2005). *The effect of print size on reading speed in dyslexia.* Journal of Research in Reading, 28: 332-349.

O'Regan JK. (1990). *Eye movements and reading.* In: Eye movements and their role in visual and cognitive processes, Kowler Ed., Elsevier, New York.

Olzak L, Thomas JP. (1986). *Seeing spatial patterns. In: Handbook of perception and human performance: Sensory processes and perception (Vol. 1),* Boff, Kaufman, & Thomas Eds., New York.

Parkes L, LundJ, Angelucci A, Solomon JA, Morgan M. (2001). *Compulsory averaging of crode orientation signals in human vision.* Nature Neuroscience, 4: 739-744.

Pelli DG, Farell B. (1999). *Why use noise?* Journal of the Optical Society of America A, 16: 647-653.

Pelli DG, Farell B, Moore DC. (2003). *The remarkable inefficiency of word recognition.* Nature, 423: 752-756.

Pelli DG, Palomares M, Majaj NJ. (2004). *Crowding is unlike ordinary masking: Distinguishing feature integration from detection.* Journal of Vision, 4: 1136-1169.

Pelli DG, Tillman KA, Freeman J, Su M., Berger TD, Majaj NJ. (2007). *Crowding and eccentricity determine reading rate.* Journal of Vision, 7 (2), 20: 1–36.

Petrov Y, Popple AV. (2007). *Crowding is directed to the fovea and preserves only feature contrast.* Journal of Vision, 7 (2), 8: 1-9.

Peyrin C, Démonet JF, N'Guyen-Morel MA, Le Bas JF, Valdois S. (2011). *Superior parietal lobule dysfunction in a homogeneous group of dyslexic children with a visual attention span disorder.*Brain and Language, 118: 128-138.

Pinon MC, Gattass R, Sousa AP.(1998). *Area V4 in Cebus monkey: Extent and visuotopic organization.* Cerebral Cortex, 8; 685-701.

Põder E, Wagemans J.(2007). *Crowding with conjunctions of simple features.* Journal of Vision, 7 (2), 23: 1-12.

Rayner K. (1986). *Eye movements and the perceptual span in beginning and skilled readers.* Journal of Experimental Child Psychology, 41: 211-236.

Rayner K, Well AD, Pollatsek A. (1980). *Asymmetry of the effective visual field in reading.* Perception & Psychophysics, 27: 537-544.

Rayner K, Well AD, Pollatsek A, Bertera JH. (1982). *The availability of useful information to the right of fixation in reading.* Perception & Psychophysics, 31: 537-550.

Rayner K, Murphy LA, Henderson JM, Pollastek A. (1989). *Selective attentional dyslexia.* Cognitive Neuropshychology, 6: 357-378.

Sagi D, Julesz B. (1984). *Detection versus discrimination of visual orientation.* Perception, 13: 619-628.

Selfridge OG. (1959). *Pandemonium: A paradigm for learning*. In: The Mechanisation of Thought Processes. H.M.S.O., London.

Sperling G. (1960). *The information available in brief visual presentation.* Psychological Monographs, 74: 1-29.

Spinelli D, De Luca M, Judica A, Zoccolotti P. (2002). *Crowding effects on word identification in developmental dyslexia.* Cortex, 38: 179-200.

Strasburger H. (2005). *Unfocused spatial attention underlies the crowding effect in indirect form vision.* Journal of Vision 5: 1024-1037.

Strasburger H, Harvey LO jr, Rentschler I. (1991). *Contrast thresholds for identification of numeric characters in direct and eccentric view.* Perception & Psychophysics, 49: 495-508.

Strasburger H, Rentschler I. (1995). *Is the crowding effect of purely attentional origin?* Perception, 24(Suppl.): 77.

Taylor SG, Brown DR. (1972). *Lateral visual masking: Supraretinal effects when viewing linear arrays with unlimited viewing time.* Perception & Psychophysics, 12(1-B): 97-99.

Thomas JP, Padilla GJ, Rourke DL. (1969). *Spatial interactions in identification and detection of compound visual stimuli.* Vision Research, 9: 283-292.

Toet A, Levi DM. (1992). *The two-dimensional shape of spatial interaction zones in the parafovea.* Vision Research, 32: 1349-1357.

Townsend JT, Taylor SG, Brown DR. (1971). *Lateral masking for letters with unlimited viewing time.* Perception & Psychophysics, 10: 375-378.

Treisman AM, Gelade G. (1980). *A feature-integration theory of attention.* Cognitive Psychology, 12: 97-136.

Tripathy SP, Cavanagh P. (2002). *The extent of crowding in peripheral vision does not scale with target size.* Vision Research, 42: 2357-2369.

Tripathy SP, Levi DM. (1994). *Long-range dichoptic interactions in the human visual cortex in the region corresponding to the blind spot.* Vision Research, 34: 1127-1138.

Tyler CW, Likova LT. (2007). *Crowding: A neuroanalytical approach.* Journal of Vision, 16: 1-9.

Vidyasagar TR. (1998). *Gating of neuronal responses in macaque primary visual cortex by an attentional spotlight.* NeuroReport, 9: 1947-1952.

Vidyasagar TR. (2001). *From attentional gating in macaque primary visual cortex to dyslexia in humans.* Progress in Brain Research, 134: 297-312.

Westheimer G, Hauske G. (1975). *Temporal and spatial interference with vernier acuity.* Vision Research, 15: 1137-1141.

Westheimer G, Shimamura K, McKee SP. (1976) *Interference with line-orientation sensitivity.* Journal of Optic Society of America, 66: 332-338.

Wilkinson F, Wilson HR, Ellemberg D. (1997). *Lateral interactions in peripherally viewed texture arrays.* Journal of the Optical Society of America A, 14: 2057-2068.

Wolford G. (1975). *Perturbation model for letter identification.* Psychological Review, 82: 184-199.

Wolford G, Shum KH. (1980). *Evidence for feature perturbations.* Perception & Psychophysics, 27: 409-420.

Yu D, Cheung SH, Legge GE, Chung STL. (2007). *Effect of letter spacing on visual span and reading speed.* Journal of Vision, 7(2), 2: 1-10.

Chapter XIV

One or More Dyslexias?

It is a matter of debate whether developmental dyslexia is a single entity characterized by variations along a continuum of lexical abilities or if it is made of different types. This is a crucial aspect since it could help to account for the different responses to the psychophysical and electrophysiological tests as well as for rehabilitative purpose.

As reminded by Stein [2001], reading requires the integration of two different stages:

- The visual recognition and integration of the letters making up the syllables and in turn the words.
- The phonological (i.e. grapheme-to-phoneme) conversion that serves the purpose of matching each syllable with the corresponding sound.

The selective or predominant alteration of one of these two processes may lead to different clinical orientations, such to make developmental dyslexia not a single, uniform entity but a set of classes. Therefore, Boder proposed to divide developmental dyslexia into three classes [Boder, 1973]:

- dyseidetic
- dysphonetic
- dysphoneidetic or mixed forms[248].

Dyseidetic dyslexics are prevented from recognizing the word as a whole, as a single orthographic configuration, as a visual *gestalt*[249]. For this reason, the only way patients have to read is via an analysis of the word letter-by-letter, i.e. by using the so-called *sublexical route*[250]. Errors concern especially phonetically irregular words[251]. Dyseidetic subjects, whose

---

[248] Dyslexics can be divided according to the classification of Boder by means of the Dyslexia Determination Test [Griffin & Walton,1987] or The Adult Dyslexia Test [Griffin et al., 1990].

[249] Gestalt can be translated as "organized whole" and refers to the phenomenon for which the global configuration has a greater value than its single constituents. For example, when presenting a drawing of a house, the house is recognized as such and not as the walls, roof and windows it is made of.

[250] See part II, chapter 6.

[251] Like the English words "laugh" or "does", which can be respectively read as "log" or "laf" and "duz".

prevalence ranges from 10 to 30%[252] [Flynn & Deering, 1989; Boder & Flynn, 1991], are claimed to suffer from a visuoperceptive impairment [Boder, 1973; Ciesielski, 1989; Flynn & Boder, 1991; Farmer & Klein, 1995].

Unlike the dyseidetic type, the dysphonetic form, whose incidence in the dyslexic population is about 55-70% [Deering & Flynn, 1989; Flynn & Boder, 1991], is affected by phonological problems [Boder, 1973; Farmer & Klein, 1995] and by the difficulty to apply the grapheme-to-phoneme conversion. Moreover, dysphonetics are prevented from analyzing the elementary constituents (the letters and then the syllables) of the words[253]. Their difficulty is particularly evident when reading unfamiliar words or the so-called non-words[254] that are meaningless configurations[255]. Non-words, indeed, cannot be inferred based on their visual configurations, but they require a systematic decoding and arrangement of their components, i.e. letters and then syllables. Now, such a combination would be defective in this class of patients.

Finally, the dysphoneidetic pattern shares characteristics belonging to the two previous subgroups and is considered the most severe form. Its prevalence is around 10% [Flynn & Deering, 1989; Flynn & Boder, 1991].

The classification of Boder requires reading performance to be measured for words and non-words: compared to the normative data, in dyseidetics the reading performance localizes beyond the second standard deviation for words, within the second standard deviation for non-words, and the difference of the two measurements has to be at least half a standard deviation.

On the contrary, the reading performance of the dysphonetics is beyond the second standard deviation for non-words and within the second standard deviation for words, with a difference between the two values of at least half a standard deviation. Finally, if the difference between words and non-words is less than half a standard deviation, the subject is expected to suffer from the mixed or dysphoneidetic forms [Boder, 1973; Lorusso et al., 2004].

The putative correspondence between these classes of dyslexia and a possible cortical impairment has been investigated (figure 1): dyseidetics would suffer from a defect in the gyrus angularis and in the parietooccipital lobe, whereas the dysphonetic type it is advanced to depend on impairment of the gyrus supramarginalis and of the insula [Roeltgen & Heilman, 1984; Ridder et al., 1997][256].

In fact, these classes cannot be so rigidly categorized so as to allow a brain mapping and a univocal correspondence with M/P impairment. Borsting tried to characterize 8 dysphoneidetic and 9 dyseidetic patients by measuring contrast sensitivity for sinusoidal gratings with spatial frequency ranging from 0.5 to 12 cycles/degree, moving with a temporal frequency of 1 Hz and 10 Hz [Borsting et al., 1996]. Surprisingly, compared to controls,

[252] Up to 34% according to Slaghuis & Ryan [1999].

[253] In 1924 Wolpert introduced the term spelling dyslexia to indicate the form that affects subjects who are compelled to decode the word letter by letter, being impossible for them the immediate perception of the shape of a word.

[254] The recognition of irregular words is preserved.

[255] Examples of non-words. in the Italian language are "graceli", "lottopra", in the English language are “bos”, “salder”.

[256] The peculiar damage of the magnocellular system in dysphonetic and dysphoneidetic subjects would lie in the insula [Ridder et al., 1997]; indeed, it is remarkable that according to a PET study the insula shows metabolic activation during the saccadic movements [Anderson et al., 1994].

contrast sensitivity was reduced by about 0.3 log units at low spatial frequencies[257] not in the dyseidetic patients but in the dysphoneidetics. Indeed, since this selective contrast sensitivity defect denotes a magnocellular impairment, this finding suggests the magnocellular visuoperceptive defect to be a marker of the dysphoneidetic dyslexia and not, as expected of the dyseidetics.

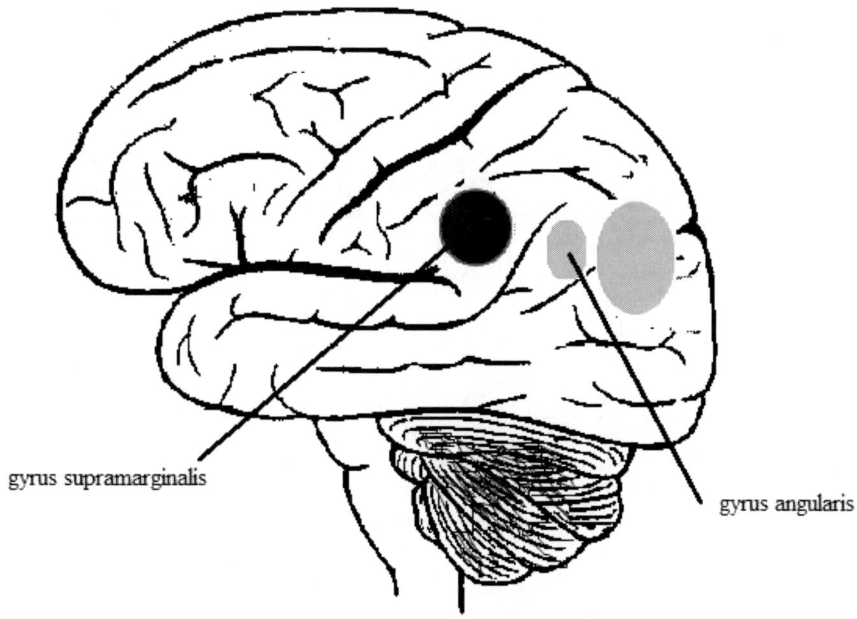

Figure 1. The brain areas putatively related to the different types of dyslexia. Gray: dyseidetic; black: dysphonetic. The insula is not shown in this figure.

The following year the experiment was repeated recruiting also 6 dysphonetic patients and the range of temporal frequency was extended to 25 Hz. The results confirmed decreased contrast sensitivity more evident at the higher temporal frequencies[258] (thence indicative of a magnocellular impairment) only in the dysphoneidetic class [Ridder et al., 1997].

In another study, the three most representative functions in the magnocellular domain, i.e. contrast sensitivity[259], coherent motion perception and vision persistence time have been measured in dyseidetic, dysphoneidetic and dysphonetic teenagers [Slaghuis & Ryan, 1999]. Contrast sensitivity in the first group turned out to be normal, while in dysphoneidetics a reduction was observed at 0.5 and 2 cycles/degree, irrespective of the temporal frequency, and at 2 and 4 cycles/degree for stationary stimuli. Contrast sensitivity in dysphonetics was defective for stationary stimuli (2 and 4 cycles/degree) and at 8 Hz (at 0.5 and 2 cycles/degree). Overall, these results are in line with those of Borsting et al. [1996]. The levels of significance are reported in Table I.

[257] From 0.5 to 2 cycles/degree.

[258] Contrast sensitivity reduced by 0.6 log unit at 25 Hz.

[259] Contrast sensitivity was measured presenting static or flashing gratings with spatial frequency ranging from 0.5 to 8 cycles/degree, at a temporal frequency of 4-16 Hz.

Table I. Levels of significance compared to a control group for different combinations of temporal and spatial contrast sensitivity in dyseidetic (DE), dysphoneidetic (DPE) and dysphonetic (DP) dyslexics. SCTR = significant compared to controls, SCTR+DE = significant compared to controls and dyseidetics. Left: data from Slaghuis & Ryan [1999]. Right: data from Borsting et al. [1996]

Temporal/spatial frequency [Slaghuis& Ryan, 1999]	DE	DPE	DP	Temporal/spatial frequency [Borsting et al., 1996]	DE	DPE
Stat 0.5 c/deg	ns	ns	ns	1Hz 0.5 c/deg	ns	ns
Stat 2 c/deg	ns	Sctr	Sctr	1Hz 1 c/deg	ns	ns
Stat 4 c/deg	ns	Sctr+DE	Sctr+DE	1Hz 2 c/deg	ns	ns
Stat 8 c/deg	ns	ns	ns	1Hz 4 c/deg	ns	ns
4Hz 0.5 c/deg	ns	Sctr	ns	1Hz 8 c/deg	ns	ns
4Hz 2 c/deg	ns	Sctr	ns	1Hz 12 c/deg	ns	ns
4Hz 4 c/deg	ns	ns	ns			
4Hz 8 c/deg	ns	ns	ns			
8Hz 0.5 c/deg	ns	Sctr	Sctr			
8Hz 2 c/deg	ns	Sctr	Sctr			
8Hz 4 c/deg	ns	ns	ns	10Hz 0.5 c/deg	ns	Sctr
8Hz 8 c/deg	ns	ns	ns	10Hz 1 c/deg	ns	Sctr
16Hz 0.5 c/deg	ns	Sctr	ns	10Hz 2 c/deg	ns	Sctr
16Hz 2 c/deg	ns	Sctr	ns	10Hz 4 c/deg	ns	ns
16Hz 4 c/deg	ns	ns	ns	10Hz 8 c/deg	ns	ns
16Hz 8 c/deg	ns	ns	ns	10Hz 12 c/deg	ns	ns

Likewise, coherent motion perception as well as visual persistence time[260] was abnormal only in the dysphonetic subjects. In conclusion, the magnocellular defect does not seem to affect the whole dyslexic population, but is restricted to a group of patients.

Unexpectedly, this group is not the dyseidetic (considered as the class affected by a visuoperceptual impairment), but the dysphonetic and especially the dysphoneidetic types [Borsting et al., 1996].

A later model classifies developmental dyslexia into two classes: *deep* or *phonological dyslexia* and *surface dyslexia* [Castles & Coltheart, 1993]. In deep dyslexia, the sequential analysis of characters and syllables when reading non-words and unfamiliar words is defective. Therefore, in deep dyslexics a decoding anomaly has been postulated [Farmer & Klein, 1995] and phonological dyslexia can be assimilated to the dysphonetic type of Boder. On the contrary, surface dyslexics are mainly prevented from reading terms that cannot be decoded via a grapheme-phoneme conversion, such as the irregular English words [Patterson et al., 1985] or the homophones[261]. Actually, to be read at best, the homophones and irregular

260 The paradigm chosen to measure the visual persistence time was the apparent movement of Ternus (Ternus, 1938: see chapter 8).

261 The homophones are words with same sound but different meanings: in the Italian language: *cieco* and *ceco, lago* and l'ago, letto and *l'etto* (*blind* and *Czech*, *Lake* and *the needle*, *bed* and the *hectogram*, respectively), In English: *buy-by; meet-meat; week-weak.*

words require, more than the local analysis, the visual processing at a global level, that is to say a correct *visual synthesis*: for this reason, surface dyslexia can be assimilated to the dyseidetic form of Boder. In general, reading rate of surface dyslexics is slow, albeit (with the exception of the homophones and irregular terms) quite accurate. The slowness is evident especially when processing words whereas for non-words reading speed is less affected [Longoni et al., 1990].

Surface dyslexia prevails in transparent languages such as German [Wimmer, 1993] and Italian [Sartori & Job, 1983; Zoccolotti et al., 1997, 1999]; on the contrary, deep dyslexia is more common among English native speakers [Castles & Coltheart, 1993,Velvet et al., 2004].

Like Borsting, Slaghuis and Ryan failed in detecting M-related contrast sensitivity defects in the dyseidetic group, so did an Italian study in a sample of patients affected by surface dyslexia[262] [Spinelli et al., 1997].

Impaired temporal rate processing[263] is supposed to be the common basis underlying abnormal reading in both subtypes, to an extent depending on the level (mainly phonological/auditory or visuoperceptive) it shows. However, the fact that the linguistic and orthographic performance of surface dyslexics is similar to that of normal readers, leads to believe that the lexical difficulty in this class comes from a simple developmental delay.

Bakker has advanced a different classification based on the imbalanced activation of the two cerebral hemispheres [Bakker, 1979, 1992]. According to this paradigm, the lexical acquisition in its early stage of development relies on the right hemisphere, which promotes the establishment of the visuoperceptive strategies required to decode the grapheme. Over time, visual decoding becomes automatic and the reading function tends to switch from the right into the left hemisphere, to match the acquired visuoperceptive strategies with the linguistic ones. If this transition is hindered, the young reader cannot do but keeping on the visuoperceptive strategy: the result is a slow and fragmented reading with many repetitions and corrections (time-consuming errors). On the contrary, if the shift is premature, the reader happens to be not yet ready to manage the complex linguistic strategies and to integrate them with the visuoperceptive decoding: in comparison with the previous case, the result is a faster but inaccurate reading with omissions, substitutions or additions (substantive errors). The persistent activation of the right hemisphere accounts for the P-type (or perceptual), while the L-form (or linguistic) would depend on the untimely activation of the left hemisphere. Mixed forms are classified as M-type [Bakker, 1979, 1992]. The reading rate in P-dyslexics is beyond -1 SD compared to the normative values, whereas in the L-type it localizes within this cutoff. The L-form would match the dysphonetic class of Boder, the P-form would fit the dyseidetic type [Licht, 1994].

Therefore, the lexical disability would stem from the imbalance between the activation of the two cerebral hemispheres. An indirect confirmation of the different activation level of the cerebral hemispheres in dyslexics is given by the interemispheric asymmetry of visual checkerboard-evoked potentials: in some patients, in fact, the electrophysiological response is weaker in the right hemisphere, in others it is lower on the left side [Mecacci et al., 1983].

Lovett classifies the dyslexics into two subtypes according as the prominent alteration affects the accuracy (*accuracy disabled*) or the reading rate (*rate disabled*) [Lovett, 1984,

---

[262] In surface dyslexics contrast sensitivity turned out to be defective at the highest spatial frequencies tested (16c/deg) for stationary gratings.

[263] See chapter 12.

1987]. Interestingly, in this second class the lexical accuracy, normal for single words, tends to worsen when reading a text, suggesting the rate disabled dyslexics to be particularly susceptible to the influence of surrounding visual elements.

Table II. The current classifications of developmental dyslexia

Classification	Class	Characteristics
Boder [1973]	Dyseidetic	Impaired recognition of the word as a whole. Use of the sublexical route. Prevalent impairment: words and irregular words.
	Dysphonetic	Prevalent impairment: non-words. M-system deficit (in the most severe cases).
	Dysphoneidetic	Impairment of words + non-words. M-system deficit. Considered the most severe form.
Castles & coltheart [1993]	Surface dyslexia	Prevalent impairment: words (especially if irregular or homophones). Tendency to turn words into non-words. Use of the sublexical route. Slow but pretty accurate reading. Delayed lexical development.
	Deep or Pholonogical	Prevalent impairment: non-words. Anatomofunctional anomaly.
Bakker [1979, 1992]	L form	Related to the dysphonetic type of Boder. Faster but less accurate reading than the P form. Higher activation of the left hemisphere.
	P form	Related to the dyseidetic type of Boder. Slower, hesitant, fragmented reading, but more accurate than the L form. Higher activation of the right hemisphere.
	M form	Features of the two previous types.
Stein & fowler [1982]	Visual	Fixation instability due to unstable dominance prevents the accurate sequential analysis of the sentence. Impairment of non-words and words (words are transformed into non-words). M-system deficit.
Lovett [1984, 1987]	Accuracy disabled	Defective word recognition. Reduced accuracy.
	Rate disabled	Decreased reading rate when reading sentences. Particular susceptibility to the surrounding visual elements (increased crowding effect?).
Valdois [1995]	Visuoattentional	Visuoattentional deficit. Prevalent impairment: non-words.
	Non visuoattentional	Lack of visuoattentional deficit.

Even the visual attention may be a discriminating criterion: patients free from attentional defects show a good ability especially when processing non-words, that (compared to words) demand a higher visuo-attentional level. On the contrary, the so-called *visuoattentional dyslexia* refers to dyslexics affected by impaired visual attention [Valdois et al., 1995].

A classification has been provided even from a visual perspective. It makes the stability of ocular dominance as the distinctive factor of the so-called *visual dyslexia* [Stein & Fowler, 1982]: when performing the Dunlop test, visual dyslexics would show unstable dominance, which affects their fixation when reading[264].

Table II resumes the aforementioned paradigms.

In summary, developmental dyslexia can be considered not as a single entity but made of at least two different subtypes, one of which is mainly characterized by a deficit of the transient system along the visual pathway. The involvement of more genes, one of them in charge of the orthographic ability, one of the phonological ability and finally one responsible for both functions, supports this position [Stein, 2001]. Therefore, equivocal results may arise when the dyslexic class of the recruited patients is not taken into consideration [Lennerstrand & Ygge, 1992]. As an example, the frequent lack of classification of the dyslexic sample could explain why even when mean differences are statistically significant, the visuoperceptive alterations never involve all the subjects under examination [Victor et al., 1993; Gross-Glenn et al., 1995; Johannes et al., 1996].

Yet, according to other researchers, developmental dyslexia represents the tail of a Gaussian distribution of the lexical skill in the general population: the peak is represented by the normal readers while the left portion includes subjects with reduced lexical ability (figure 2). The studies of Shaywitz et al. [1992], Eden et al. [1994], implicitly Demb et al. [1998] and more recently of Patching and Jordan [2005] support this point of view: dyslexia is expected to be the final part of a continuum of lexical skills, starting from a condition of good reading, passing through poor readers and ending with dyslexics. The continuity of the spectrum is suggested by the fact that not only in dyslexics but even in normal subjects the contrast sensitivity of the best readers is higher compared to the less proficient ones and this difference correlates with the reading rate.

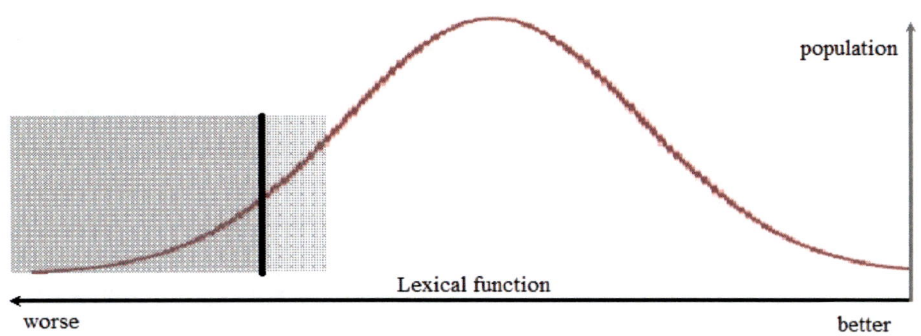

Figure 2. The distribution of the lexical ability in the population. The light grey area on the right side of the black bar refers to poor readers, the dark gray interval on the left side of the black bar identifies dyslexics. The position of the black bar corresponds to the operational definition (reading rate -2SD compared to the normative values).

[264] Visual dyslexics would be also characterized by the debated deficit of contrast sensitivity [Mason et al., 1993].

Not only contrast sensitivity but even critical fusion frequency and coherent motion perception show a consistent correlation with the lexical performance[265] (r=0.461 and 0.356, respectively), irrespective of the lexical level [Talcott et al., 1998].

The same applies to the visual attention. Visual attention has been assessed in a group of 59 normal children[266] by comparing coherent motion detection before and after adding a cue aimed at promoting the attentive orientation: in subjects whose visual attention is efficient, adding the cue would improve motion detection, otherwise it would be of no avail [Kinsey et al., 2004]. According to this paradigm, visual attention turned out to be less efficient in the poor readers than in the most skilled ones and was found to correlate to the reading ability, suggesting it could be a marker of the lexical function both in dyslexics and in normal children [Kinsey et al., 2004]. As expected, the finding (further confirmed by Talcott et al., 2002), was more evident with non-words, since non-words require higher visuo-attentional levels compared to words[267].

Therefore visual attention, contrast sensitivity, movement perception, critical frequency of fusion, dominance stability and, probably, lateral masking, in the general population are expected to follow a Gaussian distribution across the spectrum of reading ability, from normal readers to dyslexics.

Different subtypes of lexical disabilities could stem from the different combination of these functional profiles in each single case. This solution seems able to combine the two positions: dyslexia as a single clinical entity forming the tail of a continuous distribution and dyslexia as a multifaceted condition made of different classes.

By integrating each other, these abnormal functions would contribute to determine in each patient a complex pattern of abnormalities depending on the different contribution of each component: yet, the resulting patterns, albeit different, fall within the same pathological condition, that is to say developmental dyslexia (Figure 3).

Therefore, together to patients with prevalent difficulty in grapheme/phoneme conversion (dysphonetics or deep dyslexics), the left tail of the spectrum would be made of subjects who show substantial problems in the visual processing of the word as a whole, i.e. as a single configuration (dyseidetics or surface dyslexics).

Still, not only the second group but even the first could be affected by a perceptive problem. This anomaly, however, would not occur at a global level, that is to say in processing the words as single configurations but at a local level, in the analysis of the single letters and syllables.

In summary, a visuoperceptive impairment can affect reading in two different ways: on a local and global plane. The terms "phonological" or "dysphonetic" and dyseidetic are therefore misleading not only because they tend to oppose the phonological impairment to the visuoperceptive one but even because the latter is limited to the dyseidetic (global) approach without considering the analytical (local) involvement. In fact, in developmental dyslexics the phonological and the visual aspects rather than opposing, are strictly intermingled.

Upon these bases, at the end of the second part will be advanced a personal classification of the visuoperceptive component worthy to be experimentally verified.

[265] Especially referred to non-words.

[266] Aged between 8.9 and 11.8 years.

[267] Especially compared the more common words, that do not require a sequential analysis of the syllables to be recognized.

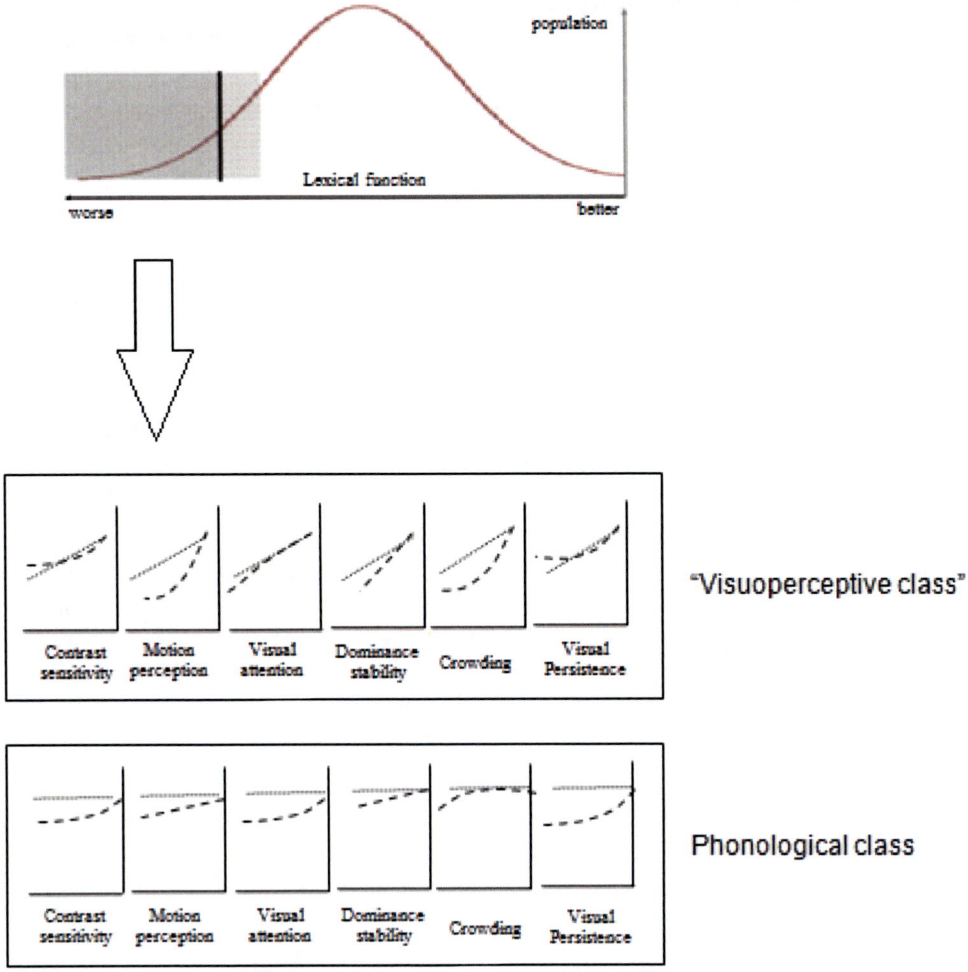

Figure 3. The contributions of the defective visuoperceptive functions in the different subtypes of development dyslexia. In the panels below the distribution frequency; the ordinate refers to the level of efficiency of the function, the abscissa to the lexical ability within the grey area. Upper panel: a *visuoperceptive class* shows the worsening of the visuoperceptive tasks as a function of the reading ability (dashed lines). However the phonological component (dotted line) is constantly present, irrespective of the amount of the impairment referred to each visuoperceptive function. Lower panel: a pure phonological class shows no worsening in the visuoperceptive domain (gray lines) as a function of the reading ability. However, in some cases the phonological component to a certain extent can be supplemented by a visuoperceptive component (dashed line) making the phonological class less "pure". For illustrative purposes in the upper panel the relation between phonological impairment and reading ability (dotted line) is linear. The shape of the curves is purely indicative.

References

Anderson TJ, Jenkins IH, Brooks DJ, Hawken MB, Frackowiak RSJ, Kennard C. (1994). *Cortical control of saccades and fixation in man. A PET study.* Brain, 117: 1073-1084.

Bakker DJ. (1979). *Hemispheric differences and reading strategies: Two dyslexias?* Bulletin of the Orton Society, 29: 84-100.

Bakker DJ. (1992). *Neuropsychological classification and treatment of dyslexia.* Journal of Learning Disabilities, 25: 102-109.

Boder E. (1973). *Developmental dyslexia: a diagnostic approach based on three atypical reading-spelling patterns.* Developmental Medicine and Child Neurology, 15: 663-687.

Borsting E, Ridder WH, Dudeck K, Kelley C, Matsui L, Motoyama J. (1996). *The presence of a magnocellular defect depends on the type of dyslexia.* Vision Research, 36: 1047-1053.

Castles A, Coltheart M. (1993). *Varieties of developmental dyslexia.* Cognition, 47: 149-180.

Ciesielski KT. (1989). *Event-related potentials in children with specific cognitive disability.* Neuropsychologia, 27: 303-313.

Demb JB, Boynton GM, Best M, Heeger DJ. (1998). *Psychophysical evidence for a magnocellular pathway deficit in dyslexia.* Vision Research, 38: 1555-1559.

Eden GF, Stein JF, Wood MH, Wood FB. (1994). *Differences in eye movements and reading problems in dyslexics and normal children.* Vision Research, 34:1345-1358.

Farmer ME, Klein RM. (1995). *The evidence for a temporal processing deficit-linked to dyslexia.* Psychonomic Bulletin Review, 2: 460-493.

Flynn JM, Boder E. (1991). *Clinical and electrophysiological correlates of dysphonetic and dyseidetic dyslexia.* In:Vision and Visual Dyslexia, Stein Ed., CRC Press, Boca Ranton, FL.

Flynn JM, Deering WM. (1989). *Subtypes of dyslexia: investigation of Boder's system using quantitative neurophysiology.* Developmental Medicine and Child Neurology, 31: 215-223.

Griffin JR, Walton HN. (1987). *Dyslexia Determination Test.* I-MED, Los Angeles.

Griffin JR, Christenson GN, Walton HN. (1990). *The Adult Dyslexia Test.* Reading and Perception Therapy Center, Culver City, CA.

Gross-Glenn K, Skottun BC, Glenn W, Kushch A, Lingua R, Dunbar M, Jallad B, Lubs HA, Levin B, Rabin M, Parke LA, Duara R. (1995). *Contrast sensitivity in dyslexia.* Visual Neuroscience, 12: 153-163.

Johannes S, Kussmaul CL, Munte TF, Mangun GR. (1996). *Developmental dyslexia: passive visual stimulation provides no evidence for a magnocellular processing defect.* Neuropsychologia, 34: 1123-1127.

Kinsey K, Rose M, Hansen P, Richardson A, Stein J. (2004). *Magnocellular-mediated visual-spatial attention and reading ability.* Neuroreport, 15: 1-5.

Lennerstrand G, Ygge J. (1992). *Dyslexia: ophthalmological aspects 1991.* Acta Ophthalmologica, 70: 3-13.

Licht R. (1994). *Differences in word recognition between P- and L-type reading disability.* In: The Balance Model of Dyslexia: Theoretical and clinical progress, Licht & Spyer Eds., Van Gorcum, Assen, NL.

Longoni AM, Scalisi TG, Sigismondi A. (1990). *Studio di un caso di dislessia evolutiva.* Rassegna di Psicologia, 7: 31-47.

Lorusso ML, Facoetti A, Pesenti S, Cattaneo C, Molini m, Geiger G. (2004). *Wider recognition in peripheral vision common to different subtypes of dyslexia.* Vision Research, 44: 2413-2424.

Lovett MW. (1984). *A developmental perspective on reading dysfunction: accuracy and rate criteria in the subtyping of dyslexic children.* Brain and Language, 22: 67-91.

Lovett MW. (1987). *A developmental approach to reading disability: accuracy and speed criteria of normal and deficient reading skill.* Child Development, 58: 234-260.

Mason A, Cornelissen P, Fowler S, Stein J. (1993). *Contrast sensitivity, ocular dominance and specific reading disability*. Clinical Vision Sciences, 8: 345-353.

Mecacci L, Sechi E, Levi G. (1983). *Abnormalities of visual evoked potentials by checkerboards in children with specific reading disability.* Brain and Cognition, 2: 135-143.

Patching GR, Jordan TR. (2005). *Spatial frequency sensitivity differences between adults of good and poor reading ability.* Investigative Ophthalmology and Visual Science, 46: 2219-2223.

Patterson KE, Marshall JC, Coltheart M. (1985). *Surface dyslexia : Neuropsychological anfd cognitive analyses of phonological reading*, Patterson, Marshall & Coltheart Eds., Erlbaum, London.

Ridder W, Borsting E, Cooper M, NcNeel B, Huang E. (1997). *Not all dyslexics are created equal*. Optometry and Vision Science, 74: 99-104.

Roeltgen DP, Heilman KM. (1984). *Lexical agraphia further support for the two-system hypothesis of linguistic agraphia*. Brain, 107: 811-827.

Sartori G, Job R. (1983). *Phonological impairment in Italian: Acquired and delopmental dyslexia.* In: The acquisition of symbolic skills. Rogers & Sloboda Eds., Plenum Press, New York.

Shaywitz SE, Escobar MD, Shaywitz BA, Fletcher JM, Makuch R. (1992). *Evidence that dyslexia may represent the lower tail of a normal distribution of reading ability*. New England Journal of Medicine, 326: 145-150.

Slaghuis WL, Ryan JF. (1999). *Spatio-temporal contrast sensitivity, coherent motion, and visible persistence in developmental dyslexia.* Vision Research, 39: 651-668.

Spinelli D, Angelelli P, De Luca M, Di Pace E, Judica A, Zoccolotti PL. (1997). *Developmental surface dyslexia is not associated with deficits in the transient visual system*. NeuroReport, 8: 1807-1812.

Stein JF, Fowler S. (1982). *Diagnosis of dyslexia by means of a new indicator of eye dominance.* British Journal of Ophthalmology, 66: 332-336.

Stein JF. (2001). *The magnocellular theory of developmental dyslexia.* Dyslexia, 7: 12-36.

Talcott JB, Hansen PC, Willis-Owen C, McKinnell IW, Richardson AJ, Stein JF. (1998). *Visual magnocellular impairment in adult develomental dyslexics.* Neuro-Ophthalmology, 20: 187-201.

Talcott JB, Witton C, Hebb GS, Stoodley CJ, Westwood EA, France SJ, Hansen PC, Stein JF. (2002). *On the relationship between dynamic visual and auditory processing and literacy skills; results from a large primary-school study*. Dyslexia, 8: 204-225.

Ternus J. (1938). *The problem of phenomenal identity.* A sourcebook of Gestalt psychology. Ellis DW Ed., Routledge & Kegan, London.

Valdois S, Gérard C, Vanault P, Dugas M. (1995). *Peripheral developmental dyslexia: a visual attentional account?* Cognitive Neuropsychology, 12: 31-67.

Vellutino FR, Fletcher JM, Snowling MJ, Scanlon DM. (2004). *Specific reading disability (dyslexia): what have we learned in the past four decades?* Journal of Child Psychology and Psychiatry, 45: 2-40.

Victor JD, Conte MM, Burton L, Nass R. (1993). *Visual evoked potentials in dyslexics and normals: failure to find a difference in transient or steady-state responses.* Visual Neuroscience, 10: 939-946.

Wimmer H. (1993). *Characteristics of developmental dyslexia in a regular writing system.* Applied Psycholinguistics, 14: 1-33.

Wolpert I. (1924). *Die Simultanagnosie: Storung der gesamtauffassung.* Zeitschrift fur die Gesamte Neurologie und Psychiatrie, 93: 397.

Zoccolotti P, Angelelli P, Colombini MG, De Luca M, Di Pace E, Judica A, Orlandi M, Spinelli D. (1997). *Caratteristiche della dislessia superficiale evolutiva nella lingua italiana.* Archivio di Psicologia Neurologia e Psichiatria, 58; 254-284.

Zoccolotti P, De Luca M, Di Pace E, Judica A, Orlandi M, Spinelli D. (1999). *Markers of developmental surface dyslexia in a language (Italian) with high grapheme-phoneme correspondence.* Applied Psycholinguistics, 20: 191-216.

Chapter XV

Visual Rehabilitation: State of the Art and Controversies

It is clear, at this point, that dyslexics may suffer even from a visuoperceptive impairment that contributes to the deterioration of the lexical function. If on the one hand dyslexia does not rely solely on a visuoperceptive deficiency, on the other hand the phonological alteration *per se* is often unable to account for all the signs and symptoms, as well as for the different lexical patterns among patients. Moreover, the visual aspect can be a relevant factor not only in the diagnostic phase but also for the rehabilitative approach: indeed, more than 30% of the patients do not respond satisfactory to the phonological treatment alone [Whiteley et al., 2007]. It is revealing that in recent decades many visuoperceptive rehabilitation protocols have been advanced and especially in the English-speaking countries the number of publications in the optometric field on the subject has been growing exponentially. And yet, many of these studies are affected by procedural irregularities, questionable statistical analysis and arguable interpretation of the results, so that authoritative organizations such as the *American Academy of Pediatrics*, the *American Association for Pediatric Ophthalmology and Strabismus and the American* Academy of Ophthalmology in 1998 and then in 2001 admonished against visual rehabilitative solutions. They stated that, to date, there is no scientific evidence that correction of subtle visual defects can alter the brain's processing of the visual stimuli and that dyslexics should avoid remedies involving eye exercises, filters, tinted lenses, or other optical devices that are lacking of scientific prove of efficacy [1998][268]. Although developmental dyslexia is conceivable as a *continuum* of lexical abilities, classifying patients is a fundamental requisite to assess correctly the results obtained in the advanced visuoperceptive treatments and, if proved effective, to customize their administration according to the subtype of dyslexia the patients belong to.

In evaluating and prescribing visuoperceptive rehabilitation programs, caution is mandatory to avoid false expectations in patients and in parents.

Since a treatment should be undertaken as soon as possible, early diagnosis is crucial [Lennerstrand & Ygge, 1992]: the development of the M-mediated visual functions is completed around 8-10 years of age [Barnard et al., 1998], so patients should be treated

[268] A firm reply to this official position was published the same year on *Optometry* [Bowan, 1998].

before this age. Still, when, that is to say at what age the treatment should be administered is a matter of debate: since many pupils suspected to be dyslexics in the first grade school demonstrated normal reading skills in the third grade [Shaywitz et al., 1992], it has been suggested to let the children develop their own lexical strategy and, in case, to treat them later (at 8 years). In this case the treatment should not be aimed at replacing their acquired lexical paradigm but at assisting it [Geiger et al., 1994; Geiger & Lettvin, 2000]. The possibility that dyslexics implement spontaneously a second and more effective reading strategy after becoming aware of the weakness of the former is suggested by the existence of the so-called *conditional dyslexics* [Geiger & Lettvin, 2000]. Conditional dyslexics are those patients (more common than it is generally believed) showing different lexical ability and different profiles of their attentional visual field (the FRF) during the day (but irrespective of the day or the week). It is as if in some moments they could put the most effective (recently acquired) strategy into practice and in others they come back to their previous one: during the "good" periods the FRF turns out to be normalized while in the "bad" times it is abnormal [Geiger et al., 1992].

Listing all the visuoperceptive rehabilitative solutions, many of which are not properly visual, would go beyond the aim of this study. The discussion will focus on the most authoritative experiences that have to do with our competences.

The visual conditions that promote reading[269] are:

- normal visual acuity.
- normal oculomotor coordination and fixation: in particular, convergence deficit often makes vision blurred and unsteady, leading to asthenopia.
- Normal accommodation.
- Neutral or suitably corrected refraction.

A failure in one or more of these factors may hamper reading and learning to read, so a complete ophthalmological and orthoptic examination (with particular attention to refraction, accommodation, convergence, phorias, fusional amplitudes, oculomotor control and ocular dominance) is recommendable in the visual assessment of dyslexic patients. In case of a convergence defect, even mild, orthoptic training has to be administered and it is advisable to correct any refractive error. However, even if ruling out problems of this type can help the lexical task, it is not a solution *per se*.

As stated by Norn, when asthenopia is treated by a great variety of corrections, this can by no means be identified with the therapy or the cure of developmental dyslexia, and if the cure is obtained, this must be due to a mistaken diagnosis. Therefore, even though visual anomalies may make reading extremely difficult, they are not the cause of developmental dyslexia. However, a careful ophthalmological examination is recommendable for dyslexic children to prevent possibly existing visual anomalies from worsening the reading disability. [Norn et al., 1969].

The visual rehabilitative techniques advanced so far can be divided into four categories (Table I): a-functional therapies. b-oculomotor training. c-visuoperceptive training. d-pharmacological therapies.

[269] But do not prevent developmental dyslexia.

Table I. The main visual rehabilitation techniques advanced for the treatment of developmental dyslexia. In the third column are the studies in support, in the last column the possible counter evidence

Functional therapies	Dominance reinforcement by monocular occlusion	Stein & Fowler, 1981, 1982, 1985; Masters, 1988; Stein et al., 1987, 1988, 2000; Stein & Talcott, 1999.	Bishop, 1989.
Oculomotor training		Coleman, 1972; Heath et al., 1976; Getz, 1980; Seiderman, 1980; Flax, 1983; Solan, 1981,1993; Williams et al., 1992.	Farr & Leibowitz, 1976; Gilberg & Gilberg, 1983; Kavale & Mattson, 1983.
Visuoperceptive training	*Training* of visual attention	Bakker & Vinke, 1985; Geiger & Lettvin, 1986; Bakker et al., 1981, 1990; Rayner et al., 1989; Bakker, 1992; Geiger et al., 1994; Geiger & Lettvin, 1999, 2000; Facoetti et al., 2003; Lorusso et al., 2005.	Fahle & Luberichs, 1995.
	Audiovisual training	Kujala et al., 2001.	
	crowding reduction and *visual span* extension	Spinelli et al., 2002.	
Pharmacological therapy	Piracetam	Di Ianni, 1985; Wilsher, 1986; Wilsher et al., 1987; Winblad, 2005.	
	Supplementation with polyunsaturated fatty acids	Stordy, 1995; Richardson & Montgomery, 2005.	
	Methylphenidate	Sheppard et al., 1999.	
Compensatory strategies	Coloured filters	Irlen, 1983, 1989, 1991; (Stein, 2003).	Hoyt, 1990; Parker, 1990; Robinson & Foreman, 1990a,b; Evans &Drasdo, 1991; Wilkins, 1994; Christenson et al., 2001.
	Mild positive lenses	Simons & Grisham, 1987; Solan, 1993.	Jennings, 2000.
	(Prisms)	Jaśkowski & Rusiak, 2005.	
	"Anisotropization" of the text	Aleci et al., 2012.	

The rehabilitative techniques must be distinguished from the *compensatory strategies*, which are not aimed at treating the visual system of the patient, but simply to improve reading, counterbalancing his/her deficient functions[270].

Functional Therapies: Monocular Occlusion

Among the advanced rehabilitative techniques based on robust scientific criteria, the monocular occlusion is one of the most promising.

The monocular occlusion aims at treating fixation instability in dyslexics, as shown since the seventies by Dunlop [1972], by enhancing the ocular dominance. Reading of patients with unstable dominance would improve after the occlusion of one eye for a few months during reading and near vision.

The results obtained in a group of 30 dyslexics with unstable dominance[271] have been published in the early eighties [Stein & Fowler, 1981, 1982]. At the end of the follow-up (six months), dominance stability and lexical performance were compared with those of 15 untreated patients. In 51% of the occluded subjects, ocular dominance turned stable, whereas in the control group the change occurred only in 24% of cases. In addition, the lexical age of the treated sample increased in average by 13.5 months compared to 4 months of the control group. In 1985 the results of another study, with a larger sample (148 patients[272]) and a placebo group[273] were published on *Lancet* [Stein & Fowler, 1985].

As previously reported[274], this method of treatment has been debated since from its rational assumptions In particular it was observed that in both experiments the average age of the children, a main factor able to bias the results of the Dunlop test, was not reported [Bishop, 1989].

Moreover, the age and the lexical level of the patients at the baseline are two variables that can affect the results of the occlusive treatment. For this reason, the data obtained from the previous study have been re-evaluated using the T-score[275] instead of the reading age,[276] since the T-score is reported not to be affected by the lexical development over time [Bishop, 1989]. By adopting the T-score, a significant correlation was found between the lexical level at the baseline and its subsequent improvement after six and twelve months: the reading improvement achieved by patients would depend, therefore, on their lexical level at the baseline: the more severe the initial lexical impairment of the child, the less likely it is for him to make consistent progress [Bishop, 1989]. Also, the correlation between development of stable reference and reading improvement would depend on the initial reading ability, so that children who developed stable reference in the first phase of the study tended to be those patients whose initial reading problems were less severe [Bishop, 1989]. This are

[270] However, some strategies like the variation of the spatial characteristics of the text could have even a positive modulatory effect on the plasticity of the cortical areas, helping over time the lexical improvement.

[271] As assessed with the Dunlop test.

[272] Of the 148 patients, 68% showed unstable dominance.

[273] As a placebo was prescribed a pair of glasses.

[274] See chapter 10.

[275] The T-score (that can be regarded as an analogous of the z-score) refers to the number of standard deviations (SD) above or below the mean reading value measured in a normal population of the same age. An

[276] Normally the lexical age matches the chronological age. Reduced lexical age compared to the chronological age is suggestive of reading disability.

considerations that tend to discredit a treatment that is expected to be equally (if not *more*) effective in the most serious situations.

Finally, the reading improvement observed after the first six months in children who developed stable dominance was not confirmed after twelve months, i.e. at the end of the second follow-up. Therefore, the putative ameliorative effect of monocular occlusion in children with unfixed reference in improving their reading scores has been questioned.

And yet, as reminded by Stein, the estimate based on T-scores has several drawbacks, since T scores are not sensitive measures of the lexical function and their use prevents from detecting the reading progress made from a consistent proportion of children after developing stable vergence control [Stein, 1989]. By adopting the more sensitive lexical age, the reading improvement of children whose vergence control became stable would become evident in dyslexic children, independently of their lexical age at the baseline or of their IQ [Stein, 1989].

It is therefore reaffirmed and underlined that:

1. a deficit of the binocular control can determine the lexical problems of a child as it makes him unable to accurately locate small visual stimuli such as letters in a word.
2. monocular occlusion, enhancing the stability of dominance, improves the convergence control and eventually helps the fixation to be stable: thereby, patients tend to read faster and better.

Even if a poor binocular control can be the consequence of linguistic difficulties, many children with reading problems do suffer from primitive fixation instability [Stein, 1989].

The effectiveness of monocular occlusion[277], has been confirmed in other experiments, with reading improvement after 6 months in 2/3 of the pathological sample [Stein et al., 1987, 1988], in line with the results published by Masters in the same period [1988].

Moreover, about ten years later in a group of 143 dominant unstable dyslexics[278] without ophthalmological or orthoptic problems, a double-masking study was performed [Stein et al., 2000]. In this investigation, only half of the sample underwent the occlusion. Dominance stability and lexical performance in this group were compared after 3, 6 and 9 months with the results measured in the control patients who received a pair of yellow lenses as a placebo. After 3 months, 59% of the occluded dyslexics and only 36% of the controls turned out to have stable dominance at the Dunlop test. After 9 months this difference turned to not significant, as the percentage of subjects who had achieved a stable dominance in the meantime had increased to a less extent in the case (occluded) group compared to the controls (5% vs. the 18% respectively). The improvement would be permanent, with no need to repeat the treatment [Stein et al., 2000]. Even if some regressions to the starting unstable fixation condition were observed among the treated dyslexics, reading ability of patients who achieved dominance stability improved, confirming the relationship between occlusive treatment and lexical progress.

The protocol is suitable to children aged between 7 and 11 years [Stein & Fowler, 1985], but it is more effective if administered within 9 years of age [Stein & Talcott, 1999]. So, the

[277] In association with orthoptic training.
[278] Age between 7 and 11 years.

scientists claimed that the oculomotor consequences of a magnocellular deficit may be solved with an early rational treatment aimed at the underlying mechanism.

In conclusion, monocular occlusion seems to be effective in improving reading in dyslexic patients affected by unstable dominance. However, before it can be definitely accepted, this rehabilitation technique requires (as usual) experimental confirmation from other laboratories.

Visual Training of the Eye Movements

Visual training can be defined as the training of the visual system aimed at obtaining the normalization of its own defective functions. In this case, the defective function is the lexical ability and visual training focuses on the eye movements. Even if the majority of the optometric literature supports the effectiveness of this technique (see for example Coleman, 1972; Flax, 1983; Seiderman, 1980; Solan, 1981, 1993, Williams et al., 1992), as a matter of fact a real improvement in the oculomotor pattern is reported in a limited number of studies [Heath et al., 1976; Getz, 1980], and even less investigations support the ameliorative effect of the training of the eye movements on the lexical function. Gillberg and Gillberg [1983] for example, while arguing that visual exercises based on oculomotor tasks can improve the eye movements, have claimed that this progress does not lead to a correspondent reading improvement. Indeed, due to the reduced size or the lack of a control group, the methodological rigor of these studies is often questionable. In many cases visual training was administered together with other rehabilitation programs so that it is difficult to establish to what extent the results depend on the experimental protocol under examination. The *American Academy of Pediatrics* [2011][279] denies any efficacy of the visual training, in line with previous reports [Farr & Leibowitz, 1976] and with a meta-analysis dating 1983 [Kavale & Mattson, 1983].

At the moment, therefore, the usefulness of the oculomotor training in the treatment of developmental dyslexia is controversial. The attempts[280] stem more from empirical and anecdotal findings than from controlled and severe clinical trials.

Visuoperceptive Training

Compared to the oculomotor training, the scientific basis of the visuoperceptive trainings advanced so far seems to be sounder. However, few studies on this topic are available, to date [281].

In a neurophtalmological perspective, the more interesting researches were addressed to the rehabilitation of visual attention, crossmodal audiovisual stimulation and lateral masking facilitation.

[279] For an exhaustive discussion see: American Academy of Pediatrics, 2011: p. 845-846.
[280] For further information refer to the specific studies.
[281] For an exhaustive (but conservative) discussion see: American Academy of Pediatrics, 2011: p. 843-848.

i-Visual Attention Rehabilitation

As previously reported, visual attention is made of two stages: attentional orientation, able to select the visual region where the target localizes [Facoetti et al., 2003] and attentional focusing, aimed at enhancing the visual processing of the target by preventing the input coming from the surrounding stimuli via inhibitory circuits [Cave & Zimmerman, 1997; Mounts, 2000].

A defect of these dynamics in dyslexics is of great importance and should deserve to be adequately treated [Brannan & Williams, 1987; Gernsbacher, 1993; Geiger & Lettvin, 1999; Klein & D'Entremont, 1999; Facoetti et al., 2003]. Indeed, the rehabilitation of the lexical function by visual attention training is shown to be promising and could be a valuable approach to investigate the role of this function on the lexical disability.

Visual Hemispheric Specific Stimulation (VHSS)

Bakker maintained that the lexical disability depends on an imbalance of the activation of the two cerebral hemispheres[282]. The preferential activation of the right hemisphere causes a slow and fragmented reading, typical of the perceptual or P-form, whereas the preferential activation of the left hemisphere that accounts for the linguistic or L-type, makes reading rapid but inaccurate. The M-type encompasses the characteristics of both L- and P-type. The *Visual Hemispheric Specific Stimulation* (*VHSS*: Bakker et al., 1990; Bakker, 1992] aims at stimulating the defective hemisphere (left in the P-type, right in the L-type) by projecting words in the contralateral visual hemifield (right hemifield for the P-type, left for the L-type)[283].

The treatment led to a reading improvement (speed and accuracy) in 35 L-type and 35 P-type dyslexic children[284], confirmed by the change of the electrophysiological potentials in the two hemispheres (Event-Related Potentials, ERP[285]). The correlation between lexical function and the electrophysiological response turned out to be significant [Bakker & Vinke, 1985]. These results are in agreement with the findings published four years earlier [Bakker, et al., 1981], and later confirmed in 26 L-type and 26 P-type dyslexics [Bakker et al., 1990][286]. The ameliorative effect of the VHSS paradigm as found in English patients applies also to the transparent idioms: the hemispheric function in P-, L- and M-type Italian dyslexics[287] was trained for about 4 months[288] [Facoetti et al., 2003]. At the end of the practice, in these patients average reading speed turned out to be significantly increased, from

---

[282] Chapter 14.

[283] In the VHSS, P-dyslexics are presented simple, high frequency words in their right hemifield while for L-patients are presented complex, low frequency words in the left hemifield. For the mixed forms (M-type) are used stimulations with complex words (L-type stimulations) for the first two months, followed by simple words (P- type stimulations) during the next two months.

[284] Average age: 10 years.

[285] The term ERP is the acronym for for *Event-Related Potential* and refers to any electrophysiological response evoked in the brain by perceptions, thoughts, stimulation, or, as in this case, lexical tasks. Visual Evoked Potentials, a useful tool for the study of the magnocellular function in dyslexics, can be regarded as a particularl type of ERP.

[286] Still, Dryer et al. [1999] found that P and L-type patients after hemispheric visual stimulation improved their lexical performance regardless of the specific (L- or R-) type of stimulation. The authors argued, therefore, that the benefit does not depend on the VHSS per se but is the result of a non-specific effect provided by the visual training.

[287] Mean age: 9.8 years.

[288] Two sessions of 45 minutes a week.

88.7 to 59.2 msec per syllable[289] whereas a control group who was given a linguistic training did not show any improvement. Similar results were obtained considering the reading accuracy, i.e. the reading errors (in average reduction from 10.6 errors to 4.3 errors in the case group after the training)[290].

Modification of the FRF

As previously described, in occidental beginner readers the right hemifield of the form resolving field, symmetrical in preverbal age, narrows progressively so as to take on the normal appearance of the skilled readers [Zegarra-Moran & Geiger, 1993; Lorusso et al., 2004]. The same happens for the left hemifield of the Hebrew pupils, since in the Hebrew writing system the direction of reading is reversed [Geiger et al., 1992]. The fact that the Form Resolving Field narrows in the direction of reading suggests that the visuo-attentional gradient is an acquired function [Geiger & Lettvin, 1987, 1989, 1993; Geiger et al., 1992], and as such liable to be modulated in developmental age [Geiger & Lettvin, 1986]. As a matter of fact, the FRF of dyslexic children is broader and more symmetric than the FRF of adult patients [Geiger et al., 1992].

Since visual training is shown to be effective in improving visual attention [Sireteanu & Rettenbach, 1995] and that visual attention is important for reading, there is reason to believe that an intervention during the plastic phase on the FRF of dyslexics could be effective in correcting its shape. For this purpose a specific rehabilitation technique has been developed. Two monitored clinical trials, the study of Tübingen and the study of Brookline, have been designed to address this topic.

In the first investigation [Geiger et al., 1994], 15 German dyslexic children[291] were recruited. The sample was divided into two groups, a control group made of patients who continued with the traditional rehabilitation protocol adopted in their school and a case group, who in addition was asked to make use when reading of a cardboard mask with a rectangular opening. The opening was large enough to allow reading the longer words while hiding the surrounding text. It was required to place the mask on the page and to read through its opening, making it slide along the sentence (Figure 1). The goal of the mask is to help focusing the visual attention. Patients were required to use the mask while reading at least half an hour a day for three months along with eye/hand coordination exercises[292]. At the end of the training period, a narrowing of the FRF on the right side was observed in the case group but not in the control sample.

Therefore, the shape of FRF in dyslexics subjected to the visual training approached that of the normal readers, as the difference on the right gradient was no longer significant. The change was associated with a significant improvement in reading rate and accuracy (1.22 equivalent degrees[293] in the treated subjects vs.0.17 in the dyslexics belonging to the control group). After other 5 months, a further (albeit more modest) reading progress was observed in the case group (0.62 equivalent degrees). At the same time a reading improvement was evident also in those patients belonging to the control group who, in the meantime, were administered the same rehabilitation protocol. The FRF instead remained unchanged.

---

[289]Corresponding Z-score: from-2.7 to -1.5 SD compared to the normative level.
[290]Corresponding Z-score: from-1.9 to-0.6 SD compared to the normative level.
[291]Mean age: 11 years.
[292]For example drawing, writing, modeling for at least half an hour a day.
[293]The equivalent degree is a unit of measure adopted in the reading tests by German researchers.

The study of Brookline [Geiger & Lettvin, 1999] was similar: 12 dyslexic children[294] were divided into an experimental group and a control group. The experimental group underwent the same rehabilitation protocol adopted in the previous study. After 3.3 months, the FRF narrowing was associated to a reading improved by 1.8 equivalent degrees, rising to 2.75 after 3.7 additional months of training. Since the progress persisted unchanged after five years, it can be regarded as definitively acquired.

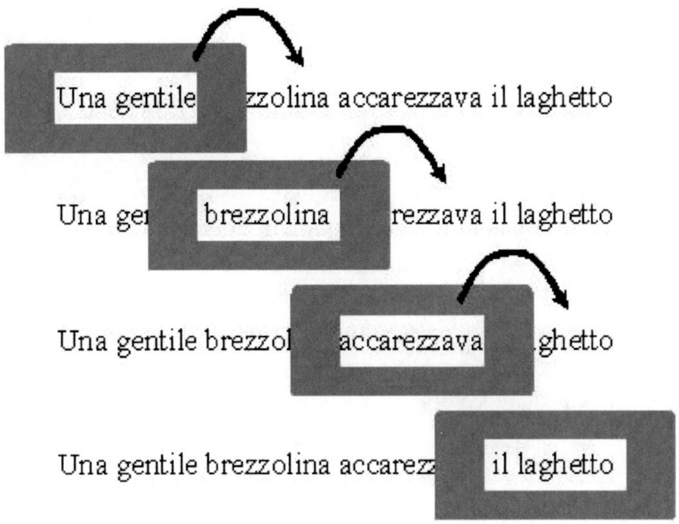

Figure 1. The masking rehabilitation technique. "A gentle breeze caressed the little lake". The patient moves a cardboard mask superimposed on the text toward the right so as to help the attentional focus and to reduce the interference of the peripheral lexical environment.

Rayner reported the case of a college professor suffering from developmental dyslexia diagnosed since he was a boy[295] [Rayner et al., 1989]. He found in this patient a specific attentional deficit characterized by the interference of the peripheral environment on the attentional focus centered on the fixation point: the outcome was a difficulty to process the letters and syllables in foveal projection caused by the masking effect of the parafoveal ones. In this case, too, the aid of a sliding mask adapted to hide the peripheral parts of the string and to expose its central portion led to a lexical improvement. These findings, albeit promising, should be critically examined. Even if the results were confirmed in a subsequent German study on 49 children subjected to a similar rehabilitative training, the improvements were not so evident: 19 patients had no advantage and the progress of the responsive ones was less than expected according to the previous findings[296] [Fahle & Luberichs, 1995]. Moreover, in the reported studies patients were not classified.

The modulation of the FRF has been obtained also by means of the VHSS paradigm. In a group of dyslexic children[297], FRF narrowing was found after VHSS training. However, the change occurred on the left side and not on the right one as expected [Lorusso et al., 2005].

[294] Mean age: 10.8 years.
[295] See chapter 11.
[296] 0.72 equivalent degrees after 2 months.
[297] Age: 8-14 years.

This peculiar result is probably due to the tachistoscopic modality of presentation[298], which would promote the orientation rather than the focusing of visual attention. If this interpretation were confirmed, the application of the VHFF paradigm with short and long presentation times would allow a double modulation of the attentional visual field, enhancing the focusing on the right slope and shifting the orientation from the left to the right side.

ii-Audiovisual Training

More complex training strategies aim at improving the temporal rate processing by joining auditory and visual stimulation. Indeed, normally the auditory input may affect the processing of the visual information [Snowden & Doyle, 2001]. A paradigm aimed at enhancing in dyslexics the plastic modulation of the neuronal structures responsible for the PST has been developed by the group of Kujala [Kujala et al., 2001]. In summary, it consists of a stimulation based on the emission of a sequence of 3-15 tones. Each tone is graphically represented on a screen as a bar whose position, length and thickness depend respectively on its pitch, duration and intensity. The subject was asked to listen to the auditory sequence while following the visual sequence on the screen and to press a key when the last sound corresponding to the last bar was emitted. In the same study, a further stimulation technique was made of two sequences of bars matching two different acoustic sequences. In this case, the task was to associate each of the two acoustic sequences to the corresponding visual sequence (figure 2).

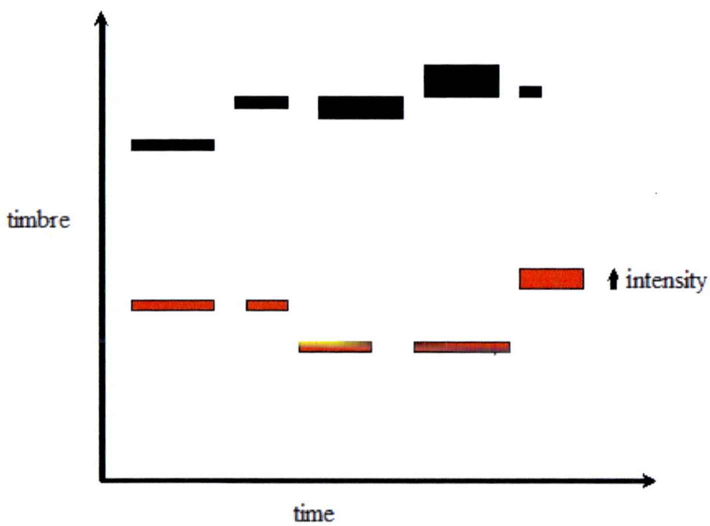

Figure 2. Example of audiovisual training. In black and red are two sequences made up of 5 tones. Visually, each tone corresponds to a bar whose shape and position on the screen depends on its pitch (vertical position of the bar), duration (length), and intensity (thickness). In the first modality, only one sequence is administered. The subject is asked to listen to the acoustic sequence combining the sound heard to the corresponding displayed bar and to press a key after the last tone of the acoustic sequence is emitted. In the second modality, two sequences of bars correspond to two different acoustic sequences. The patient is required to associate each of the two acoustic sequences to the corresponding visual sequence.

[298] Presentation time: 200 msec.

In the experiment, 34 patients underwent the audiovisual training and results were compared with those obtained in 24 untreated dyslexics of the same age (7 years).

Each training session, lasting 10 minutes, was administered twice a week for seven weeks. At the end of the training the children read faster and more accurately. In confirmation of this finding, in 11 dyslexics of the two groups the amplitude of the electroencephalographic potentials registered

during the emission of pairs of tones turned out to be wider in the treated sample.

These reports suggest that the audiovisual training has a positive effect in enhancing the temporal sequential processing and consequently the reading function of dyslexic children. As reported [Singer, 1995; Pantev et al., 1998], early treatment is recommendable and the outcome may depend on the type of dyslexia.

A technique aimed at training dyslexics suffering from TRP impairment to discriminate sequences of sounds has been described also in the auditory domain [Farmer & Klein: 1995]. Patients were required to recognize auditory sequences: at the beginning the task was made easier by increasing the duration of the sounds, then the duration was shortened until the performance of the dyslexics matched that of the normal readers.

As will be discussed in the second part, a similar paradigm could be applied in the visuoperceptive domain in order to correct the abnormal spatial relationship perception, when found in patients.

In conclusion, a growing body of evidence on the neuronal plasticity and its modulation [Ahissar et al., 1992; Näätänen et al., 1993; Recanzone et al., 1993; Elbert et al., 1995; Kraus et al., 1995; Tremblay et al., 1998; Winkler et al., 1999] makes the audiovisual training aimed at improving the temporal rate processing a solution that deserves to be further investigated.

iii-crowding Reduction and Visual Span Extension

As previously reported, positive effect on reading rate may be obtained via a rehabilitative protocol able to reduce crowding and to enlarge the visual span. For a discussion on this topic, refer to chapter 13.

Pharmacological Therapy

The cure of developmental dyslexia does not leave out the pharmacological approach. Particularly interesting are piracetam and especially dietary integration with polyunsaturated fatty acids.

i-Piracetam

Piracetam is a gamma-aminobutyric acid (GABA) derivative, effective in restoring the plasticity of the cellular membranes and in modulating the neuronal transmission. It is well tolerated even at high dosages. Initially defined *nootropic*, it helps the cognitive function without inducing sedation or excitability [Giurgea, 1972]. Piracetam enhances the neural function through the modulation and the consolidation of synaptic connections. In a double masking study, 12 weeks long piracetam treatment was found effective in improving the reading rate in a sample of 275 dyslexics [Di Ianni et al., 1985]. The finding has been confirmed in a further multicentric double-masking investigation, which involved 225 dyslexic children[299]. The improvement, in the absence of important side effects, was observed after the first 12 weeks of therapy and persisted as long as the end of the follow-up (36 weeks) [Wilsher et al., 1987]. At least two reviews [Wilsher, 1986; Windblad, 2005] confirmed the usefulness of piracetam in a wide range of conditions including developmental dyslexia. The effect of the drug on the lexical function of dyslexic children, however, is modest and in many cases takes months to show.

ii-Polyunsaturated Fatty Acids

The integration with polyunsaturated fatty acids is an interesting possibility that is recently gaining consent. Fatty acids in the form of phospholipids are the major constituents of cellular membranes. Cellular membranes are made of a double layer of these molecules in which a fatty acid is linked to the second atom of the carbon chain (position SN-2). The membrane is continually renewed by a metabolic cycle driven by the cytosolic phospholipase A2 enzyme (PLA2). The PLA2 takes off the fatty acid from the SN-2 position, renews it and places it back in the same place on the phospholipidic molecule [Horrobin et al., 1995; Horrobin & Bennett, 1999]. This process requires a large amount of polyunsaturated fatty acids, in particular arachidonic, digammalinolenic, docosahexaenoic and eicosapentaenoic acid. In the adult these substances are obtained via synthesis from precursors (α-linolenic acid and linolenic acid) while in the fetus and in the early postnatal period it is provided by the mother respectively via the placenta and mother's milk.

Polyunsaturated fatty acids, which make up 20% of the dry weight of the brain, are involved in myelinogenesis so that reduced dietary intake may result in abnormal myelination of the ganglion cells of the visual pathway [Biase & Salvati, 1997; Mayer, 1999]. This defect is functionally revealed by abnormal visual evoked potentials in preterm newborn children [Faldella et al., 1996] and the alteration of the fatty acids metabolism in dyslexic subsequent to high seric concentration of phospholipase A2 is well documented [Richardson et al., 1997;MacDonell et al., 2000]. Abnormal PLA2 levels, therefore, lead to depletion of polyunsaturated fatty acids from the neuronal membranes of neuronal cells, in particular from the large ganglion cells that, due to their size, are particularly vulnerable to such a deficiency [Ahmad et al., 2002]. Considering that the anatomofunctional deficit in these patients is found to be greatly dependent on the magnocellular system, it is worthwhile investigating why magnocells are especially vulnerable to defective fatty acids metabolism. A possible explanation is that the surface extent of the magnocellular membrane is wider compared to the parvocellular one. Therefore, the reduced availability of the structural substrate of the cellular membrane would slow the growth of the magnocells more than the parvocells. Thus, magnocells would be fewer and smaller, as found in the geniculate lateral body of dyslexics[300].

Phospholipids are involved not only in the formation of the cellular membranes, but also of the cytoskeleton[301], and the cytoskeleton is a second main factor determining the size of the cells [Olsen et al., 1998]. Due to abnormal formation of the cellular membranes and of the

---

[299] Age ranging from 6 years and 6 months to 12 years and 11 months.

[300] See chapter 9.

[301] Phospholipids interact with the so-called *microtubules associated proteins* (MAP), the main constituents of the cytoskeleton, responsible for its assembly and its stability [Fawcett et al., 1994].

cytoskeleton, a reduced amount of phospholipids is expected to make M-cells smaller during the developmental stages of the brain[302].

Indeed, it has been suggested that a depletion of polyunsaturated fatty acids, in particular ω-3 and ω-6, contribute to cause the reading difficulty in dyslexics[303] [Richardson et al., 2000; Richardson & Puri, 2002]. In fact, clinical signs attributable to their deficiency not only for the visual function but also on the auditory and on the motor level have been reported in many of these patients [Taylor et al., 2000].

In a double masked crossover investigation, the Oxford-Durham Study, 117 children aged between 5 and 12 years affected by *developmental coordination disorder (DCD)*[304] were recruited [Richardson & Montgomery, 2005]. After 3 months of ω-3[305] and ω-6[306] fatty acids supplementation, mean reading age increased by 9.5 months in the treated group versus 3.3 months in the placebo group. The progress continued with the prosecution of the treatment during the following 3 months.

After the treated/placebo crossover, the improvement was confirmed in the treated group and reading age increased by 13.5 months in the ex-placebo subjects. In the study the absence of side effects and the need to find the best ratio between ω-3: ω-6 (in this case set at 4:1) are underlined.

In addition, dietary supplementation with polyunsaturated fatty acids is found to improve dyslexics' dark adaptation [Stordy, 1995].

Interestingly, considering the role the immunity system would play in the pathogenesis of our clinical condition, the phospholipase A2 is probably modulated by immunitary reactions. In fact, PLA2 are needed to synthesize the precursors of cytokines[307] and autoimmune activity causes its mobilization from cell membranes [Stein, 2001].

iii-Methylphenidate

According to some researchers, methylphenidate (an substance analog of the amphetamines) is found to be effective to a certain extent in the treatment of some disorders often associated to developmental dyslexia: in particular the left hemi neglect typical of patients affected by attentional deficits and the hyperactivity disorder (ADHD) [Baumgaert el, 1999]. Methylphenidate seems to improve the hypoactivity of the right hemisphere responsible for this clinical condition [Sheppard et al., 1999].

Compensatory Strategies

Compensatory strategies may help dyslexics to make up for their defective visuoperceptive functions. So far, however, in most of the advanced techniques there is lack of scientific evidence.

---

[302] See Taylor and Richardson [2000] for further informations.

[303] Especially in males [Richardson et al., 2000].

[304] The DCD is a clinical condition which encompasses reading difficulty.

[305] 558 mg of eicosapentaenoic acid and 174mg of docosahexaenoic acid.

[306] 60 mg of γ-linolenic acid.

[307] Cytokines are a class of molecules (proteins, glycoproteins or peptides) involved in the immune response.

i-Rehabilitation with Tinted Lenses

In the early eighties, tinted lenses were suggested to improve the lexical function of dyslexic patients and of subjects suffering from a condition first reported in U.S. and Australia and named *Irlen syndrome*, *Meares /Irlen syndrome* or *SSS syndrome*[308] [Meares, 1980; Irlen, 1983].

Described later in England by Wilkins and Neary [1991], Irlen syndrome would be characterized by difficulty of concentration, visual discomfort, eye discomfort, photophobia, headache, defective stereopsis and visual distortion. When reading, these symptoms would be exacerbated and patients would report the sensation of moving or flickering letters, so as to make their lexical pattern similar to dyslexics. Symptoms would be triggered by serial configurations (as a sequences of letters) and tend to get worse as the reading goes on, especially in presence of bright or fluorescent light.

The aetiopathogenesis of this (supposed) clinical condition, that is claimed to affect from 12 to 14% of the general population and 46% of dyslexic subjects [Irlen, 1997], is unclear.

According to Irlen, patients' visual system would be hypersensitive to some wavelengths for inappropriate and excessive neuronal activation (cortical hyper excitability: Wilkins et al., 1999). Applying selective colored filters would filter the hypersensitive wavelengths, helping the visual processing [Irlen, 1983, 1989, 1991]. Even if the Irlen lenses have gained great popularity, their effectiveness has to be ascertained. First and foremost, the SSS syndrome is not a clinical entity admitted by the scientific community and, as pointed out by Hoyt [1990], it is based on vague and non specific symptoms stemming from anecdotal evidence. Secondly, the definition *scotopic sensitivity syndrome* suggests an alteration of the scotopic sensitivity, i.e. the visual sensitivity at low luminance levels, and assumes the functioning of the retinal rods, responsible for the scotopic vision, to be abnormal. Still, the environmental illumination level is well far from the scotopic range when reading. Therefore, even admitting the SSS syndrome does exist, its clinical pattern does not explain how the lack of sensitivity at low luminance levels can affect reading, since reading normally takes place in a floodlit environment.

As a matter of fact, the studies in support of the colored filters for the treatment of dyslexia have been defined as methodologically weak and with no solid theoretical bases[309] [Parker, 1990; Evans & Drasdo, 1991]. So far, experimental confirmations from other laboratories are missing [Christenson et al., 2001] and (when reported) the favorable results could be well due to a placebo effect. A double masked, placebo-controlled study has been published in 1994 [Wilkins et al., 1994]. The experiment investigated the effectiveness of the tinted lenses in improving the symptoms of the SSS syndrome and the lexical function in a group of children. As a result, reduced SSS-related symptoms were found in subjects wearing Irlen lenses and in the placebo, with a more pronounced effect in the former. Instead, the lexical function (assessed as reading speed and accuracy) was not affected by the treatment. Therefore, even if the effect of the colored filters on the asthenopeic symptoms may be worthy of further validation (visual discomfort reduction and slight improvement in visual search have been reported also by Wilkins & Neary, 1991), in dyslexic subjects the Irlen technique has proved to be of no avail.

---

[308] *Scotopic Sensitivity Syndrome.*

[309] As an example, see the randomized, but not double-masked study of Blaskey et al. [1990].

THE influence of the placebo effect in these studies has been pinpointed by Robinson and Foreman who tested in a group of students the effect of Irlen filters and of blue lenses on reading and other academic skills in two double-masked crossover experiments [Robinson & Foreman, 1999a, b]. After a follow-up lasting up to 20 months, results were compared with those of an untreated group. Compared to the latter, an increase of the lexical performance and of the academic skills was observed not only when wearing the Irlen filters but even with the blue lenses. Thus, the improvement can be regarded as a bias.

In conclusion, to date there is no evidence that the rehabilitative model based on the Irlen technique can really help the lexical performance of dyslexic subjects[310] [Solan & Richman, 1990]. Therefore, the rehabilitation of dyslexics by means of tinted lenses is up to now a paradigm without a plausible rational criterion and missing of solid experimental evidence. It is revealing that the choice of the optimum filter is at the discretion of the patient [Helveston, 1990, Coyle, 1995], and that the estimated number of tests required to find the most suitable color is about one thousand (sic!) [Willkins et al., 2005]. Nevertheless, the role of the wavelength on the magno- and parvocellular stimulation is well documented: a red illuminated background reduces the transient response in monkeys [Dreher et al., 1976; Kruger, 1977, Schiller & Malpeli, 1978] and in humans [Breitmeyer & Williams, 1990]. In fact, the M system is inhibited by the long light wavelengths and it is particularly responsive to the short wavelengths (blue light). On the contrary, the P system is mainly sensitive to the long wavelengths (red light) [Breitmeyer & Williams, 1990; Williams et al., 1991]. Therefore, patients affected by a defect of the transient system could benefit from the use of a short wavelength light, for example a blue illumination: actually, in this experimental condition the temporal processing rate of the visual stimuli and the comprehension of the written text in dyslexics is shown to improve [Williams et al., 1990]. In a double-masked experiment, a consistent reading improvement after wearing yellow filters for three months was found in one third of the patients: the lexical age in these subjects was grown 6 months more than in the placebo group[311]. To confirm the advantage of shifting the visual sensitivity toward lower wavelengths, in 10% of cases the positive effect was obtained with a blue filter rather than a yellow one [Stein, 2003].

In conclusion, even if the rehabilitation with the Irlen technique is not supported by any authoritative experimental confirmation (and therefore should not be used in clinical practice), it is worthwhile to provide further insight into the putative ameliorative effect of tinted lenses on the magnocellular activity and on the lexical function of dyslexic patients.

ii-Rehabilitation with Positive Lenses of Low Power

It has been argued in the optometric literature that accommodative inertia[312] can cause reading problems [Simons & Grisham, 1987; Solan, 1993], so that the use of positive lenses of low power would be helpful. However, no differences in the accommodative amplitude have been reported between dyslexics and normal readers [Olitsky & Nelson, 2003][313].

---

[310] For an exhaustive discussion of these issues see: American Academy of Pediatrics, 2011: p. 838-841.

[311] Rather than enhancing the sensitivity to the short wavelengths, these results could depend on the inhibitory effect of the yellow lenses on the long wavelengths.

[312] The *accommodative inertia* it the delay required to modify the accommodation of the eyes (i.e. the refractive power of the ocular dioptre) such as from near vision to far vision or vice versa.

[313] Chapter 5.

Therefore, the results from studies aimed at assessing the beneficial effects of low positive power lenses on the lexical function have been defined feeble [Jennings, 2000].

Therefore, there is no reason to take account of this solution.

iii-Prismatic *Rehabilitation*

Even if (as far as we know) this approach has not yet been tested in dyslexics, prisms could be effective in improving their lexical function [Jaśkowski & Rusiak, 2005]. The rationale lies on the putative presence in dyslexics of a left hemineglect[314] so that its treatment could have a positive effect on the lexical function. Actually, the use of prismatic lenses of Fresnel, aimed at shifting the visual field toward the right side, is found to be useful in patients with hemineglect [Rode et al., 2001][315] and their usefulness is worthy to be assessed in dyslexics, as well.

iv- Adaptation of the Interletter Spacing or the Spatial Relationship of the Text

As previously reported, dyslexic reading may be improved by compensatory strategies aimed at adapting and customizing the characteristics of the written text: for example by increasing interletter spacing[316]. Unfortunately, few studies on this topic are available. In the second part of this treatise the results of a compensatory paradigm consisting in the horizontal "stretch" of the visual space occupied by the lexical strings are reported. The goal of such a manipulation is to make up for the anisotropic visual unbalance along the vertical axis, as found in a group of patients.

Conclusion

Before a treatment can be declared as effective, it is paramount to make sure of its scientific validity, which naturally does not depend on its popularity but on the *evidence-based medicine*. If the evidence is scarce or feeble, then the solution cannot be shared by the scientific community. According to Swanson [Swanson et al., 1999], of the 900 papers published in 30 years of research, two-thirds have to be rejected as being not rigorous and of the remaining 25% (about 205) only 5% (about 10) meet the methodological criteria so as to make them as possible reference studies. Considering that the specific literature on visual rehabilitation in developmental dyslexia is a minority component, then the overall number of consistent studies can be counted on the fingers of one hand. Personal opinions or anecdotal cases are interesting as they can be taken as cues for new researches but do not represent scientific evidence and therefore should not be generalized. Also clinical trials have to be judged critically: in literature, valid studies mingle with less solid experiments.

To assess the effectiveness of a rehabilitation visual technique in developmental dyslexia the survey should always be designed as a double-masked crossover, recruiting two groups of

---

[314] Chapter 11.

[315] After an adaptating period, with the improvement which persisted up to 5 weeks [Frassinetti et al., 2002; Dijkerman et al., 2004].

[316] Chapter 13.

patients (better if also a control group) one of which receives the treatment under investigation while the second is given a placebo.

At the beginning and at the end of the treatment (t1), the operator, unaware of the group the patients belong to (cases or controls), submits both samples to the same battery of tests.

The rehabilitation protocol is then reversed in the two samples and at the end of this second period of treatment (t2), the difference between the improvements obtained in the two groups is checked again.

The rehabilitation technique can be retained as putatively effective if a statistically significant improvement is observed in the treated group at the end of both the first and the second phase (i.e. after the treatment switch). In addition, the experiment should be repeated and the results should be confirmed not only in the same laboratory but also in different research centers. It would be preferable to test the hypothesis with a multicentric trial, able to perform the experiment in different structures at the same time and the data should be analyzed by an independent group of experts.

Evidently, implementing this design requires a considerable amount of energies and resources. As an alternative, a meta-analysis can be performed. The meta-analysis provides a scientific overall judgment on the results obtained from the published studies on the subject, selected according to specific and stringent requirements. In this case, however, the deleterious effect of the so-called *publication bias*[317] has to be taken into consideration.

If the effectiveness of a protocol were rigorously demonstrated, the technique should be transferred to the clinical practice, paying attention to the economic cost and to the time required for the rehabilitation. In addition, it should be born in mind that the improvement is assessed on the average performance of the affected population: therefore, it is misleading to expect the paradigm works in every single case.

Above all, visual rehabilitation in dyslexic patients has to be administered within a multidisciplinary frame. Since developmental dyslexia is not a neuro-ophthalmological but a neuropsychiatric and logopedic condition, a shared commitment is mandatory.

References

Aleci C, Piana G, Piccoli M, Bertolini M. (2012). *Developmental dyslexia and spatial relationship perception.* Cortex, 48: 466-476.

Ahissar E, Vaadia E, Ahissar M, Bergman H, Arieli A, Abeles M. (1992). *Dependence of cortical plasticity on correlated activity of single neurons and on behavioral context.* Science, 257: 1412-1415.

Ahmad A, Moriguchi T, Salem N. (2002). *Decrease in neuron size in docosahexaenoic acid-deficient brain.* Pediatric Neurology, 26: 210-218.

American Academy of Pediatrics. (2011). *Joint Tecnical Report-Learning Disabilities, Dyslexia, and Vision.* Pediatrics, 127: 818-852.

Bakker DJ. (1992). *Neuropsychological classification and treatment of dyslexia.* Journal of Learning Disabilities, 25: 102-109.

[317] Studies that provide noticeable results tend to be more frequently accepted and published compared to those who fail to find a potentially interesting trend.

Bakker DJ, Moerland R, Goekoop-Hoefkens M. (1981). *Effects of hemisphere-specific stimulation on the reading performance of dyslexic boys: A pilot study.* Journal of Clinical Neuropsychology, 3, 155-159.

Bakker DJ, Vinke J. (1985). *Effects on hemisphere-specific stimulation on brain activity and reading in dyslexics.* Journal of Clinical and Experimental Neurophysiology, 7: 505-525.

Bakker DJ, Bouma A, Garden CJ. (1990). *Hemisphere-specific treatment of dyslexia subtypes: a field experiment.* Journal of Learning Disabilities, 23: 433-438.

Barnard N, Crewther SG, Crewther DP. (1998). *Development of a Magnocellular Function in Good and Poor Primary School-Age Readers.* Optometry and Visual Science, 75: 62-68.

Baumgaertel A. (1999). *Alternative and controversial treatments for attention deficit/hyperactivity disorder.* Pediatric Clinics of North America, 46: 977-992.

Bishop DV. (1989). *Unfixed reference, monocular occlusion, and developmental dyslexia-a critique.* British Journal of Ophthalmology, 73: 209-215.

Blaskey P, Scheiman M, Parisi M, Ciner EB, Gallaway M, Selznick R. (1990). *The effectiveness of Irlen filters for improving reading performance: a pilot study.* Journal of Learning Disabilities, 23: 604-612.

Bowan MD. (1998). *Learning Disabilities, Dyslexia, and Vision a Subject Review. A rebuttal, literature review, and commentary.* Optometry, 73: 553-575.

Brannan J, Williams M. (1987). *Allocation of visual attention in good and poor readers.* Perception & Psychophysics, 41: 23-28.

Breitmeyer BG, Williams MC. (1990). *Effects of isoluminat-background colour on metacontrast and stroboscopic motion: Interactions between sustained (P) and transient (M) channels.* Vision Research, 30: 1069-1075.

Cave KR, Zimmerman JM. (1997*). Flexibility in spatial attention before and after practice.* Psychological Science, 8: 399-403.

Christenson GN, Griffin JR, Taylor M. (2001). *Failure of blue tinted lenses to change reading scores of dyslexic individuals.* Optometry, 72: 627-633.

Coleman HM. (1972). *The West Warwick visual perception study, part II.* Journal of the American Optometric Association, 43: 532-543.

Committee on Children with Disabilities, American Academy of Pediatrics, American Academy of Ophthalmology, American Association for Pediatric Ophthalmology and Strabismus. (1998). *Learning disabilities, dyslexia, and vision: a subject.* Pediatrics, 102: 1219-1219.

Coyle B. (1995). *Use of filters to treat visual-perception problem creates adherents and sceptics.* Canadian Medical Association Journal, 152: 749-750.

Di Biase A, Salvati S. (1997). *Exogenous lipids in myelination and demyelination.* KaoHsiung Journal of Medical Sciences, 13:19-29.

Di Ianni M, Wilsher CR, Blank MS, Conners CK, Chase CH, Funkenstein HH, Helfgott E, Holmes JM, Lougee L,

Maletta GJ, Milewski J, Pirozzolo FJ, Rudel RG, Tallal, P. (1985). *The effects of piracetam in children with dyslexia.* Journal of Clinical Psychopharmacology, 5: 272-278.

Dijkerman HC, Webeling M, Ter Wal GM, Groet E, Van Zandvoort MJ. (2004). *A long-lasting improvement of somatosensory function after prism adaptation, a case study.* Neuropsychologia, 42: 1697-1702.

Doyle MC, Snowden RJ. (2001). *Identification of visual stimuli is improved by accompanying auditory stimuli: The role of eye movements and sound location.* Perception, 30: 795-810.

Dreher B, Fukuda Y, Rodieck R. (1976). *Identification, classification and anatomical segregation of cells with X like and Y like properties in the lateral geniculate nucleus of old-world primates*. Journal of Physiology, 258: 433-452.

Dryer R, Beale IL, Lambert AJ. (1999). *The Balance Model of dyslexia and remedial training: An evaluative study.* Journal of learning Disabilities, 32: 174-186.

Dunlop P. (1972). *Dyslexia. The orthoptic approach.* Australian Orthoptic Journal, 12: 16-20.

Elbert T, Pantev C, Wienbruch C, Rockstroh B, Taub E. (1995). *Increased use of the left hand in string players associated with increased cortical representation of the fingers.* Science, 270: 305-307.

Evans BJW, Drasdo N. (1991). *Tinted lenses and related therapies for learning disabilities: a review*. Ophthalmic and Physiological Optics, 11: 206-217.

Facoetti A, Lorusso ML, Paginoni PL, Umiltà C, Mascetti GG. (2003). *The role of visuospatial attention in developmental dyslexia: evidence from a rehabilitation study.* Cognitive Brain Research, 15: 154-164.

Fahle M, Luberichs J. (1995). *Extension of a recent therapy for dyslexia.* German Journal of Ophthalmology, 4 :350-354.

Faldella G, Govoni M, Alessandroni R, Marchiani E, Salvioli GP, Biagi PL, Spano C. (1996). *Visual evoked potentials and dietary long chain polynsaturated fatty acids in preterm infants.* Archives of Disease in Childhood - Fetal and Neonatal Edition, 75: 108-112.

Farmer ME, Klein RM. (1995). *The evidence for a temporal processing deficit linked to dyslexia.* Psychonomic Bulletin Review, 2: 460-493.

Farr J, Leibowitz HW. (1976). *An experimental study of the efficacy of perceptual-motor training.* American Journal of Optometry and Physiological Optics, 53: 451-455.

Fawcett JW, Mathews G, Houdsen E, Goedert M, Matus A. (1994). *Regenerating sciatic nerve axons contain the adult rather than the embryonic pattern of microtubule associated proteins.* Neuroscience, 61: 789-804.

Flax N. (1983). *Guest Editorial: Optometry and Dyslexia.* Journal of the American Optometric Association, 54: 593- 594.

Frassinetti F, Angeli V, Meneghello F, Avanzi S, Làvadas E. (2002). *Long lasting amelioration of visuospatial neglect by prism adaptation*. Brain, 125: 608-623.

Geiger G, Lettvin JY. (1986). *Enhancing the perception of form in peripheral vision.* Perception, 15: 119-130.

Geiger G, Lettvin JY. (1987). *Peripheral vision in persons with dyslexia.* New England Journal of Medicine, 316: 1238-1243.

Geiger G, Lettvin JY. (1989). *Dyslexia and reading as examples of alternative visual strategies*. In: Brain and reading, Von Euler, Lundberg & Lennerstrand Eds., Macmillian Press, New York.

Geiger G, Lettvin JY. (1993). *"Manifesto on dyslexia"* In: Facets of Dyslexia and Its Remediation, Wright & Groner Eds., Elsevier, Amsterdam.

Geiger G, Lettvin JY. (1999). *How dyslexics see and learn to read well.* In: Reading and Dyslexia: Visual and Attentional Processes in Reading and Dyslexia, Everatt Ed., Routledge: London, New York.

Geiger G, Lettvin JY. (2000). *Developmental dyslexia: A different perceptual strategy and how to learn a new strategy for learning.* Saggi, 26: 73-89.

Geiger G, Lettvin JY, Fahle M. (1994). *Dyslexic children learn a new visual strategy for reading: a controlled experiment.* Vision Research, 34: 1223-1233.

Geiger G, Lettvin JY, Zegarra-Moran O. (1992). *Task-determined strategies of visual process.* Cognitive Brain Research, 1: 39-52.

Gernsbacher MA. (1993). *Less skilled readers have less efficient suppression mechanisms.* Psychological Science, 4: 294-298.

Getz DJ. (1980). *Learning enhancement through visual training.* Academic Therapy, 15: 457-466.

Gillberg IC, Gillberg C. (1983). *Three-year follow-up at age 10 of children with minor neurodevelopmental disorders. Behavioural problems.* Developmental Medicine & Child Neurology; 25: 438-449.

Giurgea C. (1972). *Vers une pharmacologie de l'activité intégrative du cerveau. Tentative du concept nootrope en psychopharmacologie [Towards an integrative pharmacology of the activity of the brain. Attempt at the nootropic concept in psychopharmacology].* Actual Pharmacologie (Paris), 25: 115-176.

Heath EJ, Cook P, O'Dell N. (1976). *Eye exercises and reading efficiency.* Academic Therapy, 11: 435-445.

Helveston EM. (1990). *Scotopic sensitivity syndrome.* Archives of Ophthalmology, 108: 1232-1233.

Horrobin DF, Bennett CN. (1999). *New gene targets related to schizophrenia and other psychiatric disorders: enzymes, binding proteins and transport proteins involved in phospholipid and fatty acid metabolism.* Prostaglandins, Leukotrienes and Essential Fatty Acids., 60: 141-167.

Horrobin DF, Glen AI, Hudson CJ. (1995). *Possible relevance of phospholipid abnormalities and genetic interactions in psychiatric disorders: the relationship between dyslexia and schizophrenia.* Medical Hypotheses, 45: 605-613.

Hoyt, C.S. (1990). *Irlen lenses and reading disabilities.* Journal of Learning Disabilities, 23: 624-626.

Irlen H. (1983). *Successful treatment of learning disabilities.* Presented at the 91st Annual Convention of the American Psychologists Association, August 1983; Anaheim, California.

Irlen H. (1989). *Improving reading problems due to symptoms of scotopic sensitivity syndrome using Irlen lenses and overlays.* Education, 109: 413-417.

Irlen H. (1991). *Reading by colours.* Avery Publishing Group Ed., New York.

Irlen H. (1997). *Reading problems and Irlen coloured lenses.* Dyslexia Review, 4-7.

Jaśkowski P, Rusiak P. (2005). *Posterior parietal cortex and developmental dyslexia.* Acta Neurobiologiae Experimentalis, 65: 79-94.

Jennings AJ. (2000). *Behavioural optometry: a critical review.* Optometry in Practice, 1: 67-78.

Kavale K, Mattson PD. (1983). *"One jumped off the balance beam": Meta-analysis of perceptual-motor training.* Journal of Learning Disabilities, 16: 165-173.

Klein RM, D'Entremont B. (1999). *Filtering performance by good and poor readers.* In: Reading and Dyslexia: Visual and Attentional Processes in Reading and Dyslexia, Everatt Ed., Routledge, London, New York.

Kraus N, McGee T, Carrell TD, King C, Tremblay K. (1995). *Central auditory system plasticity associated with speech discrimination training.* Journal of Cognitive Neuroscience, 7: 27-34.

Kruger J. (1977). *The shift-effect in the lateral geniculate body of the rhesus monkey.* Experimental Brain Research, 29: 387-392.

Kujala T, Karma K, Ceponiene R, Belitz S, Turkkila P, Tervaniemi M, Näätänen R. (2001). *Plastic neural changes and reading improvement caused by audiovisual training in reading-impaired children.* Proceedings of the National Academy of Sciences of the United States of America 2001; 98: 10509-10514.

Lennerstrand G, Ygge J. (1992). *Dyslexia: ophthalmological aspects 1991.* Acta Ophthalmologica, 70: 3-13.

Lorusso ML, Facoetti A, Pesenti S, Cattaneo C, Molini m, Geiger G. (2004). *Wider recognition in peripheral vision common to different subtypes of dyslexia.* Vision Research, 44: 2413-2424.

Lorusso ML, Facoetti A, Toraldo A, Molteni M. (2005). *Tachistoscopic tratment of dyslexia changes the distribution of visual-spatial attention.* Brain Cognition, 57:135-142.

MacDonell LE, Skinner FK, Ward PE, Glen AI, Glen AC, Macdonald DJ, Boyle RM, Horrobin DF. (2000). *Increased level of cytosolic phospholipase A2 in dyslexics.* Prostaglandins, Leukotrienes and Essentially fatty Acids, 63: 37-39.

Masters MC. (1988). *Orthoptic management of visual dyslexia.* British Orthoptic Journal, 45: 40-48.

Mayer M. (1999). *Essential fatty acids and related molecular and cellular mechanisms in multiple sclerosis: New looks and old concepts.* Folia Biologica (Prague), 45: 133-141.

McConkie GW, Rayner K. (1975). *The span of the effective stimulus during a fixation in reading,* Perception & Psychophysics, 17: 578–586.

Meares O. (1980). *Figure/ground, brightness contrast, and reading disabilities.* Visibile Language, 14: 13-29.

Mounts JR. (2000). *Evidence for suppressive mechanisms in attentional selection: feature singletons produce inhibitory surrounds.* Perception & Psychophysics, 62: 969-983.

Näätänen R, Schröger E, Karakas S, Tervaniemi M, Paavilainen P. (1993). *Development of a memory trace for a complex sound in the human brain.* NeuroReport, 4: 503-506.

Norn MS, Rindziunski E, Skydsgaard H. (1969). *Ophthalmologic and orthoptic examinations of dyslectics.* Acta Ophthalmologica, 47: 147-160.

Olitsky SE, Nelson LB. (2003). *Reading disorders in children.* Pediatric Clinics of North America, 50: 213-224.

Olsen MK, Reszka AA, Abraham I. (1998). *KT5720 and U-98017 inhibit MAPK and alter the cytoskeleton and cell morphology.* Journal of Cellular Physiology, 176: 525-536.

Pantev C, Oostenveld R, Engelien A, Ross B, Roberts LE, Hoke M. (1998). *Increased auditory cortical representation in musicians.* Nature, 392: 811-814.

Parker, RM. (1990). *Power, control, and validity in research.* Journal of Learning Disabilities, 23: 613-620.

Rayner K, Murphy LA, Henderson JM, Pollastek A. (1989). *Selective attentional dyslexia.* Cognitive Neuropshychology, 6: 357-378.

Recanzone GH, Schreiner CE, Merzenich MM. (1993). *Plasticity in the frequency representation of primary auditory cortex following discrimination training in adult owl monkeys.* Journal of Neuroscience, 13: 87-103.

Richardson AJ, Calvin CM, Clisby C, Schoenheimer DR, Montgomery P, Hall JA, Hebb G, Westwood E, Talcott JB, Stein JF. (2000). *Fatty acid deficiency signs predict the severity of reading and related difficulties in dyslexic children.* Prostaglandins, Leukotrienes and Fatty Acids, 63: 69-74.

Richardson AJ, Cox IJ, Sargentoni J, Puri BK. (1997). *Abnormal cerebral phospholipid metabolism in dyslexia indicated by phosphorus-31 magnetic resonance spectroscopy.* NMR in Biomedicine, 10: 309-314.

Richardson AJ, Montgomery P. (2005). *The Oxford-Durham Study: A randomized, controlled trial of dietary supplementation with fatty acids in children with developmental coordination disorder.* Pediatrics, 115: 1360- 1366.

Richardson AJ, Puri BK. (2002). *A randomized double-blind, placebo-controlled study on the effects of supplementation with highly unsaturated fatty acids on ADHD-related symptoms in children with specific learning difficulties.* Progress in Neuro-Psychopharmacology and Biological Psychiatry, 26: 233-239.

Robinson GL, Foreman PJ. (1999a). *Scotopic sensitivity/Irlen syndrome and the use of coloured filters: a long term placebo controlled and masked study of reading achievement and perception of ability.* Perceptual & Motor Skills, 89: 83-113.

Robinson GL, Foreman PJ. (1999b). *Scotopic sensitivity/Irlen syndrome and the use of coloured filters: a long term placebo controlled study of reading strategies using miscue analysis.* Perceptual & Motor Skills, 88: 35-52.

Rode G, Rossetti Y, Boisson D. (2001). *Prism adaptation improves representational neglect.* Neuropsychologia, 39: 1250-1254.

Schiller P, Malpeli J. (1978). *Functional specificiyà of lateral geniculate nucleus laminae of the rhesus monkey.* Journal of Neurophysiology, 41: 788-797.

Seiderman, AS. (1980). *Optometric vision therapy - results of a demonstration project with a learning disabled population.* Journal of the American Optometric Association, 51: 489-493.

Shaywitz SE, Escobar MD, Shaywitz BA, Fletcher JM, Makuch R. (1992). *Evidence that dyslexia may represent the lower tail of a normal distribution of reading ability.* New England Journal of Medicine, 326:145-150.

Sheppard D, Bradshaw J, Mattingley J, Lee P. (1999). *Effects of stimulant medication on the lateralisation of line bisection judgements of children with attention deficit hyperactivity disorder.* Journal of Neurology, Neurosurgery & Psychiatry, 66: 57–63.

Simons HD, Grisham JD. (1987). *Binocular anomalies and reading problems.* Journal of the American Optometric Association, 58: 578-587.

Singer W. (1995). *Development and plasticity of cortical processing architectures.* Science, 270: 758-763.

Sireteanu R, Rettenbach R. (1995). *Perceptual learning in visual search: Fast, enduring but not specific.* Vision Research, 35: 2037-2043.

Solan HA. (1981). *A Rationale for the optometric treatment and management of children with learning disabilities.* Journal of Learning Disabilities, 14: 568-572.

Solan HA. (1993). *Dyslexia and Learning disabilities: An overview.* Optometry and Vision Science, 70: 343-347.

Solan HA, Richman J. (1990). *Irlen Lenses: a critical appraisal.* Journal of the American Optometric Association, 61: 789-796.

Stein JF. (1989). Unfixed reference, monocular occlusion, and developmental dyslexia-a critique. British Journal of Ophthalmology, 73: 319-320.

Stein JF. (2001). *The magnocellular theory of developmental dyslexia.* Dyslexia, 7: 12-36.

Stein JF. (2003). *Visual motion sensitivity and reading.* Neuropsychologia, 41: 1785-1793.

Stein JF, Fowler S. (1981). *Visual Dyslexia.* Trends in the Neurological Sciences, 4: 77-80.

Stein JF, Fowler S. *(1982). Diagnosis of dyslexia by means of a new indicator of eye dominance.* British Journal of Ophthalmology, 66: 332-336.

Stein JF, Fowler S. (1985). *Effect of monocular occlusion on visuomotor perception and reading in dyslexic children.* The Lancet, 2: 69-73.

Stein JF, Richardson, Fowler S. (2000). *Monocular occlusion can improve binocular control and reading in dyslexics.* Brain, 123: 164-170.

Stein JF, Riddell PM, Fowler S. (1987). *Fine binocular control in dyslexic children.* Eye, 1: 433-438.

Stein JF, Riddell PM, Fowler S. (1988). *Disordered vergence eye movement control in dyslexic children.* British Journal of Ophthalmology, 72: 162-166.

Stein JF, Talcott J. (1999). *Impaired neuronal timing in developmental dyslexia-the magnocellular hypothesis.* Dyslexia, 5: 59- 77.

Stordy BJ. (1995). *Benefit of docosahexaenoic acid supplementation to dark adaptation in dyslexia.* The Lancet, 346-385.

Swanson HL, Hoskyn M, Lee CM. (1999). *Interventions for students with learning disabilities: A meta-analysis of treatment outcomes.* Guilford Press Ed., New York.

Taylor KE, Richardson AJ. (2000). *Visual function, fatty acids and dyslexia.* Prostaglandins, Leukotrienes and Essential Fatty Acids, 63: 89-93.

Taylor KE, Higgins CJ, Calvin CM, Hall JA, Easton T, McDaid AM, Richardson AJ. (2000). *Dyslexia in adults is associated with clinical signs of fatty acid deficiency.* Prostaglandins, Leukotrienes and Essential Fatty Acids, 63: 75- 78.

Tremblay K, Kraus N, McGee T. (1998). *The time course of learning: Neurophysiologic changes during speech training,* NeuroReport, 9: 3357-3560.

Whiteley HE, Smith C, Connors L. (2007) *Young children at risk of literacy difficulties: factors predicting recovery from risk following phonologically based interventions.* Journal of Research in Reading, 30: 249-269.

Wilkins AJ, Baker A, Amin D, Smith S, Bradford J, Zaiwalla Z, Besag FM, Binnie CD, Fish D. (1999). *Treatment of photosensitive epilepsy using coloured glasses.* Seizure, 8: 444-449.

Wilkins, AJ, Evans BJW, Brown J, Busby A, Wingfield AE, Jeanes R, Bald J. (1994). *Double-masked placebo-controlled trial of precision spectral filters in children who use coloured overlays.* Ophthalmic and Physiological Optics 1994;14: 365-370.

Wilkins AJ, Neary G. (1991). *Some visual, optometric and perceptual effects of coloured glasses.* Ophthalmic and Physiological Optics, 11: 163-171.

Wilkins A, Sihra N, Smith IN. (2005). *Technical Note: How do precision tints have to be and how many are necessary?* Ophthalmic and Physiological Optics, 25: 269.

Williams MC, Breitmeyer BG, Lovergrove WJ, Gutierrez C. (1991). *Metacontrast with masks varying in spatial frequency and wavelength.* Vision Research, 31: 2017- 2023.

Williams MC, LeCluyse K, Bologna N. (1990). *Masking by light as a measure of visual integration time in normal and disabled readers.* Clinical Vision Sciences, 5: 335-343.

Williams MC, LeCluyse K, Rock-Faucheux A. (1992). *Effective interventions for reading disability.* Journal of the American Optometric Association, 63: 411-417.

Wilsher CR (1986). *Effects of piracetam on developmental dyslexia.* International Journal of Psychophysiology, 4: 29-39.

Wilsher CR, Bennett D, Chase CH, Conners CK, Diianni M, Feagans L, Hanvik LJ, Helfgott E, Koplewicz H, Overby P, Reader MJ, Rudel RG, Tallal P. (1987). *Piracetam and dyslexia: effects on reading tests.* Journal of Clinical Psychopharmacology, 5: 272-278.

Winblad B. (2005). *Piracetam: a review of pharmacological properties and clinical uses.* CNS Drug Reviews, 11: 169-182.

Winkler I, Kujala T, Tiitinen H, Sivonen P, Alku P, Lehtokoski A, Czigler I, Csepe V, Ilmoniemi R, Näätänen R. (1999). *Brain responses reveal the learning of foreign language phonemes*. Psychophysiology, 36: 638-642.

Zegarra-Moran O, Geiger G. (1993). *Visual recognition in the peripheral field: letters versus symbols and adults versus children.* Perception, 22: 77-90.

Part Two
Reading with their Eyes: A Phenomenological Approach

From what reported so far, what can be gatherer with a reasonable certainty is:

a) that developmental dyslexia is inheritable and its anatomopathological basis is neurological, as suggested by convincing pathological, diagnostic imaging and functional arguments.
b) that it is a multidisciplinary disease with a visuoperceptive component whose role, although subordinate to the neuropsychiatric one, probably is more important than thought up to now.
c) that the magnocellular system is most likely involved at a both the anatomical and functional level.

However, it remains to be ascertained which of the reported deficits of the M-system in the visual pathway have a real causal role and which are simply epiphenomena. In other words, it is necessary to focus on the final step of the multifaceted visuoperceptive impairment that directly contributes to affect the lexical task in developmental dyslexics.

Whatever it is, the visuoperceptive impairment we are referring to must apply to the lexical function so as to make this application able to explain the clinical picture in a direct and evident way. In an attempt to shed light on this controversial point, our considerations do not proceed from an alleged magnocellular cause to explain the symptoms. On the contrary, they start from the symptoms to formulate a hypothesis aimed at accounting the visuoperceptive causal factors.

Actually, patients find hard to process sequences of letters, whereas if characters are presented one by one their difficulty vanishes and symbols are recognized with no effort. We attributed this problem to an abnormal perception of the spatial relationships, which is to the reduced sensitivity in estimating the exact ratios or proportions of the extent of the visual configurations along the two cardinal axes.

In this second part, therefore, we have theorized that an alteration of the spatial relationship perception (SRP), leading to a perceptual distortion of the written text, provides a substantial contribution to prevent the lexical function.

Moreover, we have advanced SRP impairment to be the common functional platform for the heterogeneous visuoperceptive psychophysical findings discussed so far.

In addition, we have argued fixation instability to make worse this perceptual distortion.

Finally, a classification of the visuoperceptive components that may affect every single patient has been advanced.

Chapter XVI

Prelude to the Perceptive Shrinking

Despite the considerable experimental efforts, developmental dyslexia still escapes from a defined aetiopathogenetical framework: the theories about its origin are not exhaustive and cover the subject from too different perspectives. Dyslexia looks like a paradox, since despite its original definition of "word blindness" is an explicit hint to the sense of sight, its evaluation and treatment has always been done in the centers of neuropsychiatry, psychology, speech and phoniatric therapy, and has never involved the ophthalmological departments. The ophthalmological examination, when prescribed, serves simply the purpose to rule out refractive or binocular function disorders and manifest eye diseases.

Yet, although developmental dyslexia is not a condition of strict ophthalmological pertinence, it is evident at this point that the even the visual perception is involved to a certain extent: the sensation of characters and syllables twisting each other, overlapping or moving and the confusion between mirror syllables and letters, arouse great interest in the visual aspect of the disease. Actually, the attention on the neuro-ophthalmological side of developmental dyslexia is growing among researchers.

As reported at the beginning of this treatise, the scientific approach to dyslexia is born in the anatomopathological field. In the last decades, areas of dysplasia and ectopia have been demonstrated in the cerebral cortex of dyslexics patients, together to the subversion of the asymmetry of the planum temporale and of the operculum, the excessive development of the corpus callosum especially in its posterior part and finally the reduced trophism of the right anterior lobes of the cerebellum and of the pars triangularis of the frontal cortex.

Yet, these data do not help to cast light on the way the reading difficulty takes place: in other words, the macro-and microanatomic cerebral changes[318] cannot explain the clinical features of the dyslexic pattern.

From the phonological point of view, the defect involves the phoneme representation so that patients are unable to process slight differences between acoustically similar phonemes [Godfrey et al., 1981; Werker & Tees, 1987; Reed, 1989]. This inability is linked to reduced modulation sensitivity to the auditory frequencies [Witton et al., 1998].

[318] In addition, the anatomopathological abnormalities are related to the phonological impairment and are unable to account for the visuoperceptive signs and symptoms.

Instead, from a visual perspective the peculiar feature is the dissociation between resolution acuity and lexical performance: the patient recognizes each single letter effortlessly but cannot read as expected.

It has been documented that there are dyslexics who are lacking of evident phonological deficits[319] [Wolf & Bowers, 1999; Lovett et al., 2000], that the phonological rehabilitation sometimes does not lead to appreciable effects [Lyon & Moats, 1997; Torgersen, 2000], and that the effect of print size on the reading ability cannot be predicted upon purely phonological bases[320]. Finally, some patients (defined as *visuo-attentional dyslexics*: Valdois, 1995) make more visuoperceptive errors compared to the phonological ones.

For these reasons, a complementary solution may lie on the visuoperceptive ground. Indeed, several investigations have discovered in some patients a defect involving functions mediated by the large ganglion cells along the visual pathway: in particular contrast sensitivity, motion perception and visual persistence time. These anomalies led researchers to theorize a deficit of the magnocellular system.

Therefore, although the American Academy of Pediatrics has recently argued against the magnocellular theory [American Academy of Pediatrics, 2011], it is reasonable to assume that even the visual system has a role in the pathogenesis of developmental dyslexia and that many conflicting results are probably due to the heterogeneous nature of the clinical condition.

However, a defect of the M-system referred to the aforementioned functions evidently is not able to explain how the visual perceptive impairment accounts for the lexical disability.

Nevertheless, it has been emphasized the involvement of the M-system in the genesis and in the modulation of the saccadic movement. As a matter of fact, the M- and P-pathways are also responsible for the saccade-fixation sequence: fixations are promoted by the parvocells while the saccadic pattern is driven by the magnocells, according to the *pull-and-push* theory of Findlay and Walker.

Impaired M-system leads to weak inhibition and longer duration of the fixations, which in turn give rise to a post image of the syllable. The post image is transferred by the saccadic movement onto the fixation of the next group of letters. In addition, the saccade landing turns out to be imprecise. This abnormal situation would give rise to visual confusion, apparent movement, twisting as well as overlapping of letters, syllables and words and of course reduced reading rate and lexical errors. Literature supports this perspective but at the same time fails to confirm these alterations in the extra-lexical tasks: a plausible solution accounting for the oculomotor deficit dissociation in dyslexics is that the impaired saccadic pattern in the lexical task is not primitive but secondary to the abnormal processing of the text. As stated by the American Academy of Pediatrics, the American Academy of Ophthalmology, the American Association for Pediatric Ophthalmology and Strabismus and the American Association of Certified Orthoptists, in dyslexic readers the saccadic pattern appears to be not the cause but the result of their reading problems. Decoding difficulties (and not a primitive anomaly of the oculomotor system) are responsible for the slowness of

---

[319] The phonological aspect would be more relevant in English speaking dyslexics [Velvet et al., 2004] and less decisive in transparent ortographies like German or Italian, especially in those patients who do not show any retardation in language development. It has even been argued that Italian dyslexics without language development retardation are completely free from phonological impairment [Brizzolara et al., 2006].

[320] See part I, chapter 13.

reading, the increase of the fixation duration and the number of regression saccades [American Academy of Pediatrics, 2011].

This position is confirmed by the fact that the prevalence of dyslexia in children with primitive saccadic disorders or with congenital nystagmus[321] is not higher compared to the general population and that these patients, when the reading material is made suitable for their visual impairment, tend to read fluently [Hodgetts et al., 1998]. Therefore, eye movements are driven by the characteristics of the text. We suggest a distorted perception of the visual space occupied by the sequence of the letters in the words to be responsible for the saccadic disorder, eventually contributing to the lexical disability. As previously discussed[322], the position of the fixations depends on the landing site of the saccade. Generally, the landing sites locate between the beginning and the middle of the word. This convenient viewing position (that as such minimizes the duration of fixation) does not match exactly the optimal viewing position even in normal readers. The discrepancy is due to two main factors. First, the FEM amplitude suffers from the distance from the target: this *saccadic range effect* tends to make saccades directed toward distant words *hypometric*, so that the landing site settles on the left of the optical centre of gravity. On the contrary, saccades directed towards near words tend to be *hypermetric* so that the landing site is on the right of the optical centre of gravity[323] [McConkie et al., 1988]. In addition, the amplitude of the saccades is related to the length of the words [Radach et al., 2004]: for every extra letter, it is estimated that the landing site is displaced of about 0.2 characters towards the right. To date, it is not clear whether this *length effect* depends only on the number of letters or also on the spatial extent occupied by the word. In this last case, the abnormal perception of the spatial relationship across the page may lead to misestimate the length of the word, thereby affecting the saccadic amplitude.

In summary, a visuoperceptive distortion may bias the spacing between letters and words, affecting the saccadic amplitude and worsening the discrepancies between landing site and optimal viewing position.

When reading, the visuoperceptual effect on the oculomotor modulation occurs in the visual space surrounding the fixation point. This region corresponds to the parafoveal area at the retinal level. Syllables in parafoveal projection on the right side of the fixation point, apart from being pre-processed, are responsible for the programming of the next saccadic movement: indeed, the parafoveal information plays a decisive role in determining which syllable will be targeted by the next saccade [O'Regan, 1990; Rayner et al., 1996].

The region of the string whose processing is able to modulate the saccadic activity is defined *total perceptual span* [Radach et al., 2004], whereas the *letter identification span* is the extent of the total perceptual span that can be recognized (thus processed) at each fixation[324]. The total perceptual span can trigger three saccadic events: saccade on the same

---

[321] Congenital nystagmus is characterized by spontaneous and involuntary ocular oscillations due to abnormal oculomotor control.

[322] Part I, chapter 10.

[323] The peak of distribution of the landing site in normal readers localises on the left portion of the word because the predominant effect is the former (hypometry).

[324] According to this definition, the *letter identification span* would correspond to the perceptual span and as such it would refer to the visuoperceptive function, whereas the *total perceptual span* would refer to the visual space surrounding the fixation point able to modulate the saccadic movement.

word and on the right of the previous landing site (in case of long words), saccade on the next word, and saccade skipping the adjoining word (directed toward the subsequent word)[325].

In substance, the defective saccadic pattern in dyslexics (in particular reduced FEM amplitude: Trauzettel-Klosinski et al., 2010) could depend on an abnormal total perceptual span[326].

It is arguable that crowding is stronger in some dyslexics, since they are prevented from reading sequences of characters (that is words) whereas the recognition of single letters is normal. The reinforcement of the lateral masking could depend on an abnormal sense of space, able to widen the critical spacing: if in a normal reader the current interval between letters is large enough to avoid crowding, dyslexics suffering from a larger critical spacing need a separation between letters greater than usual, so that the ordinary interval is not wide enough.

The association between crowding reinforcement and defective oculomotor rhythm during the lexical task requires a factor that acts as common denominator. This factor could be a reduced and imbalanced sensitivity to the spatial relationship, characterized by excessive anisotropy[327]: visual dyslexics would perceive the visual space in a distorted way, that is to say *shrunk* along the horizontal axis and *stretched* along the vertical coordinate.

It can be observed in figure 1 that even if the visual system were affected by a moderate contraction of the visual space along the horizontal axis (and a concomitant dilation along the vertical one: we will refer to this condition as *vertical anisotropy*), the perceptual result would be hardly noticeable in everyday experience.

On the contrary, characters are expected to be perceived closer when reading. This scenario would promote crowding, favoring the reciprocal reversing and confusion of letters and syllables: consequently, reading would be slow and inaccurate, resembling the dyslexics' reading pattern.

Therefore, a class of dyslexics would be affected by abnormal vertical anisotropy so as to cause a "perceptive shrinking" of the written text when reading. This illusory effect would have little or no influence in everyday life but would prevent patients from reading fluently.

The hypothesis of the perceptive shrinking seems able to explain the increased crowding as well as the saccadic subversion during the lexical task, as found in developmental dyslexia. Indeed, on the one hand, vertical anisotropy would make crowding stronger, deceptively reducing the interletter distance so that characters actually beyond the critical spacing (and as such readable) would fall within this range, and be affected by lateral masking. On the other hand, such an illusory contraction of the text is expected to perturb the saccade-fixation planning making the landing site shift far from the preferred viewing location. In an attempt to compensate for this perceptual imbalance, longer fixation times and reduced saccadic amplitudes would take place. In addition, due to the illusory shortening of the string, more

---

325 These three possibilities depend not only on the parafoveal visual processing but also on the linguistic characteristics of the text [Brysbaert & Vitu, 1998]. It has been observed, in fact, that the landing site tends to localize more on the left in words whose information content is at the beginning (beginning-information) such as friendship, whereas the opposite occurs for words with information content is at the end (end-information) such as microwave [Underwood et al., 1990; Everatt & Undewood, 1992]. For this linguistic effect on the position of the fixation, the concept of cognitive landing site has been advanced [Underwood & Radach, 1998].

326 An abnormal total perceptual span would strengthen the saccadic range effect and the length effect.

327 See part I, chapter 13.

backward saccades, searching for the optimal viewing position locus (exceeded by the forward movements), are triggered.

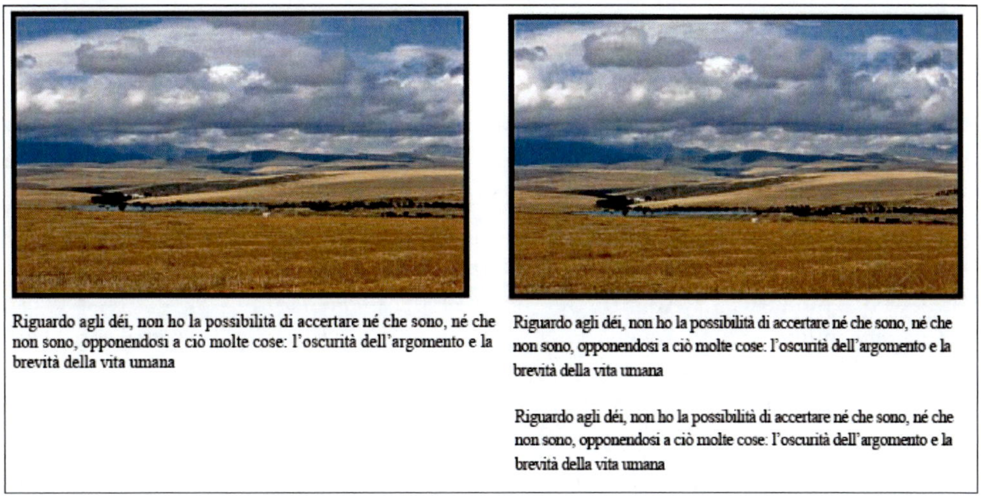

Figure 1. Effect of vertical anisotropy referred to spatial relationship perception. Simulation in the extra-lexical visual experience and during the lexical task. On the left is represented the isotropic condition, on the right a perceptual condition of vertical anisotropy is simulated (horizontal shrinking: 10%). The text on the lower right corner is "anisotropized" by 20%.
Translation of the sentence: "About gods, I have no way to ascertain neither that they are nor that they are not: many things prevent from this: the obscurity of the subject and the brevity of human life".

To investigate in this direction, the first step is to develop a technique able to evaluate the spatial relationship perception and, in case, to measure the amount of vertical anisotropy. For this purpose it is advisable to use global configurations, avoiding composite stimuli or patterns liable to activate the parvocellular system[328]. Indeed, this test, the *eidomorphometry*, measures the spatial relationship sensitivity making use of circular and elliptical targets.

References

American Academy of Pediatrics. (2011). *Joint Tecnical Report-Learning Disabilities, Dyslexia, and Vision.* Pediatrics, 127: 818-852.

Brizzolara D, Chilosi A, Cipriani P, Di Filippo G, Gasperini F, Mazzotti S, Pecini C, Zoccolotti P. (2006). *Do phonologic and rapid automatized naming deficits differentially affect children with and without a history of language delay? A study on Italian dyslexic children.* Cognitive and Behavioral Neurology, 19:141-149.

Brysbaert M, Vitu, G. (1998). *Word skipping: Implications for theories of eye movement control in reading.* In: Eye guidance in reading and scene perception, Underwood Ed., Elsevier, Oxford, UK.

Dunn-Rankin P. (1978). *The visual characteristics of words.* Scientific American, 238: 122-130.

[328] For example stimuli made up of high spatial frequency components (bars or edges).

Everatt J, Undewood G. (1992). *Parafoveal guidance and priming effects during reading: A special case of the mind being ahead of the eyes.* Consciousness and Cognition, 1: 186-197.

Godfrey JJ, Sydnal-Lasky AK, Millay KK,Knox CM. (1981). *Performance of dyslexic children on speech perception tests.* Journal of Experimental Child Psychology, 32: 401-424.

Hodgetts DJ, Simon JW, Sibila TA, Scanlon DM, Vellutino FR. (1998). *Normal reading despite limited eye movements.* Journal of the American Association for Pediatric Ophthalmology and Strabismus, 2: 182-183.

Irving-Bell L, Small M, Cowey A. (1999). *A distortion of perceived space in patients with right-hemisphere lesions and visual hemineglect.* Neuropsychologia, 37: 919–925.

Lovett MW, Steinbach KA, Frijters JC. (2000). *Remediating the core deficits on developmental reading disability: A double-deficit perspective.* Journal of Learning Disabilities, 33: 334-358.

Lyon GR, Moats LC. (1997). *Critical conceptual and methodological considerations in reading intervention research.* Journal of Learning Disabilities, 30: 578-588.

McConkie GW, Kerr PW, Reddix MD, Zola D. (1988). *Eye movement control during reading: I. The location of initial eye fixations on words.* Vision Research, 28: 1107-1118.

O'Regan JK. (1990). *Eye movements and reading.* In: Eye movements and their role in visual and cognitive processes, Kowler ED., Elsevier, Amsterdam, Holland.

Radach R, Inhoff A, Heller D. (2004). *Orthographic regularity gradually modulates saccade amplitudes in reading.* European Journal of Cognitive Psychology, 16: 27-51.

Rayner K. (1979). *Eye guidance in reading: fixation localization within words.* Perception, 8: 21-30.

Rayner K, Sereno SC, Raney GE. (1996). *Eye movement control in reading: A comparison of two types of models.* Journal of Experimental Psychology: Human Perception and Performance, 22: 1188-1200.

Reed MA. (1989). *Speech perception and the discrimination of brief auditory cues in reading disabled children.* Journal of Experimental Child Psychology, 48: 270-292.

Torgersen JK. (2000). *Individual differences in response to early interventions in reading: the lingering problem of treatment resisters.* Learning Disabilities Research & Practice, 15: 55-64.

Trauzettel-Klosinski S, Koitzsch AM, Dürrwächter U, Sokolov AN, Reinhard J, Klosinski G. (2010). *Eye movements in German-speaking children with and without dyslexia when reading aloud.* Acta Ophthalmologica, 88: 681-691.

Treutwein B. (1995). *Adaptive psychophysical procedures.* Vision Research, 35: 2503-2522.

Underwood G, Clews S, Everatt J. (1990). *How do readers know where to look next? Local information distributions influence eye fixations.* Quarterly Journal of Experimental Psychology, 42A: 39-65.

Underwood G, Radach R. (1998). *Eye guidance and visual information processing: Reading, visual search, picture perception and driving.* In: Eye guidance in reading and scene perception, Underwood G Ed., Elsevier, Oxford, UK.

Valdois S, Gérard C, Vanault P, Dugas M. (1995). *Peripheral developmental dyslexia: a visual attentional account?* Cognitive Neuropsychology, 12: 31-67.

Werker JF, Tees RC. (1987). *Speech perception in severely disabled and average reading children.* Canadian Journal of Psychology, 41: 48-61.

Witton C, Talcott JB, Hansen PC, Richardson AJ, Griffiths TD, Rees A, Stein JF, Greef GG. (1998). *Sensitivity to dynamic auditory and visual stimuli predicts nonword reading ability in both dyslexic and normal readers.* Current Biology, 8: 791-797

Wolf M, Bowers P. (1999). *The "double-deficit hypothesis" for the developmental dyslexias.* Journal of Educational Psychology, 91: 1-24.

Chapter XVII

Spatial Relationship Perception and the Eidomorphometry

The analysis of curvilinear shapes is so accurate a process to be considered a visual hyperacuity[329] [Watt & Andrews, 1982; Watt, 1984].

Indeed, to recognize environmental objects, curvatures analysis is as important as the processing of straight lines [Attneave, 1954], so that several psychophysical studies have focused on curvature discrimination [Watt & Andrews, 1982; Watt, 1984; Wilson, 1985; Fahle, 1986; Wilson & Richards, 1986; Koenderink & Richards, 1988; Fahle, 1991; Gigus & Malik, 1991; Foster et al., 1993; Whitaker et al., 1993; Kramer & Fahle, 1996; Hess, 1999] and on circular and radial patterns' perception [Wilson et al., 1997; Wilkinson et al., 1998; Wilson & Wilkinson, 1998; Loffler et al., 2003].

In these experiments, the observer generally is asked to compare the test stimulus (for example an arc of given length and curvature) with a reference stimulus. Without the presentation of a reference stimulus, the judgment and the correct recognition of configurations like ellipses with a very short focal axis can be based only on the comparison of their extent along the cardinal coordinates. In these cases, the difference in the recognition threshold for horizontally/vertically ellipses reflects the entity of the anisotropy related to the spatial relationship along the x-, y axes (*Spatial Relationship Anisotropy, SRA*). SRA is therefore an index of the imbalance of a particular function of the visual system: the *Spatial Relationship Perception (SRP).*

When dealing with quasi-circular ellipses, SRP refers to the ability to detect the difference of the extent of the configuration along the x-, y coordinates which allows making it recognizable from a configuration whose difference is 0, that is a circumference. The lower is the recognition threshold, the higher is the sensibility to the spatial extent of the configuration, and the more accurate is SRP. Irrespective of this sensibility, isotropy occurs if the recognition threshold is the same along the two coordinates, i.e. if the ability to detect a horizontal ellipse matches the ability to recognize a vertical ellipse of the same eccentricity.

---

[329] Visual iperacuity is the resolution acuity that allows to discriminate differences in the retinal position less than 5 sec arc. Examples are the Vernier acuity, which measures the vertical displacement between two lines, or the alignment task, which deals with the location of three aligned points (Daicar & Ogilvie, 1967; Wilson, 1985; Fahle, 1991; Foster et al., 1993).

On the contrary, anisotropy takes place if the threshold differs in the two kinds of configuration, revealing a preferential orientation in visual space processing.

Lower threshold (i.e. higher sensibility) for stimuli oriented along the vertical coordinate compared to the same stimuli oriented along the horizontal axis is a condition we have conventionally defined *vertical anisotropy* [Aleci et al., 2010].

In this situation, a horizontal ellipse of minimal eccentricity should appear to the observer as contracted along the x-axis and/or stretched along the y-axis, being therefore perceived as a circumference. In other words, the shrinking of the visual space along the horizontal coordinate turns the horizontal figures into circles.

Even if circular and elliptical configurations are not the only ones suitable to investigate spatial relationship perception and the related anisotropy, these stimuli have the advantage to prevent any judgment based on the angle of intersection of imaginary lines joining opposite corners, as may happen with rectangles and squares [Regan & Hamstra, 1992].

To estimate SRP and SRA, a specific psychophysical test, the *eidomorphometry*, has been devised [Aleci et al., 2010]. The eidomorphometry aims at estimating the discrimination threshold between ellipses and circles. The variable is the focal axis as well as its orientation (horizontal or vertical) while the other parameters (luminance, contrast, size) are kept constant. The eccentricity is expressed as percent *interaxis ratio (IR):*

$$IR\ (\%) = 100\ [f(x) - f(y)]\ /\ f(m_{x,y})$$

where $f(x)$ and $f(y)$ are the two axes and $f(m_{x,y})$ is the major. This way, IR measures the threshold of eccentricity required for the stimulus to be correctly recognized as elliptical. Naturally, the IR of a circumference is = 0.

Tested IR interval ranges from 36% to 1%. Each 1% matches 3.3 minarc difference between the two axes at the viewing distance (40 cm). The stimulus is displayed so that its center falls on the foveal region and its average size subtends a visual angle of 300 minarc.

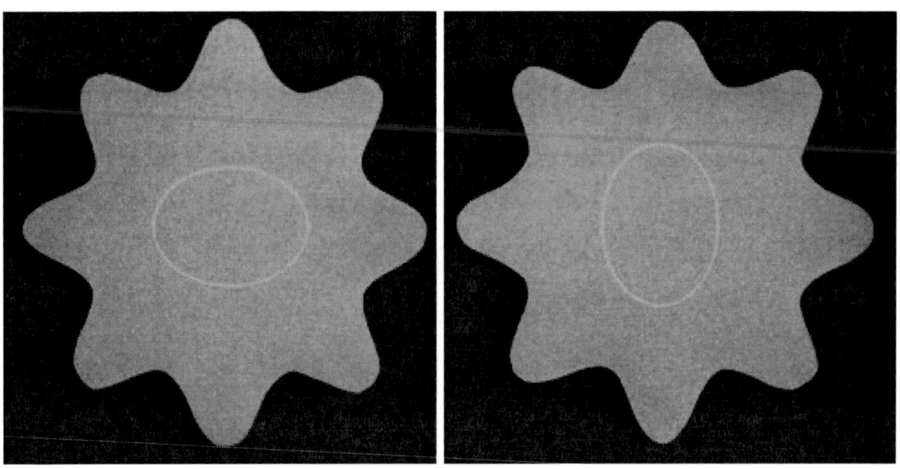

Figure 1. Eidomorphometry: two examples of elliptical stimuli. IR: ± 26% (during the examination the sinusoidal frame is barely visible).

According to Kramer & Fahle [1996], two straight lines flanking the curvilinear stimulus on both sides tend to increase the curvature detection threshold[330]. Therefore, to avoid the rectilinear edges of the screen to be used as cues for the curvature judgment of the elliptical figures, a black sinusoidal mask[331] is placed along the borders of the monitor. The very low environmental illuminance (0.15 lux) and the low luminance of the background (40 cd/m^2) make the profile of the dark mask barely visible. The luminance of the stimulus is 160 cd/m^2 and its contour 1.8 minarc wide (Figure 1).

Elliptical and circular targets are presented for 200 msec according to a triple forced choice strategy (3AFC). Stimulus eccentricity varies according to a staircase 4-2-1 procedure[332] [Dixon & Mood, 1948; Kaembach, 1991; Treutwein, 1995]. The observer is required time after time to identify the stimulus. The procedure has been devised in order to estimate separately the vertical (y-) and the horizontal (x-) orientations. In fact, even if the stimulus orientation is randomized, the answer referred to the x-ellipse affects only the next x-presentation with no effect on the IR value of the next y-stimulus and vice versa. This way the measures of the horizontal and vertical threshold (HT and VT, respectively) are independent. Their difference (HT-VT) expresses the amount of anisotropy (Spatial Relationship Anisotropy, SRA) of the visual system under examination. Conventionally,

---

[330] As long as their distance from the target is less than 10 minarc.

[331] Radial frequency: 8 cycles/360 degrees (0.022 c/deg). In the subsequent investigations the mask has been removed, since no appreciable difference was found in the threshold estimates with and without the sinusoidal profile.

[332] The staircase 4-2-1 is a psychophysical procedure widely used in perimetry to estimate the differential light sensitivity threshold in different points of the visual field and commonly adopted in other psychophysical fields. According to this paradigm, the value of the variable under observation (the luminance of a spot of light or, in our case, IR) is initially high enough to allow the detection or recognition of the stimulus (in our case the ellipse). Then, it is reduced by a pre-defined step (e.g. 4 dB or IR: 4%) after each correct answer, making the task more and more difficult. The decreasing trend carries on until the observer makes an error (i.e. after a series of correct answers [hit], the next stimulus is not detected [miss]). The trend is then reversed so that the variable is increased after each wrong response by a step that is half the pre-reversal value (e.g. 2 dB or IR: 2%). When the stimulus is recognized again, the sequence is reversed once more with a new decreasing trend (at each correct response, the value is increased by half the pre-reversal value: e.g. 1 dB or IR: 1%). The test converges at the first *miss* during the second reversal and the threshold is set as the value of the variable of the last hit. In the eidomorphometry, after each correct answer IR is lowered by 4%. After the first error the trend is reversed and after each miss the IR is increased by 2%. The first hit of this new progression is followed by a second reversal with decrease of 1% after each correct response. The IR of the last recognized ellipse is taken as the threshold value with *a prior* probability of 75%. The examination goes on with the simultaneous but independent estimate of the threshold along the two cardinal axes.

A fundamental difference between experimental and clinical psychophysical research is that the former generally tests a very small sample of normal observers who repeatedly undergo the same examination. A large amount of data is then collected from these selected subjects, accustomed to psychophysical testing, and results as average thresholds show high reliability. Evidently, in clinical field, this approach is not possible and a more conspicuous sample of observers (normal and pathological) often undergoes a single trial. A similar experimental design allows, especially in case of children, to shorten as much as possible the examination time so as to reduce the risk of attentional drops. The drawback of the method is the occurrence of large standard deviations and outliers. In the eidomorphometry, the SRP threshold estimating performed by the staircase procedure has the advantage to reduce the duration of the examination so as to avoid temporary drops of performance [Roach et al., 2004; Spry et al., 2003], which indeed are frequent in children. In accordance with Grinter et al. [2010], the method of the constant stimuli is more reliable since the final threshold estimate is based on the entire psychometric function. In addition, compared to the staircase, its outcome is more robust, as the variable of the stimulus to be displayed does not depend on the previous response and this makes the final measure less dependent from accidental errors or biases when performing the exam. Nevertheless, the constant stimuli method turns out to be time-consuming, therefore not suitable for testing children, especially if they are required to undergo a diagnostic protocol made of other tests besides eidomorphometry. Therefore, in line with other psychophysical techniques of common use in the ophtalmological clinical practice (for example perimetry), the staircase has been chosen for our purposes instead of the constant stimuli.

positive SRA (HT-VT> 0) means vertical anisotropy, therefore greater sensitivity along the vertical axis. Vertical anisotropy suggests the perceived image to be illusory "shrunk" along the horizontal axis. Figure 2 shows average VT and HT resulting from a group of 21 normal readers (12 males and 9 females), mean age 29.3 years (± 11.6), with normal visual acuity and no systemic or ophthalmological diseases, as well as serious refractive defects.

In each subject thresholds measured in one eye substantially matches the threshold measured in the other. Sensitivity to spatial relationship turned out to be high, with the vertical threshold slightly lower than the horizontal one (IR: 2.07% [± 1.25] and 3.20% [± 1.69][333] respectively).

This results suggests that the visual system of normal readers albeit highly sensitive to x-, y- differences in visual configurations, is not perfectly isotropic but suffers from a slight vertical anisotropy (SRA: 1.13% [± 2.19])[334].

The horizontal threshold ranges between 2% and 4% in 80% of the sample while in 3/4 of cases the vertical threshold is less or equal to 2%.

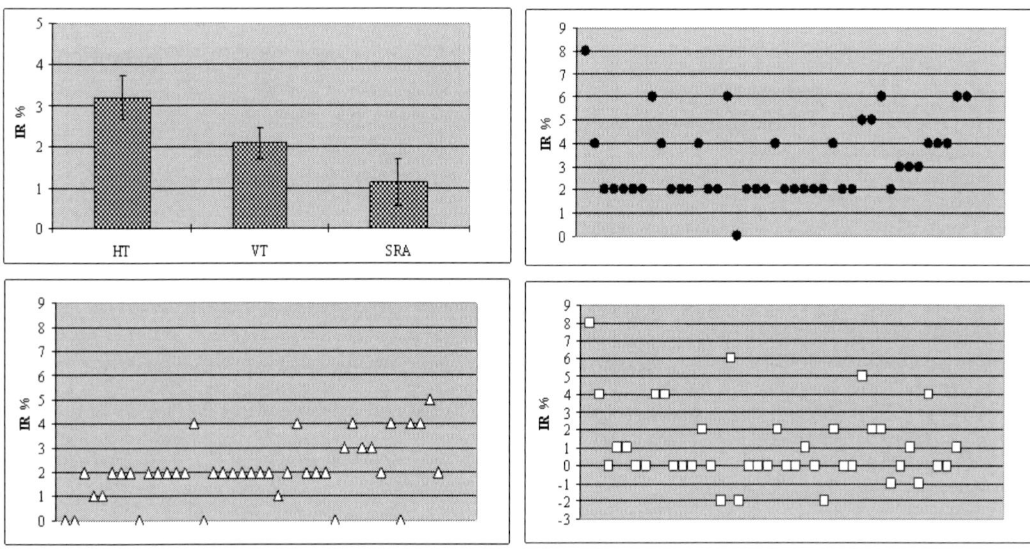

Figure 2. Spatial relationship perception: normative data in adult subjects. Top left: HT, VT, SRA (confidence interval 95%). Top right and bottom: distribution of the individual values of HT (dark circles), VT (light triangles) and SRA (light squares) in the examined population. See text for explanation.

More than half of the sample (57%) was affected by anisotropy to a certain extent. In these anisotropic subjects, vertical imbalance was found in more than 3/4 of the cases (Figure 3), even if minimal in most subjects (SRA <2% in 2/3 of the anisotropic sample and in any case seldom or never exceeding 5%).

After the technique has been tested in a reliable sample (because made of adult subjects), spatial relationship perception has been assessed in a group of normal children. The purpose was to obtain normative data to be used as a reference for the following analysis of the spatial relationship perception in dyslexic children.

[333] This proportion corresponds to a just noticeable difference (jnd) along the vertical and horizontal axis equal to 7.8 minarc, and 12 minarc, respectively.

[334] That is 4.2 minarc.

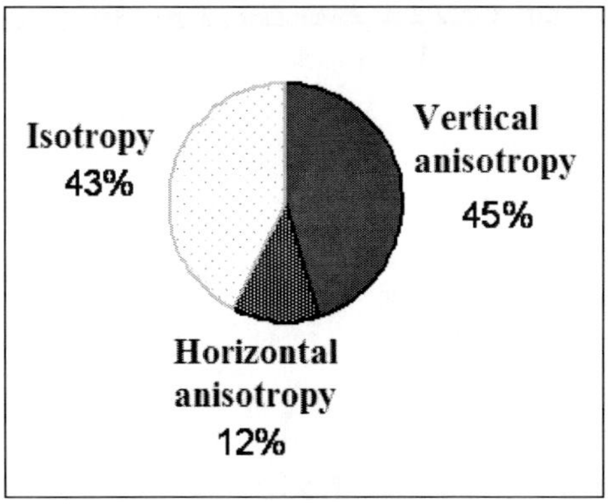

Figure 3. Isotropy and anisotropy distribution in the normal sample.

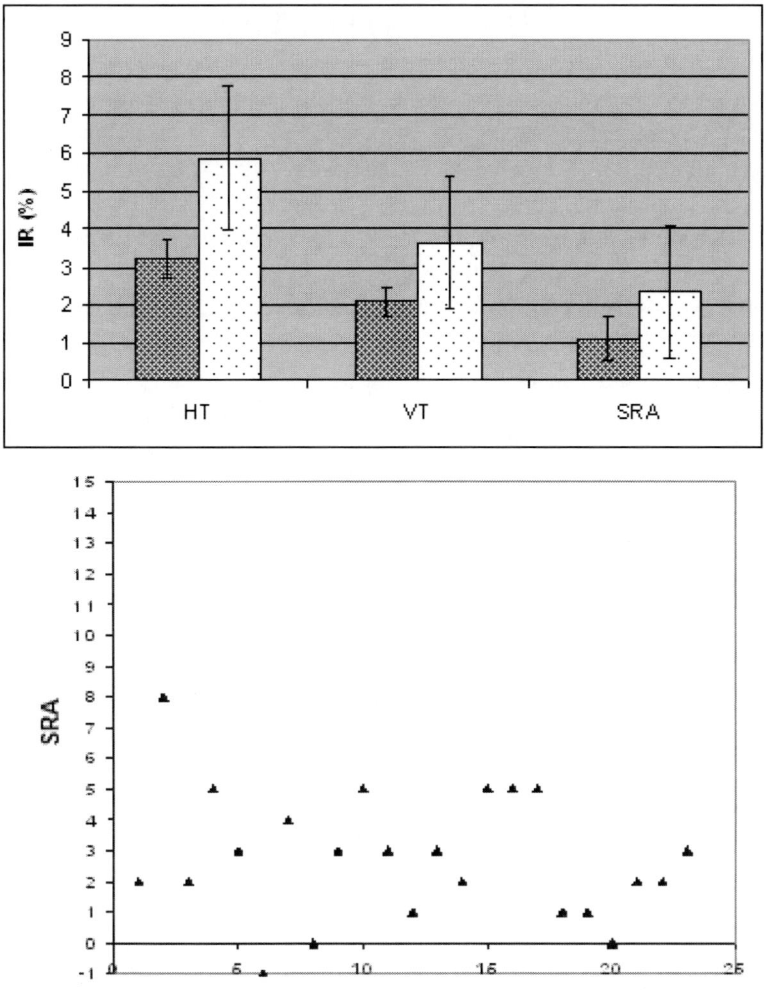

Figure 4. Spatial relationship perception: normative data in children (white dotted histograms). Upper: HT, VT, SRA (confidence interval 95%). For comparison are reported the values found in adult subjects (dark dotted histograms). Lower: distribution of the individual values of SRA in the sample.

A group of 23 pupils (mean age 9.2 ± 2.0 years) was therefore examined using the same paradigm applied to the adult sample. The results confirmed the slight lower average vertical threshold compared to the horizontal one (3.64% [± 1.75] vs. 5.86% [± 1.90[335]): thereby, even in children SRP turned out to be imbalanced (vertical anisotropy: 2.36% [± 1.75]).

By analyzing the individual data, different degrees of vertical anisotropy have been found in 87% of cases (Figure 4).

It could be argued the slightly worse performance in children compared to adults to depend on imperfect comprehension of the test in the former group, so that the SRP measurement would be biased by the cognitive development of the subject. However, this possibility is unconvincing, since no correlation is found between HT, VT, SRA and chronological age (correlation coefficient *r* respectively equal to -0.27, -0.24, -0.05, $p \geq 0.05$ in all cases).

In summary, normal readers suffer from a slight but consistent SRP anisotropy, irrespective of their age.

Indeed, in previous studies similar evidence has been provided for tasks more or less directly related to spatial relationship perception like orientation discrimination of gratings [Rovamo et al., 1982; Temme et al., 1985], spatial phase discrimination of gratings[336] [Rentschler & Treutwein, 1985; Bennet & Banks, 1987, 1991], bisection task [Yap et al., 1987], curvature perception [Fahle, 1986] and some types of Vernier acuity like the misalignment task[337] [Ludvigh, 1953; Andrews et al., 1973; Andrews & Miller, 1978, Westheimer, 2005]. Such an anisotropy at a local scale would depend on the orientation and on the shape of the receptive fields of the retinocortical pathway, from the peripheral retina (as inferred in the cat: Leventhal & Schall, 1983; Levick & Thibos, 1980; 1982) to the lateral geniculate body (as inferred in the monkey: Smith et al., 1990), up to the striate cortex (as inferred in the monkey: Bauer & Dow, 1989 and in the cat: Leventhal, 1983). Interestingly, the cortical magnification factor (the index of the cortical mapping of the retinal projections) makes the retinal representation on the cortical surface anisotropic [Hubel & Wiesel, 1977][338].

Still, compared to our technique, such perceptual tasks are performed at a local level and do not necessarily account for the anisotropic contraction of the visual space on a global scale.

As far as we know, the only study aimed at assessing the spatial relationships perception on a global scale is provided by Regan and Hamstra, and dates back 1992 [Regan & Hamstra, 1992].

In this investigation the *aspect ratio* threshold, that is to say the least *height* x *width* ratio of an ellipse that makes it recognizable from a circumference, has been measured in four normal subjects with a two-forced choice paradigm. In this study, the aspect ratio threshold was 1.014-0.995, a value in overall agreement with our measurement: in fact, the IR threshold turned into *aspect ratio* threshold ranges from 1.002 to 0.996.

---

335 The percent values correspond to a just noticeable difference of 7.8 minarc along the vertical axis and 12 minarc along the horizontal one.

336 Lower for radial orientations and higher for tangential orientations.

337 The misalignment task is a type of vernier acuity: given a triplet of points aligned along the horizontal axis, the visual system is more sensitive to the ortoaxial deviation rather than the coaxial displacement of the central point.

338 The cortical magnification factor describes the increase of the angular size of the retinal images after being transferred along the retinocortical pathway onto the cortex.

This experiment is in general agreement with our findings, confirming the slight difference in the discrimination threshold between y-/x- oriented patterns in the visual space[339].

Furthermore, the similarity between recognition threshold for elliptical stimuli and for rectangles generalizes this finding, making the SRP anisotropy not specific of curvilinear shapes. To explain the physiological mechanisms underlying the spatial relationship perception and its anisotropy on a global scale, the existence of particular neurons assigned to process the *aspect ratio* has been advanced. Such detectors would be functionally organized into two pools, the one sensitive to the vertical extent of the visual stimulus, the other to the horizontal one (the *y-pool* and *x-pool*, respectively): isotropy would result from the perfect balance between the output coming from the two pools [Regan & Hamstra, 1992].

Therefore, two factors are expected to be responsible for SRP:

-the extent of the global activation of the two quotas, which accounts for the SR overall sensitivity level: if the global activation of the two pools is low, the sensitivity is reduced to the same extent along the two axes. Thereby, the ability to detect the difference between a reference configuration (aspect ratio = 1 or IR = 0, i.e. a circle or a square) and a stimulus which develops along the x- or y-coordinates (aspect ratio ≠ 1 or IR ≠ 0, i.e. an ellipse or a rectangle), is poor irrespective of its orientation. As a consequence, VT and HT are expected to be high with no appreciable difference along the two axes, namely with no anisotropy.

- The differential activation of the two quotas, which accounts for the level of anisotropy: if the activation of the two quotas is different, the sensitivity along a cardinal axis turns out to be lower compared to the other, giving rise to SRP anisotropy. For example, if the activation of the x-pool is lower compared to y-pools, HT is expected to be higher than VT, giving rise to vertical anisotropy (SRA > 0).

It has to be ascertained whether the occurrence of anisotropy affects the overall SRP. For this purpose the sample has been divided into two groups, one isotropic (SRA=0), the other anisotropic (SRA≠0) and their relative mean thresholds have been compared [Aleci et al., 2010]. If the thresholds in the anisotropic and isotropic samples were similar, it could be stated that anisotropy has no direct effect on the overall reduction of spatial relationship sensitivity. In fact, the average threshold in the anisotropic sample turned out to be higher (4.27 [± 1.61] vs. 2.28 [± 0.67] in the isotropic group, $p < 0.01$) suggesting that anisotropic subjects suffer from worse SRP compared to the isotropic ones. Therefore, anisotropy may worsen the overall sense of the visual space.

The question remains whether, in turn, subjects with a general reduction of spatial relationship sensitivity are more likely to suffer from an imbalance along the two meridians. In this case the lack of a positive correlation between the spatial relationship threshold and the anisotropy level rules out this possibility: rather than positive, the correlation is negative, so that that the greater the overall reduction of the visual sense of the space, the smaller the anisotropic component.

Therefore, it is arguable that on the one hand the global impairment of the visual sense of the space as such does not affect its anisotropic perception, on the other hand the occurrence of anisotropy may worsen the spatial relationship perception. In summary, anisotropy affects the overall spatial relationship sensibility but the reduction of the latter does not implies the

[339] Even if the amount of the anisotropy is not reported in the study, the difference in the discrimination threshold can be deduced from figure 6 (p. 1852).

visual system to be more imbalanced along one of the two cardinal axes (Figure 5). In other terms, even if the anisotropy may impair the overall perception of spatial relationships, this general depression can occur independently from it. It follows that the occurrence of anisotropy and the global (isotropic) decay of SR sensitivity can be due to two distinct mechanisms. An anonymous reviewer suggested that the overall SRP degradation in the absence of anisotropy depends on fixation instability (therefore not to aspecific hypoactivation of the two cellular pools).

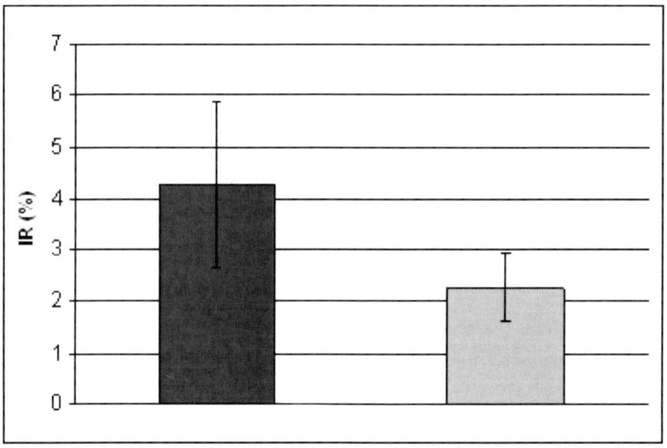

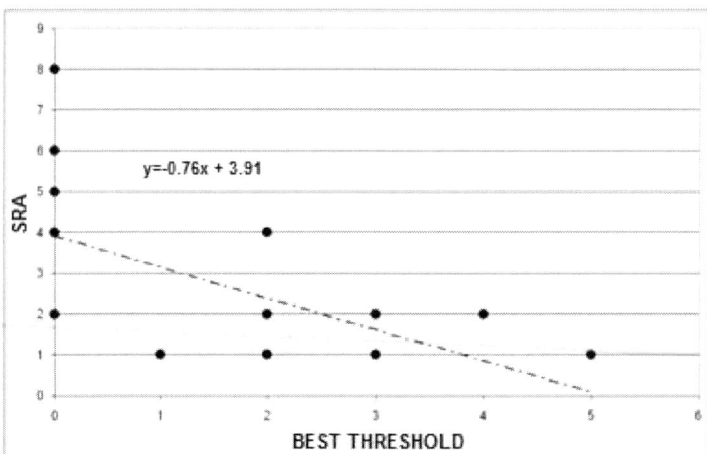

Figure 5. Upper: average threshold in the presence (dark histogram) and in the absence of anisotropy (clear histogram). Lower: correlation between SRP and SRA ($r = -0.56$, $p = 0.0063$).

In conclusion, the results obtained in normal readers (adults and children) are in substantial agreement with the investigations that have made use of local configurations and in most cases are consistent with a slight vertical anisotropy.

It is likely SRP to be a magnocellular function, since both SRP and M-system are particularly vulnerable to pathological conditions such as hemianopia [Milner & Harvey, 1995; Doricchi & Angelelli, 1999; Irving-Bell et al., 1999; Latin Corazzini et al., 2005]. This hypothesis has been supported by a study on patients affected by Williams syndrome

[Atkinson et al., 1997]. In addition, the M-system is likely to be involved in the global analysis of a visual scene [Slaghuis & Ryan, 1999]: an operation, indeed, that requires high spatial relationship sensitivity.

So if a magnocellular system impairment is expected to play a role in the onset of the visual signs and symptoms complained by the dyslexic patients, it is arguable that this impairment involves (also) the spatial relationship perception.

This is the subject we are discussing in the next chapter.

References

Aleci C, Piana G, Anselmino F. (2010). Evaluation of Spatial Anisotropy by Curvature Analysis of Elliptical Targets. *The Open Ophthalmology Journal, 4: 20-26.*

Andrews DP, Butcher AK, Buckley BR. (1973). *Acuities for spatial arrangement in line figures: human and ideal observers compared.* Vision Research, 13: 599-620.

Andrews DP, Miller DT. (1978). *Acuity for spatial separation as a function of stimulus size.* Vision Research, 18: 615-619.

Atkinson J, King J, Braddick O, Nokes L, Anker S, Braddick F. (1997). *A specific deficit of dorsal stream function in Williams'syndrome.* NeuroReport, 8: 1919-1922.

Attneave F. (1954). *Some informational aspects of visual perception.* Psychological Review, 61: 183-193.

Bauer R, Dow BM. (1989). *Complementary global maps for orientation coding in upper and lower layers of the monkey's foveal striate cortex.* Experimental Brain Research, 76: 503-509.

Bennet PJ, Banks MS. (1987). *Sensitivity loss in odd-symmetric mechanisms and phase anomalies in peripheral vision.* Nature, 326: 873-876.

Bennet PJ, Banks MS. (1991). *The effect of contrast, spatial scale, and orientation on foveal and peripheral phase discrimination.* Vision Research, 31: 1759-1786.

Dixon W, Mood A. (1948). *A method for obtaining and analyzing sensitivity data.* Journal of the American Statistical Association: 43, 109-126.

Doricchi F, Angelelli P. (1999). *Misrepresentation of horizontal space in left unilateral neglect: role of hemianopia.* Neurology, 52: 1845–1852.

Fahle M. (1986). *Curvature detection in the visual field and a possible physiological correlate.* Experimental Brain Research, 63: 113-124.

Fahle M. (1991). *Parallel perception of vernier offsets, curvature and chevrons in humans.* Vision Research, 31: 2149-2184.

Foster DH, Simmons DR, Cook MJ. (1993). *The cue for contour-curvature discrimination.* Vision Research, 33: 329-341.

Gigus Z, Malik J. (1991). *Detecting curvilinear structure in images.* UC Berkeley CSD Technical Report, 91/619.

Grinter EJ, Maybery MT, Badcock DR. (2010). *Vision in developmental disorders: is there a dorsal stream deficit?* Brain Research Bulletin, 82: 147-160.

Hess RF. (1999). *Are judgements of circularity local or global?* Vision Research, 39: 4354-4360.

Hubel DH, Wiesel TN. (1977). *Functional architecture of macaque monkey visual cortex.* Proceedings of the Royal Society of London B, 198: 1-59.

Irving-Bell L, Small M, Cowey A. (1999). *A distortion of perceived space in patients with right-hemisphere lesions and visual hemineglect.* Neuropsychologia, 37: 919–925.

Kaernbach C. (1991). *Simple adaptive testing with the weighed up-down method.* Perception & Psychophysics, 49: 227-229.

Koenderink J, Richards W. (1988). *Two-dimensional curvature operators.* Journal of the Optical Society of America, 5: 1136-1141.

Kramer D, Fahle M. (1996). *A simple mechanism for detecting low curvatures.* Vision Research, 36: 1411-1419.

Latini Corazzini L, Geminiani G, Stucchi N, Gindri P, Cremasco L. (2005). *Visual acceleration and spatial distortion in* right brain-damaged patients. Experimental Brain Research, 161: 276-284.

Leventhal AG. (1983). *Relationship between preferred orientation and receptive field position of neurons in cat striate cortex.* Journal of Comparative Neurology, 220: 476-483.

Leventhal AG, Schall JD. (1983). *Structural basis of orientation sensitivity of cat retinal ganglion cells*. Journal of Comparative Neurology, 220: 465-475.

Levick WR, Thibos LN. (1980). *Orientation bias of cat retinal ganglion cells*. Nature, 286: 389-390.

Levick WR, Thibos LN. (1982). *Analysis of orientation bias in cat retina*. Journal of Physiology, 329: 243-261.

Loffler G, Wilson HR, Wilkinson F. (2003). *Local and global contributions to shape discrimination.* Vision Research, 43: 519-530.

Ludvigh E. (1953). *Direction sense of the eye*. American Journal of Ophthalmology, 36: 139-143.

Milner AD, Harvey M. (1995). *Distortion of size perception in visuospatial neglect*. Current Biology, 5: 85-89.

Ogilvie J, Daicar E. (1967). *The perception of curvature.* Canadian Journal of Physiology, 21: 521-525.

Regan D, Hamstra SJ. (1992). *Shape-discrimination and the judgement of perfect symmetry-dissociation of shape from size.* Vision Research, 32: 1845-1864.

Rentschler I, Treutwein B. (1985). *Loss of spatial phase relationships in extrafoveal vision.* Nature, 313: 308-310.

Roach NW, Edwards VT, Hogben JH. (2004). *The tale is in the tail: an alternative hypothesis for psychophysical performance variability in dyslexia.* Perception, 33: 817-830.

Rovamo J, Virsu V, Laurinen P, Hyvärinen L. (1982). *Resolution of gratings oriented along and across meridians in peripheral vision*. Investigative Journal of Ophthalmology and Visual Science, 23: 666-670.

Slaghuis WL, Ryan JF. (1999). *Spatio-temporal contrast sensitivity, coherent motion, and visible persistence in developmental dyslexia.* Vision Research, 39: 651-668.

Smith EL, Chino Y, Ridder WH, Kitagawa K, Langston A. (1990). *Orientation bias of neurons in the lateral geniculate nucleus of macaque monkeys.* Visual Neurosciences, 5: 525-545.

Spry PGD, Johnson CA, McKendrick AM, Turpin A. (2003). *Measurement error of visual field tests in glaucoma*. British Journal of Ophthalmology, 87: 107-112.

Temme LA, Malcus L, Noell WK. (1985). *Peripheral visual field is radially organized.* American Journal of Optometry and Physiological Optics, 62: 545-554.

Treutwein B. (1995). *Adaptive psychophysical procedures.* Vision Research, 35: 2503-2522.

Watt RJ, Andrews DP. (1982). *Contour curvature analysis: hyperacuities in the discrimination of detailed shape.* Vision Research, 22: 449-460.

Watt RJ. (1984). *Further evidence concerning the analysis of curvature in human foveal vision.* Vision Research, 24: 251-253.

Westheimer G. (2005). *Anisotropies in peripheral vernier acuity.* Spatial Vision, 18 (2): 159-167.

Whitaker D, Latham K, Mäkelä P, Rovamo J. (1993). *Detection and discrimination of curvature in foveal and peripheral vision.* Vision Research, 33: 2215-2224.

Wilkinson F, Wilson HR, Habak C. (1998). *Detection and recognition of radial frequency patterns.* Vision Research, 38: 3555-3568.

Wilson HR. (1985). *Discrimination of contour curvature: data and theory.* Journal of the Optical Society of America, 2: 1191-1198.

Wilson HR, Richards WA. (1986). *Mechanisms of contour curvature discrimination.* Journal of the Optical Society of America A, 6: 106-115.

Wilson HR, Wilkinson F, Asaad W. (1997). *Concentric orientation summation in human form Vision.* Vision Research, 37: 2325-2330.

Wilson HR, Wilkinson F. (1998). *Detection of global structure in Glass patterns: implication for form vision.* Vision Research, 38: 2933-2947.

Yap YL, Levi DM, Klein SA. (1987). *Peripheral hyperacuity: isoeccentric bisection is better than radial bisection.* Journal of Optical Society of America A, 4: 1562-1567.

Chapter XVIII

Spatial Relationship Perception in Dyslexia

Based on a consistent body of evidence and in line with our findings, a general anisotropy is found to affect the processing of the visual information in normal subjects. According to the so-called *oblique effect* [Appelle 1972], for example, perception is worse along the oblique axes compared to the cardinal ones. This phenomenon, related to directional differences in the neural response, extends to contrast sensitivity [Campbell & Kulikowski, 1966; Mitchell et al., 1967], stereopsis [Mustillo et al., 1988] and vernier acuity [Saarinen & Levi, 1995; Westheiner & Beard, 1998]. In addition to the oblique effect, anisotropy along the cardinal coordinates involves contrast sensitivity and spatial resolution: both functions are better along the x-axis [Rijisdjik et al., 1980; Carasco et al., 2001], since more cortical cells are in charge of the processing along the horizontal coordinate compared to the vertical one [Li et al., 2003].

Therefore, the visual space is physiologically affected by a perceptive imbalance. On a global level, this imbalance would lead to a mild SRP-related vertical anisotropy [Aleci et al., 2010].

Indeed, in the last two decades a number of studies (in particular studies on spatial localization: Mason, 1980; Stein, 1989; Stein et al., 1989; Solman & May, 1990 and on spatial relationship representation: Pontius, 1981) has provided indirect evidence suggesting the occurrence of a visuospatial distortion in dyslexic patients.

It is therefore worthwhile investigating whether impaired spatial relationship perception and increased spatial relationship anisotropy can contribute to produce the lexical disability.

In a recent work [Aleci et al., 2012], we compared SRP in a group of 42 dyslexic children (28 males, 14 females, mean age of 8.4 + 1.9 years) with the results obtained in a sample of age-matched normal readers [see chapter 2: Aleci et al., 2010].

The inclusion criteria, consistent with those previously adopted by Stanley and Hall [1973], were lexical age reduced of at least 2.5 years with reading rate[340] and accuracy[341] below the second standard deviation compared to normal age-matched readers [Remschmidt et al., 1994], normal intellectual ability and normal or above normal IQ (according to the

[340] Reading rate assessed by the MT reading test [Cornoldi & Colpo, 1981; Cornoldi et al., 1981].

[341] I.e. number of errors.

WISC-R scale), visual acuity 60/60 and no behavioral problems or auditory impairment. Exclusion criteria were general or ophthalmological diseases, poor convergence and accommodation, latent or manifest strabismus, refractive defects greater than 2 diopters, phonological problems and poor cooperation.

In patients, both the horizontal and vertical threshold turned out to be higher than in the control group[342] (mean HT=9.16 [± 3.85] vs. 4.86 [± 1.90]; mean VT=5.73 [± 2.94] vs. 3.64 [± 1.75], $p < 0.001$ in both cases). Vertical anisotropy occurred in 85% of dyslexics: although this proportion is similar in normal readers of the same age (87%), in patients the mean level of vertical anisotropy is almost double compared to controls (4.4 ± 2.59 vs.. 2.36 ± 1.75, $p \leq 0.01$) (figure 1).

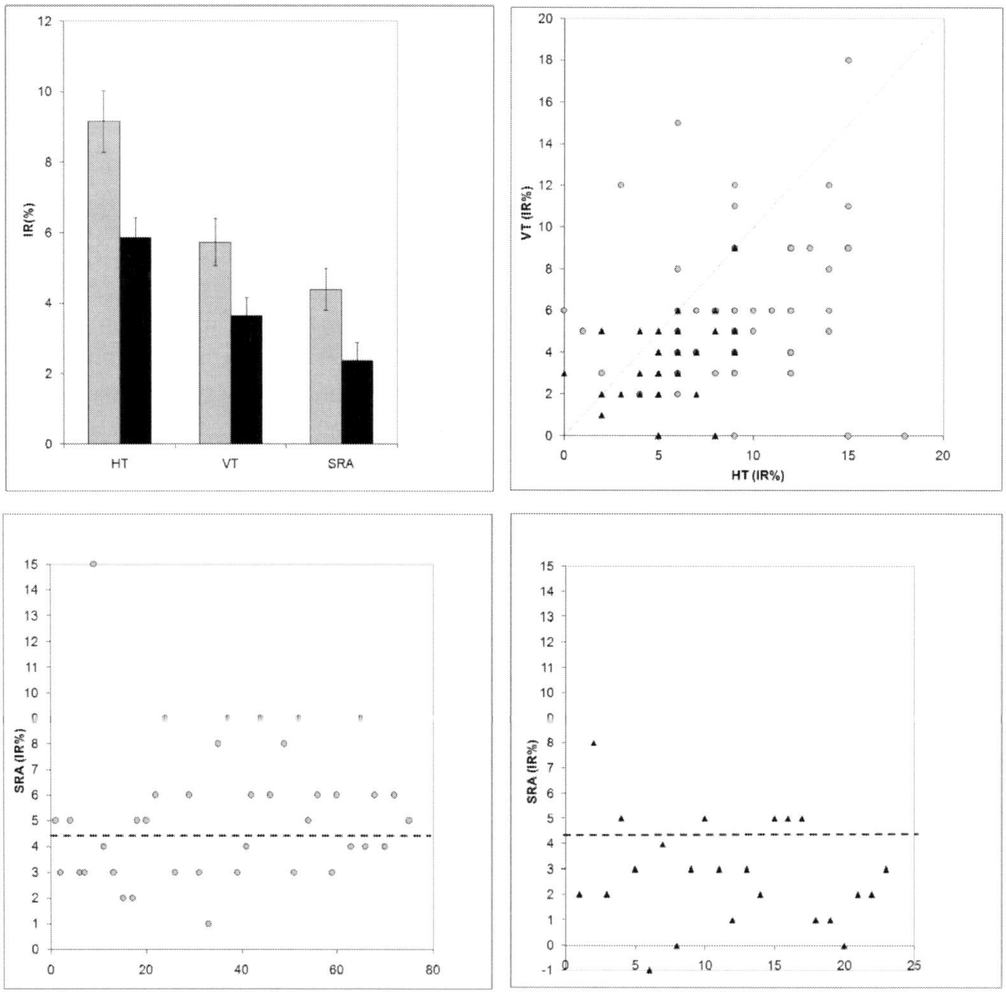

Figure 1. Top left: SRP in dyslexic children (gray bars) and in normal readers (black bars). Top right: deviation from isotropy in the dyslexic and normal sample. The circles refer to the eyes of dyslexics, the triangles to the eyes of controls. The diagonal line represents the isotropy. Bottom: distribution of anisotropy in the two groups. The dotted line represents the cut off level (average SRA of controls + 1 SD).

342 Like in normal readers, also in patients no significant threshold difference was found in the right and left eye or in the dominant and fellow eye.

Taking as a cutoff the mean SRA + 1 SD computed in normal readers[343], abnormal anisotropy was observed in 56% of dyslexics and only in 26% of the control subjects. The lack of correlation between threshold and age confirms that these results do not depend on the cognitive development.

Therefore, to a certain extent a perceptive shrinking, i.e. an anisotropic contraction of the visual space along the horizontal axis, would take place in dyslexia.

Indeed, in case of dots misalignment tasks, the visual system is more sensitive to misalignments along the vertical axis and less along the horizontal one [Westheimer, 2005; Feng et al., 2007] with a ratio between the two thresholds of 0.77 [Westheimer, 2005]. Even if it is slightly higher, this local value of anisotropy, is in substantial agreement with the global SRP anisotropy measured in our physiological sample (0.64).

However, a cause-effect link with the lexical function remains to be ascertained: indeed, it has to be verified if the spatial contraction along the horizontal coordinate can be responsible for the reading disability in patients.

The investigation is based on the putative compensatory effect of the lexical stretch along the horizontal coordinate: if dyslexics tend to perceive the words as shrunk along the *x*-axis for their anisotropic spatial relationship perception, the "stretch" of the area occupied by the lexical string should neutralize their perceptive unbalance, therefore improving their reading ability.

The lexical ability was therefore measured for different levels of dilation of the string and linear regression analysis was applied. As a countercheck, the same measurement was made after the progressive shrinking of the string, since in this case the performance is expected to worsen.

To *anisotropize* the string, the extent of the area occupied by the letters along the two cardinal coordinates was changed according to an inverse proportion[344]. The model has been subsequently implemented as a computer-assisted exam: the Reading Performance Test (REPORT).

In such experimental conditions, reading time (RTm) and reading efficiency (E) were measured in14 dyslexic and in 14 normal readers[345] [Aleci et al., 2012].

E is an index devised to account for both the reading rate and the reading accuracy. E is computed from the following equation:

$$E= (n/RTM)SQR (w/(m+1))$$

Where *n* and *w* are respectively the number of characters and words that make up the sentence[346] and *m* is the number of misspelled words (inversion of letters or syllables, mixed letters or syllables).

The words making up the reading samples were gathered from the optotype MNREAD used for near vision testing (2000, Mansfield JS Minnesota)[347].

---

343 In line with the criterion used by Spinelli [Spinelli et al., 2002].

344 The anisotropization of the strings was performed thanks to a computer hardware platform made up of a certificated LCD screen and a graphic software.

345 Mean age respectively 9.3 ± 2.3 and 9.1 ± 2.0 years.

346 Spaces between words were included.

347 The optotype MNREAD is made up of 19 sentences of the same length. The character used for the experiment subtended a horizontal angle of 24 min arc at the reading distance. The horizontal visual angle after the anisotropization ranges between 17 and 30.9 minarc.

After a short training period, subjects were asked to read aloud in binocular conditions a battery of 14 sentences displayed separately on an LCD screen. Four sentences were presented in standard conditions, six were *anisotropized* along the horizontal axis by three increasing proportions (IR=14.5%, IR=23%, IR=29%) and four by two decreasing proportions (IR=-23%, IR=-29%). The distance between the letters in the six experimental conditions, labeled H_o, $H_{+14.5}$, H_{+23}, H_{+29}, H_{-23}, and H_{-29}, were 25.92, 27.54, 28.62, 29.16, 23.76 and 22.68 min arc wide, respectively. The presentation order was randomized.

As expected, in the standard reading condition mean RTm was higher in the dyslexics compared to the controls (22.6 ± 14.9 sec vs. 10.5 ± 2.9 sec, $p < 0.05$) while E was lower (15.2 ± 9.0 versus 27.9 ± 9.5 $p < 0.05$) (figure 2).

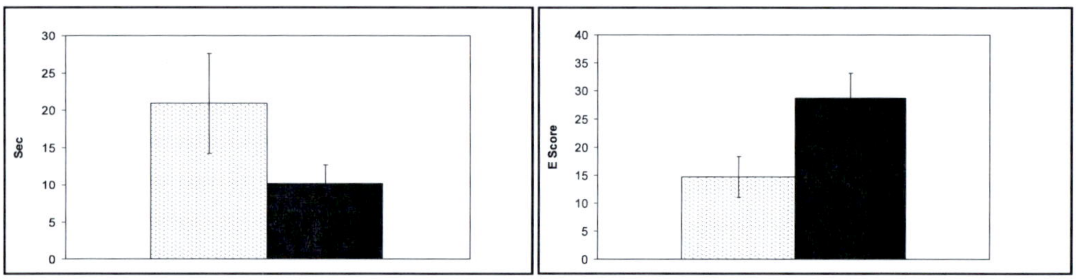

Figure 2. Reading time and efficiency in dyslexics (white bars) and controls (black bars) in standard conditions.

In figure 3 is shown the change of Rtm and E as a function of the *anisotropization* of the string in the dyslexic sample. The average reading time in patients tends to decrease with the stretch of the string ($r = -0.82$, $p < 0.05$) whereas the efficiency improves ($r = 0.89$, $p = 0.01$). On the contrary, no significant correlations are found in normal readers ($r = -0.12$ and $r = 0.43$ for RTm and E, respectively; $p > 0.05$).

In summary, more than half of the dyslexic children are found to suffer from an alteration of the spatial relationship perception characterized by anomalous vertical anisotropy. After the normalization of such a visual unbalance by stretching the sentence along the horizontal axis, the lexical performance tends to improve.

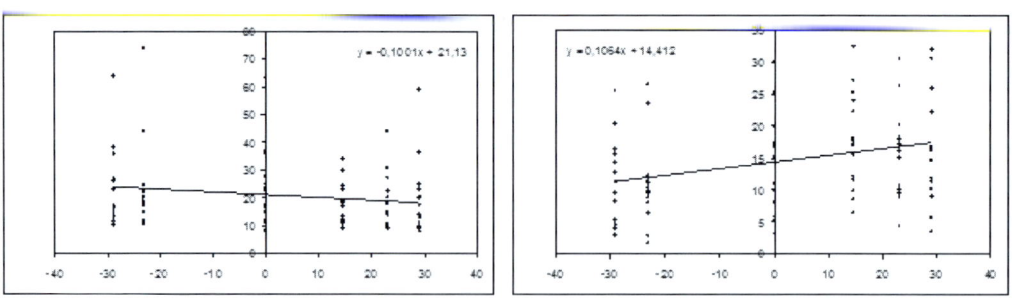

Figure 3. Correlation between the lexical function and the horizontal anisotropization of the string in dyslexic subjects. Left: RTm, right: E.

As assessed with the eidomorphometry, stimuli with prevalent horizontal development are correctly identified if the difference between their x-, y-extent is of at least 6%. Below this value the configurations are no more recognizable from the reference stimulus. This report is in line with the anisotropy highlighted in the model of Petrov and Popple [2007] and Petrov et al.. [2007] and with the anisotropy reported by Feng et al. [2007].

Recently, Greenwood et al.. [2009] measured the accuracy in evaluating the vertical displacement of the horizontal bar of a cross ("+") displayed alone or among similar distractors. The authors found a systematic and selective anisotropic positional deviation. Moreover, by adding distractors the positional threshold raised. The explanation for this detrimental effect would lie on the averaging process of the different positional estimates of the distractors, therefore able to bias the judgment focused on the stimulus-test. Likewise, the averaging of the local orientation estimates along both the more and less curved contour of an elliptical configuration would have a detrimental effect on the overall sensitivity of the stimulus. In fact, averaging tends to neutralize any curvature difference along the x-, y-axis [Watt & Andrews, 1982; Parkes et al., 2001] so that a barely elliptical shape is made perceptually indistinguishable from a circular stimulus, independently on the orientation of its focal axis.

If the visual system is anisotropic, the curvature arc whose chord is oriented along the direction of the processing unbalance is underestimated and at the same time the curvature along the perpendicular one is overestimated. In case of vertical anisotropy this *scenario* leads to perceive horizontal configurations as if they were circular patterns and circular patterns as if they were vertical ellipses. The resulting increase of the horizontal threshold (and the eventual concomitant decrease of the vertical one) quantifies such a visual distortion. It is arguable the current moderate vertical anisotropy transferred on a local scale to account for the eccentric shape of the spatial interaction zones responsible for the lateral masking. Indeed, the crowding effect on the reading task has already been discussed[348] [Bouma & Legein, 1977; Atkinson, 1991, 1993, Spinelli et al., 2002; O'Brien et al., 2005; Martelli et al., 2009] as well as the anisotropic characteristics of the spatial interaction zones [Toet & Levi, 1992][1]. It is noteworthy that the spatial interaction zones in the paracentral area are described as elliptical with the focal axis directed toward the fixation point, so that in the central visual field the critical spacing is wider for radial configurations. As a result, along the horizontal axis the recognition of characters placed side by side requires a greater separation compared to the same characters arranged vertically.

The perceptual difference depending on the spatial arrangement of the characters is in agreement with the anisotropic model described by Feng et al. [2007]: the authors, indeed, stated that in the four quadrants of the visual field lateral masking is stronger for horizontal alignments compared to vertical arrangements. Therefore, the higher integration threshold for horizontal stimuli is revealing of spatial relationship vertical anisotropy: this anisotropy would, in fact, bias the horizontal processing of the configuration and enhance the vertical one.

In summary, the main findings obtained with our investigations in dyslexics are reduced sensitivity along both cardinal axes and increased vertical anisotropy. The physiological vertical anisotropy observed at global level by means of eidomorphometry would be responsible for crowding at local level, so that the higher the vertical anisotropy, the stronger the lateral masking. The anomalous anisotropy, indeed, would result in a perceptual contraction along the horizontal coordinate of the visual space so as to cause an illusory reduction of the interletter distance: it follows that characters normally located beyond the

[348] See part I, chapter 13.

critical spacing are perceived by the patient inside this interval, and therefore turn out to be crowded. In support of this solution, in dyslexics (but not in normal readers) reading performance tends to improve as the sentence is "stretched", so as to make wider the distance between the adjoining letters.

Indeed, Liu and Arditi found that in crowded conditions the string seems shortened so that the observer tends to underestimate the number of letters it is made of [Liu & Arditi, 1996, 2000]. This experiment is interesting since it supports a link between crowding and the illusory contraction of the lexical string, as expected in presence of vertical anisotropy. The phenomenon, observed in normal readers, should be more evident in dyslexics affected by abnormal vertical anisotropy.

Due to this perceptual distortion and in agreement with the results of a recent study [Martelli et al., 2009], critical spacing in dyslexics appears broader than in normal readers. The widening of the critical spacing in dyslexics affects the lexical function via reduction of the visual span size, according to the aforementioned model [Legge et al., 2001][349].

Interestingly, the perceptual unbalance would involve even the auditory domain, as the vocal reaction time after the dilation of the interletter distance is found to be reduced in about half of the patients [Spinelli et al., 2002].

This paradigm helps to explain the reading errors made by patients, in particular those involving mirror letters and syllables. Noteworthy, in the peripheral visual field the discrimination threshold for mirror (or antiphase) gratings (spatial phase shifted by 180°) is higher compared to non-mirror gratings [Bennett & Banks, 1987, 1991] and this phenomenon is found to be markedly anisotropic. Since the same effect also applies to mirror letters, especially if presented close to other characters, it can be argued lateral masking involving mirror letters to be particularly strong [Chung, 2010].

Therefore, for the reduced coding efficiency of the spatial phase in the peripheral visual field [Braddick, 1981; Julesz, 1981; Rentschler & Treutwein, 1985], recognition threshold for mirror letters and syllables is higher and increases faster with eccentricity compared to non-mirror characters/syllables [Rentschler & Treutwein, 1985; Bennett & Banks, 1987, 1991, Chung, 2010][350].

In conclusion, due to the anisotropic compression of the visual space and the consequent crowding reinforcement along the horizontal axis, in dyslexic subjects the coding of the spatial phase (thereby the processing of mirror letters and syllables) in extrafoveal projection are made similar to the level expected in the peripheral field of normal readers. This could be the reason why the positional exchange of mirror letters in patients is pathognomonic[351]. However, the anisotropic trend has been observed only in a certain (although significant) proportion of dyslexics. In our investigation, SR anisotropy was found to be normal in 44% of the recruited patients. On the other side, about 20% of the controls showed increased levels of vertical anisotropy. Probably, in these subjects some compensatory mechanism may have preserved the lexical function from the effect of the visual space distortion. Likewise, other studies about crowding have established that only 31-32% of dyslexics suffer from abnormal

---

[349] See Part I, chapter 13.

[350] This effect does not depend on the resemblance between letters but is specific for the symmetry axis [Chung, 2010].

[351] Interestingly, Pontius found that 4/5 of the patients are prevented from solving a figure rotation, associating this feature to the frequent confusion of mirrored letters along the two cardinal axes as "p", "b", "q", or "d" (Pontius, 1981].

lateral masking [Atkinson, 1993; Spinelli et al., 2002]. These data confirm that the distortion of the visual space is not the only factor responsible for the reading disability in developmental dyslexia and that patients differ in the proportion between the linguistic-phonological involvement and the visual impairment.

The perceptual effect of the increased vertical anisotropy on the lateral masking and eventually on the lexical ability have driven our investigations: it is possible *"[...] that our visual environment is intrinsically more horizontally than vertically correlated [...]* "[Feng et al., 2007].

Therefore, the alleged role of the abnormal vertical anisotropy on the reading difficulties of dyslexics has guided the development of some specific tests[352] recently introduced in our clinical practice.

References

Ahn SJ, Legge GE, Luebker A. (1995). *Printed cards for measuring low-vision reading speed.* Vision Research, 35: 1939-1944.

Aleci C, Piana G, Anselmino F. (2010). *Evaluation of spatial anisotropy by curvature analysis of elliptical targets.* The Open Ophthalmology Journal, 4: 20-26.

Aleci C, Piana G, Piccoli M, Bertolini M. (2012). *Developmental dyslexia and spatial relationship perception.* Cortex, 48: 466-476.

Appelle S. (1972). *Perception and discrimination as a function of stimulus orientation: The oblique effect in man and animals.* Psycholgical Bulletin, 78: 266-278.

Atkinson J. (1991). *Review of human visual development: crowding and dyslexia.* In: Vision and Visual Dyslexia, Stein Ed., MacMillian Press, London, UK.

Atkinson J. (1993). *Vision in dyslexics: Letter recognition, acuity, visual crowding, contrast sensitivity, accommodation, convergence and sight reading music.* In: Facets of dyslexia and its remediation, Wright & Groner Eds., Elsevier, Amsterdam, NL.

Bennett PJ, Banks MS. (1987). *Sensitivity loss in odd-symmetric mechanisms and phase anomalies in peripheral vision.* Nature, 326: 873-876.

Bennett PJ, Banks MS. (1991). *The effect of contrast, spatial scale, and orientation on foveal and peripheral phase discrimination.* Vision Research, 31: 1759-1786.

Bouma H, Legein CP. (1977). *Foveal and parafoveal recognition of letters and words by dyslexics and by average readers.* Neuropsychologia, 15: 69-80.

Braddick OJ. (1981). *Is spatial phase degraded in peripheral vision and visual pathology?* Documenta Ophthalmologica Proceedings Series, 30: 255-262.

Campbell FW, Kulikowski JJ. (1966). *Orientational selectivity of the human visual system.* Journal of Physiology, 187: 437-445.

Carrasco M, Talgar CP, Cameron EL. (2001). *Characterizing visual performance fields: Effects of transient covert attention, spatial frequency, eccentricity, task, and set size.* Spatial Vision, 15: 61-75.

[352] These tests, which make up the TETRA™ platform, evaluate motor and sensorial ocular dominance (Domitest-M and Domitest-S, respectively), spatial relationship perception (Eidomorphometry) and reading rate as a function of the anisotropization level of the visual space. Refer to www.visualeci.com for further explanations on the TETRA analyzer.

Chung ST. (2010). *Detection and identification of crowded mirror-image letters in normal peripheral vision.* Vision Research, 50: 337-345.

Cornoldi C, Colpo G. (1981). *La verifica dell'apprendimento della lettura.* Organizzazioni Speciali Ed., Firenze, Italy.

Cornoldi C, Colpo G, Gruppo MT. (1981). *La verifica dell'apprendimento e prove oggettive MT di lettura.* Organizzazioni Speciali Ed., Firenze, Italy.

Feng C, Jiang Y, He S. (2007). *Horizontal and vertical asymmetry in visual spatial crowding effects.* Journal of Vision, 7 (2): 1-10.

Greenwood JA, Bex PJ, Dakin SC. (2009). *Positional averaging explains crowding with letter-like stimuli.* Proceedings of the National Academy of Sciences, 106: 13130-13135.

Julesz B. (1981). *Textons, the elements of texture perception, and their interactions.* Nature, 290: 91-97.

Legge GE, Mansfield JS, Chung ST. (2001). *Psychophysics of reading. XX. Linking letter recognition to reading speed in central and peripheral vision.* Vision Research, 41: 725–743.

Li B, Peterson MR, Freeman RD. (2003). *Oblique effect: A neural basis in the visual cortex.* Journal of Neurophysiology, 90: 204-217.

Liu L, Arditi A. (1996). *Letter confusion observed under small interletter spacings.* Investigative Ophthalmology & Visual Science, 75(Suppl.): 201.

Liu L, Arditi A. (2000). *Apparent string shortening concomitant with letter crowding.* Vision Research, 40: 1059-1067.

Martelli M, Di Filippo G, Spinelli D, Zoccolotti P. (2009). *Crowding, reading, and developmental dyslexia.* Journal of Vision, 9 (4): 1-18.

Mason M. (1980). *Reading ability and the encoding of location information.* Journal of Experimental Psychology: Human Perception and Performance, 6: 89-98.

Mitchell DE, Freeman RD, Westheimer G. (1967). *Effect of the orientation on the modulation sensitivity for interference fringes on the retina.* Journal of the Optical Society of America, 57: 246-249.

Mustillo P, Francis E, Oross S, Fox R, Orban GA. (1988). *Anisotropies in global stereoscopic orientation discrimination.* Vision Research, 28: 1315-1321.

O'Brien BA, Mansfeld JS, Legge GE. (2005). *The effect o print size on reading speed in dyslexia.* Journal of Research in Reading, 28 (3): 332-349.

Parkes L, Lund J, Angelucci A, Solomon JA, Morgan M. (2001). *Compulsory averaging of crowded orientation signals in human vision.* Nature Neuroscience, 4: 739-744.

Petrov Y, Popple AV. (2007). *Crowding is directed to the fovea and preservers only feature contrast.* Journal of Vision, 7 (2): 8, 1-9.

Petrov Y, Popple AV, McKee SP. (2007). *Crowding and surround suppression: not to be confused.* Journal of Vision, 7 (2): 12, 1-9.

Pontius AA. (1981). *Geometric figure-rotation task and face representation in dyslexia: role of spatial relations and orientation.* Perceptual & Motor Skills, 53: 607-614.

Remschmidt H, Schmidt M, Poustka F. (1994). *Multiaxiales Klassifikationsschema für Psychische Storüngen des Kindes-und Jugendalters nach ICD-10 der WHO.* SWI: Verlag Hans Huber Ed., Bern, Switzerland.

Rentschler I, Treutwein B. (1985). *Loss of spatial phase relationships in extrafoveal vision.* Nature, 313: 308-310.

Rijsdijk JP, Kroon JN, van der Wilt GJ. (1980). *Contrast sensitivity as a function of position on the retina.* Vision Research, 20: 235-241.

Saarinen J, Levi DM. (1995). *Orientation anisotropy in vernier acuity.* Vision Research, 35: 2449-2461.

Solman RT, May JG. (1990). *Spatial localization discrepancies: A visual deficiency in poor readers.* American Journal of Psychology, 103: 243-263.

Spinelli, De Luca M, Judica A, Zoccolotti PL. (2002). *Crowding effects on word identification in developmental dyslexia.* Cortex, 38: 179-200.

Stanley G and Hall R. (1973). *Short term visual information processing in dyslexics.* Child Development, 44: 841-844.

Stein J. (1989). *Visuospatial perception and reading problems.* Irish Journal of Psychology, 10: 521-533.

Stein J, Riddel P, Fowler S. (1989). *Brain and Reading.* Von Euler, Lundberg & Lennerstrand Eds., Stockton, New York.

Toet A, Levi DM. (1992). *The two-dimensional shape of spatial interaction zones in the parafovea.* Vision Research, 32: 1349–1357.

Watt RJ, Andrews DP. (1982). *Contour curvature analysis: hyperacuities in the discrimination of detailed shape.* Vision Research, 22: 449-460.

Westheimer G. (2005). *Anisotropies in peripheral vernier acuity.* Spatial Vision, 18: 159-167.

Westheimer G, Beard BL. (1998). *Orientation dependency for foveal line stimuli: Detection and intensity discrimination, resolution, orientation discrimination, and vernier acuity.* Vision Research 38: 1097-1103.

Chapter XIX

Does Vertical Anisotropy Lead to a Perceptive Distortion of the Characters?

The effect of abnormal vertical anisotropy on the lexical string may not be limited to the widening of the critical spacing, but could modify the perception of the elementary constituents of the letters as well, giving rise to configurations that do not belong to the alphabetical samples imprinted in the mind. Therefore, in addition to the deterioration of the positional coding and of the recognition of the characters (which are the main results of the reduction of increased critical spacing), the perceptual distortion of the shape of the characters could be a second obstacle to their correct processing.

Font Decoding

The perception and recognition of a letter occurs independently on the print style (or font). But how can the visual system recognize letters printed with different fonts, i.e. alphabetical configurations that apart from their identical informational content have different stylistic characteristics? A letter is perceived as a set of elementary constituents (set of feature units), each coded by specific detectors (the cortical receptive fields). The integration of the detectors' responses referred to each feature belonging to a given character allows coding the configuration matching that letter. And yet, the adequate coding of the letter configuration is not enough for it to be recognized as *that particular* letter: its recognition, indeed, takes place when its main characteristics match those encoded in a set of elementary or abstract alphabetical configurations, defined by Sanocki *set of letter units* [Sanocki, 1987]: this operation can be called *mapping of different fonts in the abstract alphabetical set of configurations*[353].

This way, for a given print style the visual information of a character is arranged on two levels: the first (deep) level concerns the salient features of the letter (its abstract

[353] See.Sanocki [1987] for references.

configuration) and typifies it; the second (superficial) level refers to the stylistic characteristics of that particular font, which enriches the abstract configuration of the shape and *serifs*[354] typical of *that* font.

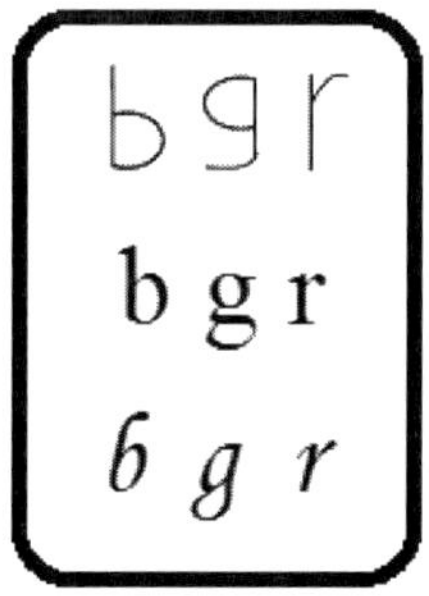

Figure 1. The two levels of the visual information of a character. Top: the abstract configuration of three letters: "b" (vertical bar with a semi-circle in the lower right corner), the "g" (vertical bar with an arc on the bottom left and a semi-circle on the top left) and the "r" (vertical bar with an arc on the top right). Middle and bottom: the same letters enriched of the characteristics of two different fonts.

For example, the letter "F" is made up of three elementary components: a vertical bar, a high upper right horizontal bar, and a right horizontal bar at the midpoint: this is the abstract or elementary configuration (F) of the letter "F ".

All the other features of the letter enrich the elementary configuration without adding further salient information, requiring the font to be mapped (decoded) within the abstract alphabetical code. Therefore, the originality of a font compared to another is given by the features that are added to the abstract configuration while its regularity (the *harmony* of the shape of the letters belonging to the same font) depends on the fact that these graphic characteristics are added according to common procedures and criteria shared for each letter. The crucial point is this: in which way is the visual system able to make a particular font fit the correspondent set of abstract alphabetical configurations, so that the font can be recognized as the letter it represents? In other words, in which way the mapping of different fonts into the abstract alphabetical code takes place? And eventually in which way the recognition of a character printed with different font can be univocal? To answer these questions simple and more complex models have been theorized, the latter defined *network models*. Both paradigms are based on the same decoding mechanism: as explained by Sanocki [1987]: the abstract alphabetical configurations are described by five categories of elementary constituents arranged in different ways[355]. The decoding task of the visual system is to bring the font configuration back to the respective abstract configuration.

Simple models theorize the detectors responsible for the recognition of the elementary constituents to work independently [Keren & Baggen, 1981, Townsend & Ashby, 1982], filtering out all the details[356] that characterize a particular style so as to focus on the

[354] *Serifs* are details like bars, segments or other little signs added to one or more features to give the letter a particular aesthetic connotation.

[355] The five categories are: vertical stroke (stroke), horizontal bar (bar), curved section (loop), corner, point. In a given character each category takes a position (for example, in the letters "p" and "q" the stroke is respectively on the left and on the right) or an intrinsic characteristic (for example, in the letters "p" and "o" the loop can subtend respectively180 or 360 degrees).

[356] For example the serifs.

informational content (i.e. the abstract alphabetical code proper of the letter) that as such is common to each font referred to that character. Additionally, the network model presumes that the detectors interact reciprocally [Palmer, 1977; Oden, 1979], so as to allow a mutual modulation that gradually improves and makes the decoding process more and more precise and fast. The network model expects the letters of the same font to be constantly related to each other by virtue of their common characteristics (such as size, shape and serif). The most interesting feature of the network model is precisely this “visuoperceptive self-modulation”, “fine-tuned” on a specific style so that the recognition strategy employed for a character made of particular features is adopted for the recognition of the next characters of the same font. This operation triggers a facilitatory loop that makes the decoding process referred to that particular font more and more easy and fluent. This process is experimentally confirmed by the fact that a sequential characters recognition is better when the letters are made up of the same font and worse in case of different fonts [McClelland, 1976; Adams, 1979; Sanocki, 1987]. The self-modulation, therefore, consists in the adjustment of the acquired parameters to decode a font so as to make it increasingly suitable to the corresponding abstract alphabetical configuration. If the font does not change along the string, the adjustment process for the previous character is acquired also for the next ones, which in fact share the same characteristics.

On the contrary, if the string is made of letters of different fonts, this self-modulation is no more available and the adjustment strategy has to be re-programmed character after character, so that the processing time of the string becomes longer: the more different is the style of each letter, the longer is the recognition time [Sanocki, 1987][357]. Such a decoding process of the fonts may rely also on the attentional focus, which acts promoting the activation of some neural pathways instead of others, depending on acquired (because previously codified) configurations[358].

Yet, a more plausible theory is claimed to be the so-called *network relaxation minima* [Tyler & Likova, 2007]. According to this hypothesis, the elementary configurations continually enhance the neural decoding system. The neural decoding system, based on the abstract alphabetical configuration, develops some states of “relaxation” when dealing with the most frequent fonts. In the presence of a given font, it "relaxes" itself to be as compatible as possible with that configuration, it *assimilates* it, and coming back to the previous state of

---

[357] Consider also that the letters recognition is quicker for certain fonts (eg Minimal compared to Serif: Sanocki, 1987): therefore there are fonts that are more readable than others. This element must be taken into consideration when preparing lexical material suitable for dyslexic patients.

[358] Pylyshyn [1999] has suggested that the attentional focus acts selecting the characteristics of a configuration. These features would then be compared with the abstract alphabetical set not on a visuospatial basis but on a descriptive (propositional) one. So, a configuration described as "below horizontal, vertical top left" codes the letter "L".

Compared to the visuoperceptive coding, a descriptive coding has the merit of drastically reducing the number of possible combinations, since a description can have different meanings, and yet the ambiguity is resolved by the context. For example, the propositional coding "below horizontal, vertical top left" can refer not only to the letter "L", but also the Roman number “fifty” ("L"), yet the lexical context within which the configuration is inserted prevents from erroneous coding (personal consideration).

As pointed out by Tyler & Likova [2007], it is after all the method used by the popular search engine *Google*. The problem in this case consists in the difficulty to describe this "propositional" approach in anatomophysiological terms and to reconcile it with the tendency to make use of the visual memory to differentiate or identify objects (including the letters).

normal efficiency decodes the font and recognizes it as corresponding to a configuration already acquired in the past[359].

In this model, too, the attentional focus would play a role of fundamental importance, selecting the relevant visual information and preventing the whole lexical context from being simultaneously analyzed.

It is worthwhile wondering whether crowding may affect also the decoding process of the lexical configuration[360] [Tyler & Likova, 2007]. Indeed, besides strengthening the spatial integration of the elementary constituents of the letters, it is possible that lateral masking affects even the mapping of the different print fonts within the abstract alphabetical code, in view of the topographical congruence between these two processes. In fact, not only the integration of the features making up a character but even the ability to label the sign "A" as the letter A resides in neuronal structures placed at a higher cortical level compared to the visual areas responsible for the simple recognition of that configuration: that is in V3 or V4. Considering the theory of the *network relaxation minima*, lateral masking may hamper the decoding of a configuration by preventing the neural system during the relaxation phase from being in a compatible state with that configuration (in fact crowded configurations are virtually configurations *nonsense*). The result is the lack of a solution when the neural system comes back to the pre-relaxation state, so that the alphabetical configuration cannot be assigned its correspondent abstract configuration. Alternatively, the configuration *nonsense* can redirect the neural system in the relaxation phase towards a wrong solution. Therefore, the effect of crowding at the decoding level of the lexical configurations would lead to an uncertain or incorrect identification of the letter. In summary, the lateral masking reinforcement occurring in many dyslexics could affect not only the recognition of the letters configuration but even the self-modulation of the decoding process.

References

Adams MJ. (1979). *Models of word recognition.* Cognitive Psychology, 11: 133-176.

Huckauf A, Nazir TA. (2007) *How odgcrnwi becomes crowding: Stimulus-specific learning reduces crowding.* Journal of Vision, 7: 1-12.

Keren G, Baggen S. (1981). *Recognition models of alphanumeric characters.* Perception & Psychophysics, 29: 234-246.

McClelland JL. (1976). *Preliminary letter identification in the perception of words and nonwords.* Journal of Experimental Psychology: Human Perception and Performance, 2: 80- 91.

Oden GC. (1979). *A fuzzy logical model of letter identification.* Journal of Experimental Psychology: Human Perception and Performance, 5: 336-352.

[359] It is argued [Huckauf & Nazir, 2007] that the generalization of the ameliorative effect of the visual training (when it transfers to other locations in the visual field, to different inter letter distances, and especially to lexical configurations other than those used during the practice), is the sign that the lexical experience tends to make the visual representation of the lexical configurations more tolerant with respect to their numberless combinations (such as spacing between letters, font or size).

[360] In other words, the lateral masking not only prevents from recognizing a configuration made of a vertical segment and three horizontal bars, but even from identifying that configuration as the letter "E".

Palmer SE. (1977). *Hierarchical structure in perceptual representation.* Cognitive Psychology, 9: 441-474.

Pylyshyn Z. (1999). *Is vision continuous with cognition? The case for cognitive impenetrability of visual perception.* Behavioural and Brain Science, 22: 341-423.

Sanocki T. (1987). *Visual knowledge underlying letter perception: Font-specific, schematic tuning.* Journal of Experimental Psychology, 13: 267-278.

Townsed JT, Ashby FG. (1982). *Experimental test of contemporary mathematical models of visual letter recognition.* Journal of Experimental Psychology: Human Perception and Performance, 8: 834-864.

Tyler CW, Likova LT. (2007). *Crowding: A neuroanalytical approach.* Journal of Vision, 16: 1-9.

Chapter XX

Dialectical Suggestions

Can spatial relationship anisotropy explain the heterogeneous visuoperceptive defects found in dyslexics? This is a question worthy to be addressed.

Here are some considerations useful as a cue for further insights.

Anisotropy and Contrast Sensitivity

It is stated that reading rate is not affected from the contrast reduction of the characters across a wide range of values but depends on the visual span. The visual span, too, is largely independent of contrast sensitivity at the current contrast level, i.e. for contrast values at least 4 times greater than the threshold (which is equal to 0. 01). On the contrary, below this cutoff (0. 04) the visual span narrows progressively till to zero as contrast approaches the threshold: between the threshold and 0. 04, even if single letters are still recognizable, words are no more readable [Legge, 2007, Legge et al., 2007]. It is remarkable that in normal readers the contraction of the visual span due to the enlargement of the critical spacing occurs for very low contrast levels, whereas in dyslexics it may take place even at (quasi) ordinary values [Pelli et al., 2004]. Therefore a contrast sensitivity deficit, even if it is too slight to prevent the patient from recognizing every single character, can contribute to narrow the visual span. Actually, in order to read ten-letter words dyslexics need a contrast of about 0.3 log units higher than required for single letters, while in the normal readers the value remains the same[361] [Martelli et al., 2009]. This finding seems to confirm that dyslexics need higher contrast than normal readers in order to preserve their visual span.

Therefore, to a certain extent even contrast sensitivity can indirectly contribute to affect the ability to read a sentence. Indeed, this detrimental effect is not related to reduced detection of the single letters, but to the visual span narrowing: the slightly lower contrast sensitivity as found in many patients, in fact, would make the visual span more susceptible to narrow.

[361] This difference is observed in mesopic conditions (28 cd/m2) for tachistoscopic presentations (presentation time: 200 msec) and disappears as the stimulus duration is delayed to 2000 msec. Longer stimulus duration would allow longer fixations. In this case longer fixations could be the compensatory attempt to stem the lateral masking reinforcement.

In conclusion, even if the contrast sensitivity reduction does not affect directly the lexical function in dyslexics, it could enhance the effect of the vertical anisotropy in shrinking the visual span via a strengthening of the lateral masking.

It is an interesting speculative line but requires validations.

Anisotropy and Motion Perception

The alteration of the spatial relationship perception may affect even motion sensitivity. In normal subjects motion perception is anisotropic and better along the cardinal axes compared to the oblique orientations [Coletta et al., 1993; Loeffler & Orbach, 2001], with greater sensitivity along the horizontal coordinate [Van de Grind et al.., 1993; Raymond, 1994][362]. Motion threshold is therefore higher in the vertical direction[363], and the slower is the movement, the more evident is this vertical/horizontal difference [Van de Grind et al., 1993].

As a result, iso-threshold curves referred to motion sensibility are elliptical with their focal axis oriented horizontally [Van de Grind et al.., 1993]: a pattern resembling the shape of the spatial interaction zones along the x-axis [Toet & Levi, 1992]. The analogy between the shape of the spatial interaction zones and of the iso-threshold curve referred to motion perception, leads to argue that the modest and physiological anisotropy of the spatial relationship perception can be the basis not only of the lateral masking but also of the motion perception asymmetry in normal readers.

Thereby, the increased SR-related vertical anisotropy found in many dyslexics could extend to the time domain: in substance, patients' reduced motion sensitivity could stem even from their abnormal vertical anisotropy, since the horizontal shrinking of the visual space would make motion perception less accurate along the horizontal coordinate.

It has been argued that reduced motion perception is the sign of defective spatial encoding [Cornelissen et al., 1998]. Indeed, in patients the ability to locate the respective position of the characters is impaired. Solman & May [1990] have shown that the accuracy to localize a letter is reduced as a function of the eccentricity and this inaccuracy is more evident in dyslexics. The study involved 20 normal reader children and 20 aged-matched dyslexics[364]. In both groups the discrepancy between the real and the estimated position of the letters was found to increase starting from 1.5 till to 6.5 degrees from the fixation point, but from 2.16 degrees of eccentricity the localization accuracy of patients turned out to be lower compared to normal readers. The authors considered this finding as suggestive of M system deficit.

In conclusion, in dyslexics the spatial localization discrepancy, which is believed to depend on a magnocellular deficit, would be related to impaired motion perception. Impaired motion perception, in turn, might stem from visual space distortion: it follows that even the positional coding of the stimulus would be biased by the anisotropic spatial relationship perception.

---

[362] This findings are referred to coherent motion perception.

[363] At low and medium speeds near the vertical meridian.

[364] Mean age: 8.5 years.

Anisotropy and Visual Attention

As reported in the first part[365], the attentional gradient aims at neutralizing the peripheral visual analysis in order to enhance the attentional focus on the central processing. The reduced attentional gradient in dyslexics involves an enlargement of the Form Resolving Field, affecting the attentional hierarchy between center and periphery. SR anisotropy could contribute to determine such an attentional subversion. In fact, for the illusory contraction of the visual space along the horizontal coordinate the more eccentric characters, located beyond the limit of the attentional field, appear shifted toward the fixation point, falling within its boundary. As a consequence, the focus tends to widen, making the attentional gradient of the FRF less steep (Figure 1).

Vertical anisotropy therefore increases the ratio FRF width/sentence length, so that the more peripheral characters, normally excluded, turn out to affect the central processing, leading to visual confusion.

In summary, according to this suggestions the anisotropic contraction of the visual space may hamper reading both in the peripheral part of the processing window and in the region surrounding the fixation point.

In the peripheral region of the processing window the spatial anisotropy widens the attentional field. Since the widening of the attentional field enhances the detrimental influence of the end portions of the string, dyslexics are predisposed to visual confusion.

In the region surrounding the fixation point vertical anisotropy makes the lateral masking stronger, narrowing the extent of the visual span.

The consequences of this phenomenon are not limited to the lexical function but can cast light on other findings, such as those referred to motion perception. It is intriguing that like the aforementioned motion iso-threshold curve and the spatial interaction zones, even the shape of the attentional focus is elliptical with the focal axis oriented horizontally [Pan & Eriksen, 1993][366].

In relation to motion sensibility, the maturation of the dynamic perception found in the first grade children compared to the kindergarten is argued to be the consequence of the attentional process refining, in turn obtained via lexical training [Boets et al., 2011]. As a matter of fact, there is evidence in support of the modulatory effect of visual attention on motion perception [Atkinson, 1991; Cornelissen et al., 1998, Raymond, 2000, Kinsey et al., 2004], to the extent that the magnocellular damage in the mediotemporal area is believed to be responsible not only for the reduced ability to process dynamic stimuli but also for the attentional impairment [Iles et al., 2000][367].

Therefore defective visual attention, supposedly depending also on anisotropic spatial relationship perception, seems to be pivotal not only in the genesis of the lexical disability but also for the comprehension of other M-mediated epiphenomena like the alteration of motion perception.

---

[365] Chapter 11.

[366] See also Cave and Bichot [1999] for a review.

[367] See part I, chapter 11.

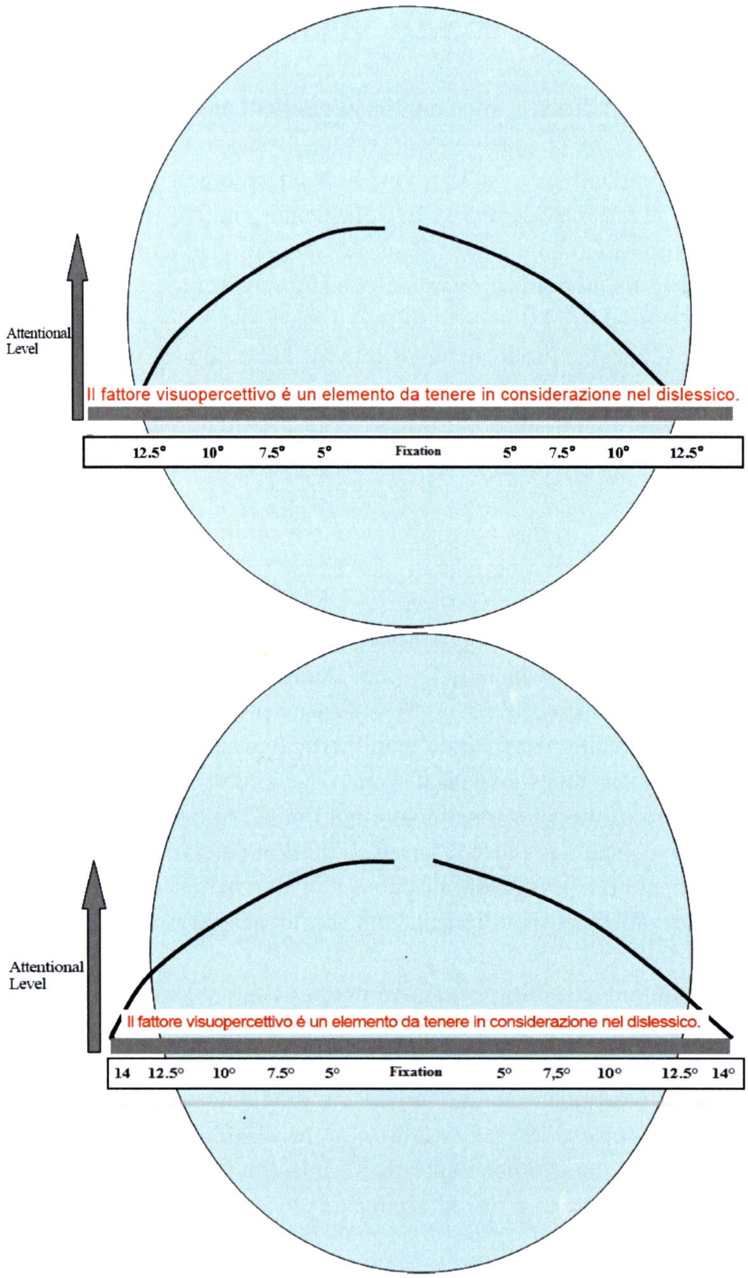

Figure 1. Apparent enlargement of the FRF compared to the extent of the lexical string as a result of abnormal vertical anisotropy. Top panel: the FRF extends up to about 12.5 degrees from the fixation center. The visual attention encompasses the central portion of the sentence and excludes the first and the last word. Bottom panel: vertical anisotropy leads to a contraction of the sentence: as a result, the whole string falls within the boundaries of the FRF. It follows that the apparent extent of the FRF compared to the length of the sentence is increased.
"*The visuoperceptive factor is an element to be taken into account in dyslexics*".

Anisotropy and Oculomotility

i- Saccadic Hypometry

It has been previously reported that the visual processing around the fixation point affects the saccadic programming, which in fact varies according to the perceptive characteristics of the text [Ehrlich & Rayner, 1981; Kerr, 1992].

About this topic, the saccadic pattern in normal and dyslexics readers as a function of the length of the words (therefore of the extent of the lexical stimulus around the fixation point) has been investigated [De Luca et al., 2002]. Subjects were presented words and non-words made of 4-5 or 8-10 characters. The saccadic amplitude was taken as the index of the modulatory effect of the lexical configuration extent on the oculomotor pattern. In normal subjects, in fact, FEM amplitude increases with the length of the string[368]: the saccadic system self-modulates based on the length of the words so as to make wider saccades for longer strings. On the contrary, in dyslexics the elongation of the string does not lead to a proportional saccadic widening. It is as if in patients the extent of long strings tends to be underestimated. This misperception would be due to the effect of the illusory shrinking, mainly evident with long words. As a consequence, the oculomotor system would fail to detect the length difference between shorter and longer strings so that the normal self-modulation gets lost. Since a primitive alteration of the saccadic pattern in dyslexics has been ruled out, the illusory spatial contraction of the string would explain why FEMs tend to land in advance.

Really, decreased saccadic amplitude during reading in dyslexics is well documented[369]. The perceptive anomaly would be responsible not only for the occurrence of hypometric forward saccades but also for the increased number of backward saccades and for a general disarticulation of the saccade-fixation sequence. The source of these phenomena go beyond the lexical domain: as previously discussed[3], the landing site differs from the *optimum viewing location*. Indeed, landing site and *optimum viewing location* are not restricted to the lexical domain but extend to any other visual stimulus, even the most basic as a pair of spots. As a matter of fact, given a configuration made of two simple and equivalent targets, the landing site matches the optimum viewing location and localizes in the middle between the two targets. On the contrary, in a more complex configuration, such as a word, the landing site depends on the visuoperceptive properties of its features. In this case the landing site tends to differ from the preferred viewing location [Findlay, 1982; Ottes et al., 1984].

The landing site has been investigated in a group of 10 adult dyslexics[370] when performing a non-lexical task [Crawford & Higham, 2001]. Subjects were asked to look at one or two simple targets displayed in the paracentral area and the position of the fixation at the end of the saccadic movement was recorded by means of an infrared technique. It was found that for a single target the landing site in dyslexics matched the landing site in normal subjects. On the contrary, when a pair of stimuli were displayed, in patients the landing site did not locate to an intermediate position between the two stimuli, i.e. to the *optimum viewing*

---

[368] This effect is found both with words and non-words, but it is greater with the former. A possible explanation is that the saccadic modulation is affected by the linguistic content of the lexical configuration.

[369] See Part I, chapter 10.

[370] Mean age: 27 years.

location of this composed (because made of two elements) configuration, but closer to the proximal target (i.e. to the less eccentric one)[371].

The result is interesting since it suggests that a contraction of the visual space along the horizontal axis takes place in dyslexics; this contraction, indeed, would be responsible for the triggering of hypometric saccades. The saccadic amplitude reduction even in the absence of lexical tasks (as found in this experiment) would make such an anisotropic distortion a global misperception of the visual space. In summary, increased vertical anisotropy tends to compress the visual space along the horizontal axis, hindering the self-modulation of the saccadic amplitude when reading and predisposing to the triggering of hypometric FEMs. It has been suggested that the anatomical region responsible for the *optimum viewing location* localizes in the deep layers of the superior colliculi [Glimcher & Sparks, 1993]. These structures are made of large, probably M-type receptive fields, suitable for processing and integrating global configurations [Findlay, 1982; Mcllwain, 1982]. Therefore, both saccadic pattern and visuospatial positional coding dysfunctions would stem from magnocellular impairment.

In the lexical retardation, the link between oculomotor imbalance and spatial perception distortion is more evident considering that the narrowing of the visual span, dependent on the horizontal contraction of the string, leads to reduced reading rate also for a compensatory increase of the number and duration of fixations and of FEMs [McConkie & Rayner, 1975]. The saccadic pattern as a function of the visual span extent confirms the dependence of the former on the perceptive characteristics of the sentence [Hochberg, 1970][372].

ii- Unstable Fixation

As previously reported in this section[373], the perceptive effect of the averaging of the local orientations estimates along the more and less curved contour of an elliptical stimulus tends to turn it into a circle. Indeed, due to abnormal vertical anisotropy, normalization of the horizontal configurations within a circular pattern and emphasis of vertical configurations are expected. In this case the horizontal threshold would increase and the vertical threshold would decrease. Yet, in many dyslexics who showed such anisotropic enhancement the threshold for vertical ellipses was higher compared to normal readers.

An unstable fixation may clarify this apparent paradox.

Especially thanks to Stein we know that 50-60% of patients suffer from unstable fixation due to unstable dominance[374]. Fixation instability affects not only the saccadic triggering [Biscaldi et al., 1998] but also the visual processing [Nazir et al., 1992]. Fixation instability would affect even the spatial relationships perception, reducing its overall sensitivity, i.e. increasing the SR threshold along both cardinal axes. This interpretation may explain why the

[371] And yet, in some dyslexics (approximately 20%) the correspondence between the landing site and the optimal viewing location was preserved in this experimental condition.

[372] Kwon et al. [2007] investigated whether the oculomotor pattern and in particular the fixation stability is the responsible of the size of the visual span and whether its widening with the development of the child is due to the progressive reinforcement of the dominance stability (which starts at the age of 4 and continues until the age of 15: Ygge et al., 2005). However, after applying a simulation analysis, the authors concluded that this solution is improbable.

[373] Part II, chapter 3.

[374] Part I, chapter 10.

increase of the vertical anisotropy in dyslexics is not always associated with the expected reduced vertical threshold compared to the vertical threshold recorded in normal readers: fixation instability would explain the overall deterioration of SRP in dyslexics in addition to their abnormal anisotropic perception.

In conclusion, according to the theoretical framework advanced in this chapter, SRP alteration could be the common basis of crowding, oculomotor pattern, contrast sensitivity, motion perception, and visual attention impairment.

The multimodal involvement of the attentional function suggests that this dialectical perspective does not limit itself to the visuoperceptive domain. It is reported, in fact, that due to a magnocellular deficit along the auditory pathway [Galaburda et al., 1994] a sluggish attentional shift makes the processing of rapid sequences of sounds abnormal in patients. Not only the orienting, but even the filtering attentional deficit extends beyond the visual space to encompass the auditory system [Taub et al., 1994; Asbjornsen & Bryden, 1998].

As a matter of fact, the hypothesis of the temporal sequential processing deficit states that dyslexics suffer from a *pan sensorial* anomaly for fast sequences of stimuli [Tallal et al., 1993; Stein & Walsh, 1997; Stein, 2001: part I, chapter [12]. In fact, the source both of the visual and the auditory attention is located in the posterior parietal cortex [Farah et al., 1989], where specific cells are in charge for the crossmodal integration [Anderson et al., 1995]. It follows that the management of the attentional process takes place in integrated (visual and auditory) modality. The analogy between visuoperceptive and auditory-phonological field is evident also for the spatial relationship perception. Tallal & Piercy [1975] have shown that in dysphasic dyslexics the processing of syllables in rapid transition (40 msec) improves if the duration of the transition is artificially increased (85 msec), whereas it worsens if it is reduced. Also McAnally and Stein [1996] reported in patients a worse performance for faster modulations of auditory stimuli.

This aspect is supported by electrophysiological findings: in dyslexics the electrophysiological potentials evoked by auditory contrasts (*da-ga*) are reduced compared to controls but normalize if the transition time between the stimuli is delayed to 80 msec [Bradlow et al., 1999]. In addition, training by means of phonemes with slowed frequency modulation was found to improve the linguistic function in children with a language delay [Merzenich et al., 1996] and the same may occur even in dyslexics[375].

The compensatory mechanism is therefore a sort of auditory temporal expansion, resembling the anisotropic spatial expansion in the visual domain.

In conclusion, dyslexics would suffer from a generalized sensorial impairment. This *pan sensorial* deficit makes our condition the result of a global dysfunction of the entire magnocellular system, whose the visuo-spatial and phono-temporal relationship perception are peculiar elements.

Indeed, such impairment is found to go beyond the sensorial domain to encompass even the motor domain.

Evidently, as a *magnosystem* pathology developmental dyslexia cannot do without the interdisciplinary approach.

---

[375] In dyslexics Tallal [1980] reported a reduced performance when asked to discriminate auditory transients. In order to distinguish a pure pitch from a frequency modulated one, in dyslexics the frequencies that make up the modulated sound must vary to a greater extent compared to normal readers [McAnally & Stein, 1996, Baldeweg et al., 1999]. Interestingly, like contrast sensitivity in the visual domain, even in the auditory domain patients' frequency modulation sensitivity for the high frequencies (240 Hz) is spared [Stein, 2001].

References

Anderson RA, Essick GK, Siegel RM. (1995). *Encoding of spatial location by posterior parietal neurons.* Science, 230: 456-458.

Asbjornsen AE, Bryden MP. (1998). *Auditory attentional shifyts in reading-disabled students: quantification of attentional effectiveness by the Attentional Shift Index.* Neuropsychologia, 36: 143-148.

Atkinson J. (1991). *Review of human visual development: crowding and dyslexia.* In: Vision and visual dyslexia, Stein Ed., MacMillian Press, Houndmills, London, UK.

Baldeweg T, Richardson A, Watkins S, Christine F, John Gruzelier J. (1999). *Impaired auditory frequency discrimination in dyslexia detected with mismatch evoked potentials.* Annals of Neurology, 45: 495–503.

Biscaldi M, Gezeck S, Stuhr V. (1998). *Poor saccadic control correlates with dyslexia.* Neuropsychologia, 36: 1189-1202.

Boets B, Vandermosten M, Cornelissen P, Wouters J, Ghesquiére P. (2011). *Coherent motion sensitivity and reading development in the transition from prereading to reading stage.* Child Development, 82: 854-869.

Bradlow AR, Kraus N, Nicol TG, Mcgee TJ, Cunnigham J, Zecker SG. (1999). *Effects of lengthened formant transition duration on discrimination and neural representation of synthetic CV syllables by normal and learning-disabled children.* Journal of the Acoustical Society of America, 106: 2086-2096.

Cave KR, Bichot NP. (1999). *Visuospatial attention: Beyond a spotlight model.* Psychonomic Bulletin & Review, 6: 204-223.

Coletta NJ, Segu P, Tiana CLM. (1993). *An oblique effect in parafoveal motion perception.* Vision Research, 33: 2747-2756.

Cornelissen P, Hansen PC, Gilchrist I, Cormack F, Essex E, Frankish C. (1998). *Coherent motion detection and letter position encoding.* Vision Research, 38: 2181-2191.

Crawford TJ, Higham S. (2001). *Dyslexia and the centre of-gravity effect.* Experimental Brain Research, 137: 122-126.

De Luca M, Borrelli, Judica A, Spinelli D, Zoccoletti P. (2002). *Reading words and pseudo-words :an eye movement study of developmental dyslexia.* Brain and Language, 80: 617-626.

Ehrlich SF, Rayner K. (1981). *Contextual effects on word perception and eye movements during reading.* Journal of Verbal Behaviour, 20: 641-655.

Farah MJ, Wong AB, Wong MA, Monheit MA, Morrow LA. (1989). *Parietal lobe mechanisms of spatial attention: modality-specific or supramodal?* Neuropsychologia, 27: 461-470.

Findlay JM. (1982). *Global vision processing for saccadic eye movements.* Vision Research, 22: 1033-1045.

Galaburda AM, Menard MT, Rosen GD. (1994). *Evidence for aberrant auditory anatomy in developmental dyslexia.* Proceedings of the National Academy of Sciences of the United States of America, 91: 8010-8013.

Glimcher PW, Sparks DL. (1993). *Representation of averaging saccades in the superior colliculus of the monkey.* Experimental Brain Research, 95: 429-435.

Hochberg J. (1970). *Components of literacy: Speculations and exploratory research.* In: Basic studies on reading, H. Levin & Williams Eds., Basic Books, New York.

Iles J, Walsh V, Richardson A. (2000). *Visual search performance in dyslexia.* Dyslexia, 6: 163-177.

Kerr WK. (1992). *Eye Movement Control During Reading: the Selection of Where to Send the Eyes (Word Skipping).* Dissertazione di dottorato, università dell'Illinois ad Urbana-Champaign, USA.

Kinsey K, Rose M, Hansen P, Richardson A, Stein J. (2004). *Magnocellular-mediated visual-spatial attention and reading ability.* NeuroReport, 15: 1-5.

Kwon M, Legge GE, Dubbels BR. (2007). *Developmental changes in the visual span for reading.* Vision Research, 47: 2889-2900.

Legge GE. (2007). *Pychophysics of reading in normal and low vision.* Erlbaum Ed., Mahwah, NJ.

Legge GE, Cheung, SH, Yu D, Chung STL, Lee H-W, Owens DP. (2007). *The case for the visual span as a sensory bottleneck in reading.* Journal of Vision, 7 (2): 1-15.

Loffler G, Orbach HS. (2001). *Anisotropy in judging the absolute direction of motion.* Vision Research, 41: 3677-3692.

Martelli M, Di Filippo G, Spinelli D, Zoccolotti P. (2009). *Crowding, reading, and developmental dyslexia.* Journal of Vision, 9 (4), 14: 1-18.

Mc Anally KI, Stein JF. (1996). *Auditory temporal coding in dyslexia.* Proceedings of the National Academy of Sciences of the United States, 263: 961- 965.

McConkie GW, Rayner K. (1975). *The span of the effective stimulus during a fixation in reading,* Perception & Psychophysics, 17: 578–586.

Mcllwain JT. (1982). *Lateral spread of neural excitation during microstimulation in intermediate gray layer of cat's superior colliculus.* Journal of Neurophysiology, 47: 167-178.

Merzenich MM, Jenkins WM, Johnston P, Schreiner C, Miller S, Tallal P. (1996). *Temporal processing deficits of language-learning impaired children ameliorated by stretching speech.* Science, 271: 77-81.

Nazir TA, Heller D, Sussmann C. (1992). *Letter visibility and word recognition: the optimal viewing position in printed words.* Perception & Psychophysics, 52: 315-328.

Ottes FP, Van Gisbergen JAM, Eggermont JJ. (1984). *Metrics of saccades responses to visual double stimuli: two different modes.* Vision Research, 24: 1169-1179.

Pan K, Eriksen CW. (1993). *Attentional distribution in the visual field during same-different judgements as assessed by response competition.* Perception & Psychophysics, 53: 134-144.

Pelli DG, Palomares M, Majaj NJ. (2004). *Crowding is unlike ordinary masking: Distinguishing feature integration from detection.* Journal of Vision, 12: 1136–1169.

Raymond JE. (1994). *Directional anisotropy of motion sensitivity across the visual field.* Vision Research, 34: 1029-1037.

Raymond JE. (2000). *Attentional modulation of visual motion perception.* Trends in Cognitive Science, 2: 42-50.

Solman RT, May JG. (1990). *Spatial localization discrepancies: A visual deficiency in poor readers.* American Journal of Psychology, 103: 243-263.

Stein J. (2001). *The magnocellular theory of developmental dyslexia.* Dyslexia, 7: 12-36.

Stein JF, Walsh V. (1997). *To see but not to read: the magnocellular theory of dyslexia.* Trends in Neurosciences, 20: 147-152.

Tallal, P, Miller S, Fitch RH. (1993). *Neurobiological basis of speech: A case for the preeminence of temporal processing.* Annals of the New York Academy of Sciences, 682: 27-47.

Tallal P, Piercy M. (1975). *Developmental aphasia: the perception of brief vowels and extended stop consonants.* Neuropsychologia, 13: 69-74.

Tallal P. (1980). *Auditory temporal perception, phonics, and reading disability in children.* Brain & Language, 9: 182-198.

Taub CF, Fine E, Cherry RS. (1994). *Finding a link between selective auditory attention and reading problems in young children: a preliminary investigation.* Perceptual & Motor Skills, 78: 1153-1154.

Toet A, Levi DM. (1992). *The two-dimensional shape of spatial interaction zones in the parafovea.* Vision Research, 32: 1349-1357.

Van de Grind WA, Koenderink JJ, Van Doorn AJ, Milders MV, Voerman H. (1993). *Inhomogeneity and anisotropies for motion detection in the monocular visual field of human observers. Vision Research*, 33: 1089-1107.

Ygge J, Aring E, Han Y, Bolzai R, Hellstrom A. (2005). *Fixation stability in normal children.* Annals of the New York Academy of Sciences, 1039: 480-483.

Chapter XXI

Advancing a Visuoperceptive-based Classification of Developmental Dyslexia

In the first part of the book, the current classifications of developmental dyslexia have been reported, highlighting the problematic dualism between the major phonological component and the visuoperceptive one.

The lack of a commonly accepted classification helps to account for the inconsistency of many experimental results: not only the dyslexic subgroups behave differently or antithetically when undergoing psychophysical tests, but classes labeled as dysphoneidetic and dysphonetic (or phonological) paradoxically show defects involving the visual domain, whereas dyseidetic dyslexics, who are expected to be affected by visuoperceptive anomalies, are found to be immune.

As a matter of fact, the prevalence of the dyseidetic type among the dyslexic population (10-30%)[376] [Flynn & Deering, 1989; Flynn & Boder, 1991] does not fit the estimate of Slaghuis & Lovegrove (1985) and Lovegrove et al. [1986, 1990], who found a visuoperceptive deficit (M-mediated) in more than 75% of patients.

Probably, these contradictory elements are due to the fact that to a certain extent and in different ways the neuro-ophthalmological alteration permeates even the classes of dyslexia considered to be free from the visuoperceptive anomaly, so that the cutoff among the different subtypes is not sharp. Classifying some developmental dyslexics as "dysphonetics" (or "phonological") implies they are affected by a pure linguistic/phonological deficit, denying they may suffer to a less extent also from visuoperceptive impairment: this is a position that, as shown, can no longer be sustained.

Within the neuro-ophthalmological boundary, it is therefore necessary to re-consider the current models of classifications.

Any classification that sets dyseidetic or surface patients against dysphonetic or phonological dyslexics should be avoided and the visuoperceptive impairment (if present) should be typified in every single patient, beyond the antagonism between the phonological and the visuoperceptive domain.

---

[376] Up to 34% according to Slaghuis & Ryan [1999].

Clearly, the scope of this proposal is not to annihilate the linguistic-phonological factor, which is undoubtedly predominant, but to characterize the concomitant visual component according to the way it affects the lexical processing.

The starting point is the paradigm called *Dual Route model*[377].

According to the Dual Route Model, the lexical processing follows two strategies: during the development of the reading function the two strategies are sequential, after its consolidation they may work in parallel:

-the sublexical route assigns a sound to a written symbol, i.e. maps the graphemic code into a phonetic map. In ordinary conditions, the sublexical route is used when facing with unknown words, in experimental conditions in presence of non-words. The sublexical strategy provides for an analysis of the words after having "cut" them into their elementary constituents, syllables and letters. The analysis of the elementary constituents of the words is the main reading strategy adopted for the first 12-18 months of schooling and takes place in the right hemisphere [Bakker, 1992; Facoetti et al., 2003].

-the lexical (or orthographic) route is responsible for the recognition of words considered as global configurations when, after being fully acquired and memorized, become common terms. Compared to the sublexical route, the lexical route, which relies on the left hemisphere [Bakker, 1992], requires greater phonological/linguistic ability.

The sublexical route is therefore the first to develop in the beginner reader. In fact, to the beginner reader each word is a new term, a *non-word*, and as such it requires complete decoding and analytical processing [Facoetti et al., 2005]. Since it is based on the visual processing of the elementary constituents (that is of the letters that make up syllables and of the syllables that make up words) the sublexical route may be affected by visuoperceptive alterations. These defects would depend on the fixation instability, on the lateral masking reinforcement and eventually on the anisotropic spatial relationship perception [Aleci et al., 2012]. Now, the dysphoneidetic or the phonological dyslexics are affected by a prevalent impairment of the sublexical route, even if they are traditionally considered as free from any visuoperceptive connotation [Borsting et al., 1996, Slaghuis & Ryan, 1999]. This consideration may help to shed light on the reason why the finding of alterations of some magnocellular function in the visual domain has been found in these classes.

Defective sublexical route leads to reading slowdown, with non-words which are more affected than words.

Contrary to the sublexical route, in the lexical route the word is learned as such, as a global shape: reading is no more provided by sequential analytical operations, but by a synthetic process into a visual gestalt, a holistic learning, and as such it is carried out on a global level. Elective impairment on this level would cause reading slowdown and difficulties especially with homophone words [Castles &Coltheart, 1993]. Instead, the lexical impairment for non-words is expected to be less evident, as non-words are processed via the sublexical route.

In order to make clearer how this double strategy can be imagined in a visuoperceptive perspective, the meaning of *local processing* and *global processing* of a visual configuration are briefly described.

---

[377] See Coltheard et al. [2001] for a review.

Local Processing and Global Processing

A visual stimulus has global and local properties. For example, a pearl necklace consists of a circular global configuration which is the necklace itself and at the same time it is made up of local constituents, which are the pearls. As it is believed that the global properties are resolved in the low spatial frequencies and the local properties are resolved in the high spatial frequencies [Navon, 1977; Antes & Mann, 1984; Shulman & Wilson, 1987; Badcock et al., 1990; Hughes et al., 1990; Lagasse, 1993], it follows that the M-system, responsible for the low spatial frequencies, is in charge of the global properties of the visual configuration whereas the P-system provides for the local analysis of the individual constituents. It is known that the transient system is well represented in the peripheral (paracentral) region of the visual field: its peripheral distribution, indeed, fits the ability to learn the global shape of the stimulus, whose extent falls well beyond the fixation point.

On the contrary, parvocells are more represented in the fovea, which is responsible for the analysis of the local characteristics (fine details) of the stimulus. The recognition of a configuration requires both phases, but there is no agreement on which is the first to occur. A group of researchers has claimed that the visual processing moves from the global to the local level, so that the M-mediated apprehension of the configuration of the stimulus as a whole precedes the analysis of its individual constituents [Kinchla, 1974; Navon, 1977; Navon & Norman, 1983; Amirkhiabani & Lovegrove, 1996; Keen & Lovegrove, 2000][378].

The precedence of the global processing has been attributed to earlier and faster activity of the transient channels compared to the sustained ones or to the inhibitory effect of the low spatial frequency components of the configuration on the sustained channels [Navon, 1977; Hughes et al., 1990]. As an alternative, the temporal order of the global-local processing is suggested to depend on the size and on features of the stimulus [Kinchla & Wolfe, 1979].

The double stage of the visuoperceptive processing takes place even in the reading task: during reading, the word is the global configuration and the syllables→ letters→ features it is made up are the local configurations [Rudnicky & Kolers, 1984; Healy et al., 1987; Allen et al., 1995; Chase, 1996]. Since dyslexics are claimed to suffer from a defect of the magnocellular pathway, the global level processing is expected to be impaired while the ability to capture the details should be undamaged. Still, in many patients anomalies of the right parietal cortex have been reported [Stein & Walsh, 1997, Hari & Koivikko, 1999] and the right parietal cortex is shown to be the region responsible for the global processing [Sergent, 1982; Robertson et al., 1988; Martinez et al., 1997; Fink et al., 1996, 1999; Proverb et al., 1998; Evans et al., 2000; Weber et al., 2000; Yamaguchi et al., 2000; Han et al., 2002; Lux et al., 2004][379].

Keen & Lovegrove [2000] investigated this aspect with an extra lexical task. Eighteen dyslexics on the one hand were asked to detect the orientation of a stimulus in the shape of "C" (global configuration) made up of small circular ("o") elements (local configurations), on

---

378 The analysis of local configurations and their synthesis within a global configuration can be investigated by means of the figures of Navon. The figures of Navon are global configurations formed in turn by configurations on a small scale (local): for example, a letter whose contour is made up of small letters that can be identical or different with respect to the big one [Navon, 1977].

379 Lesions in the right cerebral hemisphere prevent the global processing while spare the local analysis. On the contrary, lesions affecting the left cerebral hemisphere affect the local processing [Delis et al., 1986; Robertson et al., 1988; Lamb et al., 1990; Doyon & Milner, 1991].

the other hand were required to detect the orientation of small elements the shape of a "c" (local configurations) making up a circular stimulus ("O", global configuration)[380] (Figure 1).

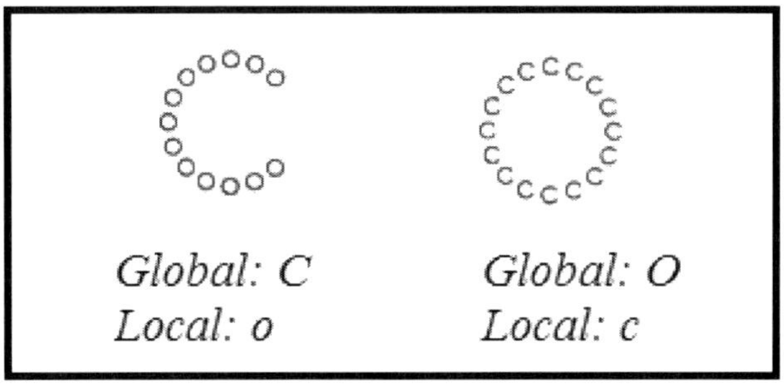

Figure 1. Example stimuli liable for the evaluation of global and local processing.

Results were compared with those obtained in normal readers. Although in dyslexics the recognition threshold turned out to be worse at both levels, even in patients (as well as in normal readers) the global configuration was processed more rapidly than the local ones, contrary to what expected [Keen & Lovegrove, 2000].

In conclusion, to date there is no evidence of a processing deficit on a M-mediated global scale in dyslexics, but only a nonspecific impairment both at the global and the local level[381]. However, since the recruited group had not been classified, it is likely that some of the patients were deficient mainly in the global processing while for others the critical factor was the local analysis.

Furthermore, local analysis impairment does not imply defective parvocellular function: as a matter of fact, threshold recognition for individual letters is not compromised in patients, suggesting their parvo-mediated ability in detecting fine details is preserved.

Instead, the anomaly would lie:

- in the *analysis* of the global configuration, i.e. in the ability to *extract* from a global configuration the local configurations, so as to process the latter individually, ruling out any interference from the adjoining stimuli, or/and:
- in the *synthesis* of the local configurations, i.e. in the subsequent integration of the features making up the global configuration.

Contour integration is the function which best accounts for the transition of the visuoperceptive processing from the local to the global level: from the pearls to the necklace, from every single aligned dot making up the outline of a form to the form itself.

Contour integration in this sense requires not only the normal functioning of the cortical receptive fields able to *analyze* the visual configuration at a local level, and therefore

380 Luminance of the target: 7.2 cd/m^2, presentation time:100 msec.

381 Some features need to be considered: first, given the large overlapping of P- and M- activity, stimuli adopted to investigate the visuoperceptive function at a global level may be not so specific as to isolate the magnocellular activity. The assumption that large configurations can be considered low frequency stimuli and small targets high frequency stimuli could be misleading: as the segments making up a large configuration are high spatial frequency components [Antes & Mann, 1984], patterns putatively suitable to evaluate selectively the global processing would carry high frequency components able ingage the parvocellular function, therefore biasing the outcome.

sensitive to the orientation of lines or edges [Hubel & Wiesel, 1968], but also and especially their arrangement at a global level, i.e. their adequate integration (*synthesis*) into a contour[382]. Contour integration is based on long-range connections of specific neurons that project their axons across the visual cortex reaching a large amount of receptive fields; this way these specialized cells are able to assemble the elementary constituents of the visual information [Gilbert et al., 1990; Ts'o et al., 1990] on a large scale, that is across wide regions of the visual field.

If detectors responsible for the *recognition* of an elementary stimulus are called receptive fields, the functional units responsible for the *integration* of a series of elementary stimuli (local configuration) within a global configuration have been defined *association fields* [Field et al., 1993]. Even reading requires the integration of local configurations (every character and syllable) into the word (the global configuration): after the investigation of Keen and Lovegrove on the ability to process local and global configurations in dyslexics, the following year Simmers and Bex [2001] focused on the transition from the first to the second level. The starting hypothesis is that impaired integration of the local configurations within a global configuration accounts for the perceptual distortions reported in many patients and eventually for their lexical difficulty: therefore, patients would suffer from a special case of abnormal contour integration. The authors measured contour integration function in a sample of adult dyslexics[383] presenting a pattern made of a series of aligned Gabor patches[384] (4 to 6), each of them with a given difference in orientation compared to the previous and the following one.

Patients turned out to be 2-3 times less sensitive than normal readers in identifying the aligned pattern made of local elements, suggesting an integration processing defect in the transition from local to global visuoperceptive level. This deficit affects the reading task, too, therefore helping to characterize the anomalous visuoperceptive behavior of a subtype of dyslexic subjects.

In summary, two basic visuoperceptive operations are required to read fluently: - The ability to recognize (with or without appropriate aids) the features making up the single letters (normal visual acuity): this function, mediated by the P-system is undamaged in patients. - The analytical subdivision of the global configurations (words) in their local features (letters and syllables) and their subsequent synthesis. Even if no evidence is available so far, since both operations involve the visual processing of global configurations it is likely to be driven by the magnocellular system.

When facing with unknown words in beginner readers or with non-words in experimental conditions, the reading task can rely only on the analytical approach: indeed, this strategy occurs when the reader can not directly access the global configuration, so as the sublexical route is the only way to decode the word, whereas the lexical route is precluded.

On the contrary, in case of common words, readers can directly access the global configuration via the lexical route. This way the laborious analysis process typical of the analytical strategy is bypassed and reading time is reduced.

---

[382] Interestingly, contour integration is not fully developed in young children [Kovacs, 2000] and its impairment has been reported also in amblyopic subjects [Hess et al., 1997; Kovacs et al., 2000; Mussap & Levi, 2000].

[383] Mean age: 24.3 years.

[384] The Gabor patches are the product of a sinusoid with a given orientation (*carrier*) enveloped in a Gaussian function (*envelope*). In the bidimensional space a Gabor patch can be described by the expression $G(x, y) = s(x,y)\, e(x,y)$ where $s(x,y)$ is the complex sinusoid and $e(x,y)$ is the Gaussian-shaped function.

Bakker's classification in some way fits this difference: type-P dyslexics make extensive use of the analytical approach (relying mainly on the sublexical route) and are prevented from using the synthetic strategy (i.e. the lexical route) because the transfer from local to global processing is impaired. As a consequence, their reading is slow and fragmented, albeit not so inaccurate. The type-L dyslexics on the other hand use too much the synthetic strategy (i.e. over-rely on the lexical route) and too little the analytical approach. The hindrance of the local analysis and their focusing exclusively on the global processing make the L-dyslexics reading fast but inaccurate.

This paradigm has the advantage to implicitly take into account the visuoperceptive imbalance between the local and the global processing of the lexical material, which is to say between the analytical and the synthetic approach to reading. And yet, anchoring the P-form to the perceptive domain and the L-form to the phonological-linguistic one, it gets stuck with the dualism we intend to overcome.

Therefore, based on the dual route model and on the differentiation between the local and global processing of the lexical configurations, the visuoperceptive anomalies often found in developmental dyslexics can be divided into two types:

1. alteration of the *analysis* of the local configurations (features of letters and letters), responsible for the component that can be defined as *dysanalytical*.

   Due to the alteration of the local analysis, in the dysanalytical dyslexics the worst performance would involve non-words, since non-words cannot be directly decoded by the global processing of the configuration. On the other hand since global processing is expected to be normal, the recognition of common words is expected to be less compromised.

   Therefore, reading in dysanalytical dyslexics is expected to be slow and inaccurate, as the result of a more laborious and imprecise analytical process, respectively. These anomalies should be more evident for non-words.

   Dysanalytical dyslexics would be affected by:

   - reinforcement of the lateral masking as a result of SRP alteration.
   - fixation instability able to prevent the spatial position encoding of letters, as proposed by Stein. Indeed, the visual classification of Stein is reinterpretable in this new perspective: fixation instability due to unstable ocular dominance makes visual dyslexics more prone to errors when reading letter sequences, frequently turning words into non-words. This would occur since fixation instability prevents from the accurate analysis of the terms (especially in case of unknown words or non-words), i.e. from correct separation into their elementary constituents (letters).
2. alteration of the *synthesis* of the features into the global configuration (the word itself), responsible for the component that can be defined as *dyssynthetical.*

The alteration of the dyssynthetical dyslexic does not involve the sequential analysis at the local level. On the contrary, it is characterized by difficulty in the transition from the local to the global level and ultimately for the synthesis and eventually the processing of the global configuration. Being impossible the direct processing of word as a whole, the only strategy available is the local analysis via the sublexical route so that (common) words and non-words (or uncommon words) are processed in the same manner, i.e.by means of local analytical strategies. In these cases, since the local analysis is spared, reading is expected to be slow and fragmented but substantially accurate both for words and non-words[385].

In the dyssynthetical class, the difficulty in the transition from local to global level would be responsible for abnormal contour integration. Table I shows schematically this proposal of visuoperceptive-based classification in dyslexics.

Table I. The personal advanced classification of the visuoperceptive impairment in developmental dyslexia

	Type of deterioration	Level of deterioration	Expected preferential lexical target	Expected lexical pattern	Pathogenetical motive
Dysanalytical component	defective local analysis (letters and syllables)	Local level -abnormal sublexical route	Worse performance for non-words	Non-words reading: - slow and fragmented -inaccurate	-Lateral masking reinforcement caused by abnormal SRP - fixation instability - Attentional deficit
Dyssynthetical component	Defective synthesis into the global configuration (words)	Global Level -abnormal lexical route	Similar performance for words and non-words (worse for homophones)	Words and non-words reading: -slow and fragmented -quite accurate (inaccurate reading of homophones)	-Disruption of *contour integration* -Attentional deficit

Of course, this classification has been devised within a purely theoretical framework: therefore, it has to be verified in experimental designs, as well as in clinical practice. Even if it presumes the two classes to be pure, in clinical practice misanalysis is expected to occur to a certain extent in dyssynthetical subjects and vice versa.

This point is supported by the so-called length effect, for which vocal reaction time tends to increase with the lengthening of the word.

The effect, negligible in normal readers [Zoccolotti et al., 1999], would be the sign of prominent use of the local analytic approach, and seems to characterize to some extent the whole dyslexic population, independently from their class. Reading time measured in German patients[386] is found to increase depending on the length of the word at a rate up to 10 times higher than in normal subjects[387] [Landerl et al., 1997; Wimmer, 1993].

This result has been confirmed in another German study. In this investigation, instead of words, strings of digits of variable length (2, 4 and 6 elements) were presented to dyslexic children and the presentation time needed for the correct recognition of a number of the

[385] In case, accuracy is expected to be worse for words and especially for homophones: in fact, in order to read a common word, the subject would be tempted to rely on the global processing that, being impaired, would necessarily make him prone to errors.

[386] German is a transparent language.

[387] 30-50 msec per letter in normal readers, up to 300 msec in dyslexics.

sequence was estimated. For each series of numbers, patients required a longer presentation time compared to controls. Moreover, the additional time required by the increase of the sequence was proportionally longer in dyslexics than in normal readers [Hawelka & Wimmer, 2005].

The analytical strategy makes reading slow also because it requires the triggering of multiple saccades on the same word [MacKeben et al., 2004]. Actually, number of saccades and analytical processing threshold seem to be related [Hawelka & Wimmer, 2005]. In addition, increased lateral masking consequent to the SR anisotropic distortion of the visual space may contribute to further delay reading of long words in dysanalytical dyslexics. This assumption would explain why longer words (whose letters are surrounded by a greater amount of peripheral distractors, therefore subjected to stronger crowding) are read worse than the shorter ones [Shapiro et al., 1990]. For this reason, too, dyslexics are particularly prevented when facing a text: indeed, this is a perceptual condition which makes foveal processing affected by a large amount of peripheral information [Hill & Lovegrove, 1993].

The advanced classification of the visuoperceptive defect in dyslexics focuses on the phase of the lexical symbol apprehension and does not consider the grapheme-to-phoneme conversion. Still, each of the two visuoperceptive types contains a phonological component whose effect in determining the lexical disability, according to the common opinion, is predominant. This phonological factor is thus a further, crucial problem: crucial but neither exclusive nor necessarily alternative to the visuoperceptive one, since a growing body of evidence suggests that in some patients a visuoperceptive component associated to a variable degree to the phonological one can worsen the lexical task. The orthographic differences in languages determine different degrees of combinations: the phonological factor appears predominant in English dyslexics[388], probably less important in transparent languages such as Italian [Sartori& Job, 1983] or German [Wimmer, 1993]

Li reported in 19 Chinese dyslexics[389] shorter saccades [Li et al., 2009]. Unlike western patients, this finding was evident in extralexical tasks. According to the authors, this anomaly is the result of a visuoperceptive impairment (since it reflects defective fixation), more evident in eastern dyslexics than in western patients[390].

Table II shows a comparison between our paradigm and the current classifications.

[388] The phonological component in the English-speaking countries would be responsible for up to 75% of cases of dyslexia.

[389] Age 9:54 ±1.4 years.

[390] Studies on Chinese dyslexics are of particular interest, since their language does not depend on the grapheme-to-phoneme conversion: differently from the characters and syllables of the alphabetic idioms, mapped into the corresponding phonemes, Chinese ideograms refer directly to meanings and as such do not require the sequential analysis of the text. This aspect together with the wealth of homophones, makes Chinese reading a task that requires adequate visuoperceptive processing mainly at the global level. A recent psychophysical and electrophysiological investigation on16 Oriental dyslexics has found a main magnocellular defect [Wang et al., 2010]. This result confirms that visual M-mediated damage affects the holistic perception of the lexical configuration: this way it would reduce the reading ability without an additional impairment of the phonological function (and in fact in Chinese readers the phonological function is not prevalent). On the contrary, Walter-Muller [1995] did not find evident magnocellular anomalies in German mother tongue dyslexics. In this case, for the high correspondence between grapheme and phoneme, reading requires even the integrity of the phonological function.

In summary, these findings seem to confirm that the traditional approach, which oppose the phonological domain to the visuoperceptive one, is not the most suitable to classify patients.

Table II. The advanced classification of the visuoperceptive impairment in developmental dyslexia and its relationship with the current classifications

Classification	Class	Reported and presumed characteristics	Type of preponderant visuoperceptive component
Boder (1973)	Dyseidetic	Defective processing of the word as a single configuration. Prevalent use of the sublexical route. Predominant impairment: words and irregular words.	*Dyssynthetical*
	Dysphonetic	Predominant impairment: non-words. M-system deficit.	*Dysanalytical*
	Dysphoneidetic	Impairment of words + non-words. M-system deficit.	*Mixed*
Castles & Coltheart (1993)	Surface dyslexia	Predominant impairment: words (especially irregular or homophones). Prevalent use of the sublexical route. Slow and fragmented reading, but pretty accurate. Cause: reading development retardation.	*Dyssynthetical*
	Deep or phonologic	Predominant impairment: non-words. Cause: anatomofunctional anomaly.	*Dysanalytical*
Bakker (1979, 1992)	L-type	In connection with the dysphonetic type of Boder. Faster reading but less accurate than the P-type. Greater activation of the left hemisphere.	*Dysanalytical*
	P-type	In connection with the dyseidetic type of Boder. Slower reading, hesitant, fragmented but more accurate than the L-type. Greater activation of the right hemisphere.	*Dyssynthetical*
Stein (1982)	Visual	Impairment of non-words and words (that are read as non-words). Fixation instability in convergence which prevents the lexical sequential analysis. Deficit of the magnocellular system.	*Dysanalytical*

Table II. (Continued)

Classification	Class	Reported and presumed characteristics	Type of preponderant visuoperceptive component
Lovett (1984, 1987)	*Accuracy disabled*	Defect in word recognition. Reduced reading accuracy.	*Dyssynthetical*
	Rate disabled	Reduced reading rate. Particular vulnerability to the surrounding visual elements (increased crowding effect).	*Dysanalytical*
Valdois classification (1995)	*Visuo-attentional*	Predominant impairment: non-words.	*Dysanalytical*
	Non *visuo-attentional*		?

The visuoperceptive classification on the one hand fits most of the models advanced thus far, on the other hand goes beyond the opposition between phonolinguistic and visuoperceptive factor since it is focused on the difficulty of the patient in visual decoding (analysis and/or synthesis of the lexical configuration) regardless of the group he/she belongs to.

The synthetic and analytical consolidation during the reading development of the child probably occur in two different moments, earlier for the analysis, later for the synthesis. Normal reading development first of all relies on the consolidation of the analytical approach (the sublexical route), since the analytical strategy is the first step for the direct learning of the holistic (synthesized) term. This interpretation may help to explain the ubiquity of the phonological deficit in the dyslexic population, since it would be strictly dependent on the sublexical route, that is on the analytical strategy. The term *phonological* subtends the conversion of the graphic configuration into its correspondent sound, after the adequate analysis of its visual features or the direct synthetic apprehension of the whole word has been accomplished. Such a connection between graphemic visual processing and subsequent phonemic conversion would account for the close relationship expected between the dysanalytical component and dysphonetic or phonological dyslexics. Interestingly, the functional anomalies typical of the dysanalytical form seem to affect also the auditory-phonological domain, as proved by some indirect experimental evidence [Tallal & Piercy, 1975; Bradlow et al., 1999; De Martino et al., 2001].

Evidently, the final purpose of this paradigm is to allow customized rehabilitation programs: dyslexics whose visuoperceptive component is compromised at the local level (dysanalytical), should undergo a visuoperceptive treatment aimed at improving the analytical process (in addition to the phonological approach); on the contrary, patients with visuoperceptive impairment at a global level should be trained to strengthen their synthetic visuoperceptive ability.

In an attempt to help the transition from the analytical to the synthetic reading strategy and to improve the global analysis of the lexical configurations (words), a visuoperceptive protocol has been devised and administered to a group of surface dyslexics [Judica et al., 2002].

According to this paradigm, subjects were asked to read single words of different length displayed tachistoscopically. The lexical task was made more and more difficult by increasing the length of the words (from 2 up to 8 letters) and the reduction of their presentation time (from 150 to 60 msec). Each training session aimed at increasing up to 60-70% the percentage of words read correctly. Results obtained in 9 dyslexic children[391] were compared with 9 age-matched normal readers. At the end of the training, improved reading rate and accuracy was observed[392] either for words and non-words, although in patients the lexical performance did not reach the normality level. In addition, after the treatment, the normalization of the fixation duration was observed. Still, the persistence of the length effect suggests that the protocol failed to shift the reading processing from the local (analytical strategy) toward the global (synthetic strategy) level[393].

Further works are requested to assess the effect of such kinds of visual training after patients have been classified according to the nature of their visuoperceptive impairment.

References

Aleci C, Piana G, Bertolini M. (2012). *Developmental dyslexia and spatial relationship perception.* Cortex, 48: 466-476.

Allen PA, Wallace B, Weber TA. (1995). *Influence of case type, word frequency and exposure duration on visual word recognition.* Journal of Experimental Psychology: Human Perception and Performance, 21: 914–934.

Amirkhiabani G, Lovergrove JW. (1996). *Role of eccentricity and size in the global precedence effect.* Journal of Experimental Psychology: Human Perception and Performance, 22: 1434-1447.

Antes R, Mann SW. (1984). *Global-local precedence in picture processing.* Psychological Research, 46: 246-259.

Badcock JC, Whitworth FA, Badcock DR, Lovergrove WJ. (1990). *Low-frequency filtering and processing of local-global stimuli.* Perception, 19: 617- 629.

Bakker DJ. (1992). *Neuropsychological classification and treatment of dyslexia.* Journal of Learning Disabilities, 25: 102-109.

Borsting E, Ridder WH, Dudeck K, Kelley C, Matsui L, Motoyama J. (1996). *The presence of a magnocellular defect depends on the type of dyslexia.* Vision Research, 36: 1047-1053.

Bradlow AR, Kraus N, Nicol TG, Mcgee TJ, Cunnigham J, Zecker SG. (1999). *Effects of lengthened formant transition duration on discrimination and neural representation of synthetic CV syllables by normal and learning-disabled children.* Journal of the Acoustical Society of America, 106: 2086-2096.

[391] Mean age: 11 years; treatment duration: 5 months with two sessions a week. Duration of each session: 1 hour.

[392] By means of the DDE battery [Sartori et al., 1995].

[393] Similar results have been reported in English-speaking surface dyslexics [Seymour & Bunce, 1994; Broom & Doctor, 1995].

Broom YM, Doctor EA. (1995). *Developmental surface dyslexia: a case study of the efficacy of a remediation programme.* Cognitive Neuropsychology, 12: 69-110

Castles A, Coltheart M. (1993). *Varieties of developmental dyslexia.* Cognition, 47: 149-180.

Chase CH. (1996). *A visual deficit model of developmental dyslexia.* In:. Developmental Dyslexia: Neural, Cognitive, and Genetic Mechanisms. Chase, Rosen, Sherman Eds., Timonium, MD: York Press, New York.

Coltheart M, Rastle K, Perry C, Langdon R, Ziegler J. (2001). *DRC: a dual route cascaded model of visual word recognition and reading aloud.* Psychological Review, 108: 204-256.

Delis DC, Robertson LC, Efron R. (1986). *Hemispheric specialization of memory for visual hierarchical stimuli.* Neuropsychologia, 24: 205-214.

De Martino S, Espesser R, Rey V, Habib M. (2001). *The "temporal processing deficit" hypothesis in dyslexia: New experimental evidence.* Brain Cognition, 46: 104-108.

Doyon J, Milner B. (1991). *Right temporal-lobe contribution to global visual processing.* Neuropsychologia, 29: 343-360.

Evans MA, Shedden MJ, Hevenor SJ, Hahn MC. (2000). *The effect of variability of unattended information on global and local processing: Evidence for lateralization at early stages of processing.* Neuropsychologia, 38: 225-239.

Facoetti A, Lorusso ML, Paginoni PL, Umiltà C, Mascetti GG. (2003). *The role of visuospatial attention in developmental dyslexia: evidence from a rehabilitation study.* Cognitive Brain Research, 15: 154-164.

Facoetti A, Lorusso ML, Cattaneo C, Galli R, Molteni M. (2005). *Visual and auditory attentional capture are both sluggish in children with developmental dyslexia.* Acta Neurobiologiae Experimentalis, 65: 61-72.

Field DJ, Hayes A, Hess RF. (1993). *Contour integration by the human visual system. Evidence for a local "association field".* Vision Research, 33: 173-193.

Fink GR, Halligan PW, Marshall JC, Frith CD, Frackowiak RS, Dolan RJ. (1996). *Where in the brain does visual attention select the forest and the trees?* Nature, 382: 626-628.

Fink GR, Marshall JC, Halligan PW, Dolan RJ. (1999). *Hemispheric asymmetries in global/local processing are modulated by perceptual salience.* Neuropsychologia, 37: 31-40.

Flynn JM, Boder E. (1991). *Clinical and electrophysiological correlates of dysphonetic and dyseidetic dyslexia.* In:Vision and Visual Dyslexia, Stein Ed., CRC Press, Boca Ranton, FL.

Flynn JM, Deering WM. (1989). *Subtypes of dyslexia: investigation of Boder's system using quantitative neurophysiology.* Developmental Medicine and Child Neurology, 31: 215-223.

Gilbert CD, Hirsch JA, Wiesel TN. (1990). *Lateral interactions in the visual cortex.* Cold Spring Harbor Symposia on Quantitative Biology, 55: 663-677.

Han S, Weaver JA, Murray SO, Kang X, Yund EW, Woods DL. (2002). *Hemispheric asymmetry in global/local processing: Effects of stimulus position and spatial frequency.* Neuroimage, 17: 1290-1299.

Hari R, Koivikko H. (1999). *Left side mini-neglect and attentional sluggishness in dyslexic adults* [Abstract]. Society for Neuroscience, 25: 1634.

Hawelka S, Wimmer H (2005). *Impaired visual processing of multi-element arrays is associated with increased number of eye movements in dyslexic reading.* Vision Research, 45: 855-863.

Healy AF, Oliver WL, McNamara TP. (1987). *Detecting letters in continuous text: effects of display size.* Journal of Experimental Psychology: Human Perception and Performance, 13: 279–290.

Hess RF, McIlhagga W, Field DJ. (1997). *Contour integration in strabismic amblyopia: the sufficiency of an explanation based on positional uncertainty.* Vision Research, 37: 3145-3161.

Hill R, Lovegrove WJ. (1993). *One word at a time: A solution to the visual deficits in SRDs?* In: Facets of dyslexia and its remediation, Wright, Groner & Kauffman-Hayoz Eds., Elsevier, Amsterdam.

Hubel DH, Wiesel TN. (1968). *Receptive fields and functional architecture of monkey striate cortex.* Journal of Physiology, 195: 215-243.

Hughes HC, Fendrich R, Reuter-Lorentz PA. (1990). *Global versus local processing in the absence of low spatial frequencies.* Journal of Cognitive Neuroscience, 2: 272-282.

Judica A, De Luca M, Spinelli D, Zoccolotti PL. (2002). *Training of developmental surface dyslexia improves reading performance and shortens eye fixation duration in reading.* (2002). Neuropsychological Rehabilitation, 12: 177-197.

Keen AG, Lovergrove WJ. (2000). *Transient deficit hypothesis and dyslexia: examination of whole-parts relationship, retinal sensitivity, and spatial and temporal frequencies.* Vision Research, 40: 705-715.

Kinchla RA. (1974). *Detecting target elements in multielement arrays: a confusability model.* Perception and Psychophysics, 15:149-158.

Kinchla RA, Wolfe J. (1979). *The order of visual processing: "Top down," bottom up," or middle out".* Perception & Psychophysics, 25: 225-231.

Kovacs I. (2000). *Human development of perceptual organization.* Vision Research, 40: 1301-1310.

Kovacs I, Polat U, Pennefather PM, Chandna A, Norcia AM. (2000). *A new test of contour integration deficits in patients with a history of disrupted binocular experience during visual development.* Vision Research, 40: 1775-1783.

LaGasse IL. (1993). *Effects of good form and spatial frequency on global precedence.* Perception & Psychophysics, 53: 89-105.

Lamb MR, Robertson LC, Knight RT. (1990). *Component mechanisms underlying the processing of hierarchically organized patterns: Inferences from patients with unilateral cortical lesions.* Journal of Experimental Psychology: Learning, Memory, and Cognition, 16: 471-483.

Landerl K, Wimmer H, Frith U. (1997). *The impact of otghographic consistency on dyslexia: A German-English comparison.* Cognition, 63: 315-334.

Li XH, Jing J, Zou XB, Huang X, Jin Y, Wang QX, Chen XB, Yang BR, Yang SY. (2009). *Picture perception in Chinese dyslexic children: an eye-movement study.* Chinese Medical Journal, 122: 267-271.

Lovegrove WJ, Garzia RP, Nicholson SB. (1990). *Experimental evidence for a transient system deficit in specific reading disability.* Journal of the American Optometric Association, 61: 137-146.

Lovegrove WJ, Martin F, Slaghuis W. (1986). *A theoretical and experimental case for a visual deficit in specific reading disability.* Cognitive Neuropshychology, 3: 225-267.

Lux S, Marshall JC, Ritzl A, Weiss PH, Pietrzyk U, Shah NJ, Zilles K, Fink GR. (2004). A functional magnetic resonance imaging study of local/global processing with stimulus presentation in the peripheral visual hemifields. Neuroscience, 124: 113-120.

MacKeben M, Trauzettel-Klosinski S, Reinhard J, Dürrwächter U, Adler M, Klosinski G. (2004). *Eye movement control during single-word reading in dyslexics.* Journal of Vision, 4: 388-402.

Martinez A, Moses P, Frank L, Buxton R, Wong E, Stiles J. (1997). *Hemispheric asymmetries in global and local processing: evidence from fMRI.* NeuroReport, 8: 1685-1689.

Mussap AJ, Levi DM. (2000). *Amblyopic deficits in detecting a dotted line in noise.* Vision Research, 40: 3297-3307.

Navon D. (1977). *Forest before trees: the precedence of global features in visual perception.* Cognitive Psychology, 9: 353-383.

Navon D, Norman J. (1983). *Does global precedence really depend on visual angle?* Journal of Experimental Psychology: Human Perception and Performance, 7: 955-965.

Proverbio AM, Minniti A, Zani A. (1998). *Electrophysiological evidence of a perceptual precedence of global vs. local visual information.* Cognitive and Brain Research, 6: 321-334.

Robertson LC, Lamb MR, Knight RT. (1988). *Effects of lesions of temporal parietal junction on perceptual and attentional processing in humans.* The Journal of Neuroscience, 8: 3757-3769.

Rudnicky AI, Kolers PA. (1984). *Size and case of type as stimuli in reading.* Journal of Experimental Psychology: Human Perception and Performance, 10: 231–249.

Sartori G, Job R. (1983). *Phonological impairment in Italian: Acquired and delopmental dyslexia.* In: The acquisition of symbolic skills. Rogers & Sloboda Eds., Plenum Press, New York.

Sartori G, Job R, Tressoldi PE. (1995). *Batteria per la valutazione della dislessia e della disortografia evolutiva.* Organizzazioni Speciali Ed., Firenze, Italia.

Seymour PH, Bunce F. (1994). *Application of cognitive models to remediation in cases of developmental dyslexia.* In: Cognitive neuropsychology and cognitive rehabilitation, Riddoch MJ & Humphreys GW Eds., Lawrence Erlbaum Associates Ltd, Hove, UK.

Sergent J. (1982). *The cerebral balance of power: confrontation or cooperation.* Journal of Experimental Psychology, 8: 253-272.

Shapiro KL, Ogdel N, Lind-Blad F. (1990). *Temporal processing in dyslexia.* Journal of Learning Disabilities, 23: 99-107.

Shulman GL, Wilson J. (1987). *Spatial frequency and selective attention to local and global information.* Perception, 16: 89-101.

Simmers AJ, Bex PJ. (2001). *Deficit of visual contour integration in dyslexia.* Investigative Ophthalmology & Visual Science, 42: 2737-2742.

Slaghuis WL, Lovergrove WJ. (1985). *Spatial-frequency-dependent visible persistence and specific reading disability.* Brain and Cognition, 4: 219-240.

Slaghuis WL, Ryan JF. (1999). *Spatio-temporal contrast sensitivity, coherent motion, and visible persistence in developmental dyslexia.* Vision Research, 39: 651-668.

Stein JF, Walsh V. (1997). *To see but not to read: the magnocellular theory of dyslexia.* Trends in Neurosciences, 20: 147-152.

Tallal P, Piercy M. (1975). *Developmental aphasia: the perception of brief vowels and extended stop consonants.* Neuropsychologia, 13: 69-74.

Ts'o DY, Frostig RD, Leike EE, Grinvald A. (1990). *Functional organization of primate visual-cortex revealed by high resolution optical imaging.* Science, 249: 417-419.

Walther-Muller PU. (1995). *Is there a deficit of early vision in dyslexia?* Perception, 24: 919-936.

Wang J, Bi H, Gao L, Wydell TN. (2010). *The visual magnocellular pathway in Chinese-speaking children with developmental dyslexia.* Neuropsychologia, 48: 3627- 3633.

Weber B, Schwarz U, Kneifel S, Treyer V, Buck A. (2000). *Hierarchical visual processing is dependent on the oculomotor system.* NeuroReport, 11: 241-247.

Wimmer H. (1993). *Characteristics of developmental dyslexia in a regular writing system.* Applied Psycholinguistics, 14: 1-33.

Yamaguchi S, Yamagata S, Kobayashi S. (2000). *Cerebral asymmetry of the "top-down" allocation of attention to global and local features.* Journal of Neuroscience, 20: RC72.

Zoccolotti P, De Luca M, Di Pace E, Judica A, Orlandi M, Spinelli D. (1999). *Markers of developmental surface dyslexia in a language (Italian) with high grapheme-phoneme correspondence.* Applied Psycholinguistics, 20: 191-216.

Chapter XXII

Rehabilitating Spatial Relationship Perceptions: *Avant-gardes* and Working Hypotheses

Nothing prevents from supposing that the anisotropic contraction of the visual space could be successfully rehabilitated. The problem can be tackled under two different points of view: the compensatory approach and the training based on neuronal plasticity.

Compensatory Approach

The supposed compensatory effect that the horizontal widening of the string can have in patients who suffer from crowding reinforcement has been previously reported[394]. Abnormal spatial relationships perception and in particular the anisotropic contraction along the horizontal axis, on the one hand strengthens the lateral masking between adjoining characters, on the other hand breaks up the saccadic programming, accounting for the impaired oculomotor pattern when reading. Widening the inter letter spacing by means of the horizontal anisotropization of the text (or by increasing the print size), would therefore improve patients' fixation instability. In fact, stretching the lexical string implies that the abnormally wide critical spacing tends to be compensated.

According to this perspective, the reading rate in eccentric position is expected to match the reading rate at the foveal level by simply widening proportionally the distance between letters. Indeed, on the basis of the radial/tangential anisotropy typical of the spatial interaction zones, it is recommendable to stretch the text along the horizontal axis to enhance eccentric reading [Toet & Levi, 1992].

Yet, although peripheral reading can improve to a certain extent with such a manipulation, it cannot be normalized. In fact, even if the horizontal stretch of a word is able to neutralize the critical spacing of the more proximal letters, it "pushes" the distal letters more peripherally, therefore makes them subjected to a stronger lateral masking, i.e. to a

[394] See Part I, chapter 13.

wider critical spacing[395]. Since the critical spacing across the word is narrower for the proximal letters and more and more larger for the distal ones, crowding is not uniform across the string but increases towards the periphery.

Therefore, interletter distance between the distal letters has to be larger compared to the proximal ones: for this reason extra-interletter widening is required for the former. Since the more the interletter spacing is widened, the more peripherally the distal letter are shifted, crowding cannot be won: peripheral reading rate cannot improve beyond a given level as the larger is the interletter distance, the narrower is the visual span.

For this reason, it is wrong to believe that peripheral crowding (as well as abnormal parafoveal crowding in dyslexics) can be completely neutralized by widening the interletter distance so as to make it greater than the critical spacing: in theory this is not possible because the critical spacing increases with the distance from the fixation point, so that the compensatory enlargement of the interval between the letters displaces the distal character towards the periphery. Thereby, the distant characters require larger and larger spacing. Unlike the peripheral crowding reinforcement found in ordinary conditions, in dyslexic children abnormal crowding is shown to occur at the paracentral level of the visual field. Therefore, in this case the visual span turns out to be narrowed leading to reduced reading rate.

In theory the optimal solution could be the horizontal anisotropization of the string (i.e. the "stretch" along the horizontal axis) not constant across the string but varying according to an incremental gradient, so as to reduce the detrimental side-effect of the compensation of the critical spacing that affects the distal characters and thereby the visual span.

Evidently, in order to obtain the maximum result from this paradigm, it is crucial to know precisely to what extent the area occupied by the sentence has to be expanded: under dimensioned widening does not allow to completely exploit the benefit, over dimensioned widening may further worsen the saccadic pattern.

For this reason the psychophysical test we have devised, the Reading Performance Test (REPORT), aims at providing an estimate of the best anisotropization value that allows an improvement of the lexical function (see Appendix C).

In summary, this type of rehabilitation strategy deserves consideration, since it could improve the analytical process in the lexical task of those dyslexic patients who show an evident increase of the critical spacing.

Training Based on the Neuronal Plasticity

It is now established that the plastic properties of the human brain typical of the early years of childhood, to some extent extend even in adulthood [Gilbert, 1998] and that the visual anisotropic properties can be modulated by the experience [Karim & Kojima, 2010a]: for example the better sensitivity of the lower compared to the upper visual hemifield presumably stems from the preferential development of visual attention across the lower sectors of space [He et al., 1996, 1997; Intriligator & Cavanagh, 2001].

[395] According to the Bouma's law.

Interestingly, the effect visual training has for stimuli presented along the cardinal coordinates is greater compared to the advantage obtained with the stimulation along the oblique axes. This phenomenon is described for Vernier acuity [Karim & Kojima, 2010b] and is related to the higher number of cortical neurons modulated for the cardinal orientations [Coppola et al., 1998; Furmanski & Engel, 2000; Li et al., 2003]. In line with these assumptions, there is some evidence suggesting lateral masking can be reduced with adequate practice[396], since it has to be regarded as an active filtering [Geiger & Lettvin, 1986] and not as a fixed feature of visuocortical detectors, as originally believed by Bouma [1970]. So, a rehabilitation strategy aimed at reducing the critical spacing and enlarging the visual span may be effective in improving reading in dyslexic children suffering from abnormally strong lateral masking. In normal adult readers, a significant reduction of the critical spacing has been observed after a training based on the visual presentation in peripheral position of triplets of letters [Chung et al., 2004, Chung, 2007]. After the practice, the peripheral reading rate was improved by 41% as a consequence of the enlargement of the visual span. Indeed, considering its effectiveness in enlarging the visual span, thereby in improving the peripheral reading rate in normal readers, such a rehabilitation strategy is worthwhile to be investigated in dyslexic children.

By virtue of the crossmodal impairment that characterizes our clinical condition, a similar approach has been reported even in the auditory domain [Farmer & Klein, 1995]. In this case the training is made of auditory patterns made easier via temporal dilation, then more difficult by gradually reducing the duration of the sound. The same approach could be adopted in the visual domain, starting from a value of horizontal anisotropization which makes easier the visuoperceptive processing of the text and progressively shrinking the spatial extent of the lexical string.

References

Bouma H. (1970). *Interaction effects in parafoveal letter recognition.* Nature, 226: 177–178.

Chung STL. (2007). *Learning to identify crowded letters: does it improve reading speed?* Vision Research, 47: 3150-3159.

Chung STL, Legge GE, Cheung SH. (2004). *Letter recognition and reading speed in peripheral vision benefit from perceptual learning.* Vision Research, 44: 695-709.

Coppola DM, White LE, Fitzpatrick D, Purves D. (1998). *Unequal representation of cardinal and oblique contours in ferret visual cortex.* Proceedings of the National Academy of Sciences of the United States of America, 95: 2621-2623.

Farmer ME, Klein RM. (1995). *The evidence for a temporal processing deficit-linked to dyslexia.* Psychonomic Bulletin Review, 2: 460-493.

Furmanski CS, Engel SA. (2000). *An oblique effect in human primary visual cortex.* Nature Neuroscience,3: 535-536.

Geiger G, Lettvin JY. (1986). *Enhancing the perception of form in peripheral vision.* Perception, 15: 119-130.

Gilbert CD. (1998). *Adult cortical dynamics.* Physiological Reviews, 78: 467–485.

[396] Part I, chapter 13.

He S, Cavanagh P, Intriligator J. (1996). *Attentional resolution and the locus of visual awareness*. Nature, 383: 334-337.

He S, Cavanagh P, Intriligator J. (1997). *Attentional resolution.* Trends in Cognitive Sciences, 1: 115-121.

Intriligator J, Cavanagh P. (2001). *The spatial resolution of visual attention.* Cognitive Psychology, 43: 171-216.

Karim AK, Kojima H. (2010a). *The what and why of perceptual asymmetries in the visual domain.* Advances in Cognitive Psychology, 6: 103-115.

Karim AK, Kojima H. (2010b). *Configurational asymmetry in vernier offset detection.* Advances in Cognitive Psychology, 6: 66-78.

Levi DM. (2008). *Crowding-An essential bottleneck for object recognition: A mini-review.* Vision Research, 48: 635-654.

Li B, Peterson MR, Freeman RD. (2003). *Oblique effect: A neural basis in the visual cortex.* Journal of Neurophysiology, 90: 204-217.

Toet A, Levi DM. (1992). *The two-dimensional shape of spatial interaction zones in the parafovea.* Vision Research, 32: 1349-1357.

Conclusion

The multidisciplinary nature of developmental dyslexia is indisputable: even if it is a syndrome of neuropsychiatric and logopedic competence, its management requires the continuous confrontation with other professionals, neuro-ophthalmologist and orthoptist included.

Naturally, such a global approach is not dictated *a priori*, but depends on the deep link among the elements that characterize our condition: because of this peculiarity, evaluating and dealing with an aspect of the syndrome without taking into account the possible effects on the others, can only lead to deceptive and potentially dangerous results.

Although the visuoperceptive factor is not the key of the problem, a large body of evidence does not allow any longer to ignore its existence. Even if (as reminded by Stein) oral language is an instinct rooted in our genetic map, reading depends on a cultural invention, therefore its acquisition is not an event given for granted.

The ability to communicate verbally dates back to the dawn of mankind. The invention of the alphabet dates back to the Phoenicians about some three thousand years ago. The substantial difference between the oral and the written communication is that the latter requires to turn a series of symbols, that is, letters that make up syllables, into a sequence of sounds.

As an essential prerequisite for this process, letters and their relative positions have to be recognized and properly coded in their relative spatial position and this is undoubtedly a visual task: only after the visual processing of the word has taken place it is possible to turn it into a sound.

Since the perceptive factor precedes the phonological one (even in dyslexics with a predominant phonological impairment), it is necessary to make sure that there is no obstacle in the visual learning of the lexical material. In the light of the increasing acquisitions, these two elements for too long considered separately and antithetical, must be regarded as the sides of the same coin, stemming from development anomalies of the central nervous system, probably caused by a damage occurred during the gestational life. Apart from the controversial hypothesis of testosterone, the relationship among dyslexia, immunological diseases and macro-and microanatomical cerebral anomalies is consistent with a disruption of the large ganglion cells system. We have discussed about the implication of the chromosome 6 in the pathogenesis of the disease and in the modulation of the immune system through a gene responsible for the major histocompatibility complex. It is remarkable that magnocells express on their specific surface antigens able to evoke an autoimmune response [Hockfield & Sur, 1990] and that during pregnancy an autoimmune reaction with the production of maternal antibodies directed against fetal magnocellular neurons has been postulated in the pathogenesis of dyslexia [Vincent et al., 2000]. The production of these autoantibodies, driven by the major histocompatibility complex, would be the factor underlying the magnocellular brain damage and the allergic and autoimmunologic diathesis in patients. By means of a specific monoclonal antibody (CAT 301), magnocellular antigens have been documented not only along the visual pathway but also along the auditory, the somesthetic and the motor pathway, as well as in the cerebellum: this ubiquity supports the concept of dyslexia as a global *pathology of the magnosystem* [Hockfield & Sur, 1990]. As pointed out by Laycock and Crewther [2008], reading is first of all a spatial task that requires the processing of syllables and words in a sequential manner. For this reason an essential prerequisite is an efficient oculomotor scanning.

Still, efficient oculomotor scanning is of no avail without normal temporal sequential processing (TSP), whose alteration in dyslexics would mainly produce sluggish visuo-attentional orientation [Brannan & Williams, 1987; Renvall & Hari, 2002]. This anomaly, M-mediated [Yantis &Jonides, 1984, 1996; Steinman et al., 1997], is found to involve other sensory modalities (especially the auditory one: Renvall & Hari, 2002), in agreement with the multimodal alteration suggested in the immunological studies. The attentional orientation slowdown is expected to affect the automatism of the sequential analysis of letters and syllables, eventually disturbing the saccadic pattern: so, dyslexics are prevented from distracting and redirecting the attention from the fixated syllable to the next, parafoveal one. As a result, reading turns out to be slow and fragmented. The oculomotor alterations are found during the lexical tasks because the properties of a written text require a very accurate time sequential processing. The anatomical center in charge of the attentional orientation is placed in the right parietal cortex, particularly in the inferior parietal lobule [Chambers et al., 2004]. Considering that this area, assisted by the Frontal Eye Field [Neggers et al., 2007], is also responsible for the saccadic programming, it is easy to figure out the close relationship between visual attention and FEMs [Biscaldi et al., 1998]. Evidently, the saccadic programming and the rhythmic alternation of attentional focus and defocus, being dynamic functions, contribute to the temporal sequential processing of the visual stimulus. Yet, visual attention and saccadic sequence interact with the processing of letters, syllables and words. Since the source of such a processing locates in the visual cortex and has to do with the spatial vision, it is comprehensible the close (magnocellular-modulated[397]) link between the parietal and the visual areas. This connection allows the signal to be continuously and mutually modulated [Gandhi et al., 1999; Martinez et al., 2001] and represents the anatomical *trait d'union* between the visuotemporal and the visuospatial aspect of the lexical function.

Is has been claimed that are the temporal and not the spatial aspects of reading to be compromised in developmental dyslexia [Eden et al., 1995]. If this statement refers to the estimate of the visual configuration change over time, it is hard to reconcile this point of view with the static characteristics of the written text. If it means that dyslexics suffer from sluggish visuospatial processing, the assumption may have a justification. In fact, even if spatial relationships perception, which has nothing to do with the analysis of dynamic configurations, is often deficient in patients, nevertheless the tachistoscopic presentations

[397] Morandi et al., 2007.

adopted in the eidomorphometry could prevent subjects with defective magnocellular functions from adequately perceive the sense of the space as required during the examination[398]. Concerning this, it is revealing that the time limit at disposal to process each syllable corresponds to a few hundreds of milliseconds, namely to the fixation time.

According to this interpretation, the impaired functions in the temporal domain (in agreement with the TSP deficit theory) transfer on the visuospatial level, where the lexical function actually takes place.

Functionally, the convergence point between temporal and spatial vision in developmental dyslexia consists in the link between the disruption of the normal saccadic pattern together to TSP –related defective visuo-attentional function on the one hand and the SRA-related crowding reinforcement on the other hand. It is a relationship based on strategies made of an extremely complex feedback. Such a complexity requires the lexical elaboration to be driven by a real cortical *servomechanism* involving the cortex as a whole. The defective TSP would be one of the main results of the input slowdown along this complex magnocellular network [Laycock & Crewther, 2008].

An impairment involving one of the stations placed along the neural network can affect the feed forward and feedback circuitry, destabilizing the entire process. Within this global framework, defective spatial relationship perception cannot absolutely be ignored. Indeed, it has been recently argued that even the visuoperceptive element is causally involved in developmental dyslexia [Laycock & Crewther, 2008], in accordance with a previous statement of Stein and Walsh, the visual impairment is an important component of developmental dyslexia, and every attempt to understand the problem which does not consider the basic visual processing is incomplete [Stein & Walsh, 1997].

A salient characteristic of developmental dyslexia is the dissociation between the saccadic sequence when reading and its normal pattern in extra lexical tasks. This dichotomy decisively contributes to discredit the concept of oculomotor imbalance as a primary cause of this clinical condition and makes the visual space distortion a plausible solution. In fact, FEM alteration when reading (and not in other conditions) could be the sign of a visuoperceptive anomaly chiefly evident in the lexical task (see Rayner, 1998 for a systematic review).

It has been demonstrated that in normal readers the saccadic pattern varies according to the characteristics of the written text: for example, reversing the order of the letters in a word, reversing the words in a sentence or finally turning the string of 180 degrees, the saccades amplitude decreases, till to fall below 30 minarc [Kowler & Anton, 1987]. This reduction in amplitude depends on the fact that the modified text requires the systematic fixation of every single letter and not just the fixation of the characters close to the perceptive centre-of-gravity of the word. In the third experimental condition the inversion of the reading direction (from left→right to right→left) produces an increase of the backward saccades up to 60% of the total FEMs. This experiment suggests that the lexical organization of the visual space is able to change the saccadic structure, which in its turn demonstrates a remarkable ability to spatial adaptation. In any case the outcome is reduced reading rate.

With regard to the aforementioned study of MacKeben [MacKeben et al., 2004],[399] it is remarkable the correlation between amplitude of the forward saccades and word length: the

[398] Spatial relationship perception tends to improve if the presentation time is delayed from 50 up to 500-1000 msec (Aleci, 2003: personal communication).

[399] See chapter 10.

model is linear in the control group while in the dyslexics it is better described by a second order polynomial function, which reaches the “ceiling” for saccadic amplitudes of approximately 60 minarc (namely 2 interletter spaces at the normal reading distance[400].

In agreement with the hypothesis of Kowler and Anton, the linear correlation would reveal normal adaptation of the saccadic width to the length of the words; the lacking of this modulation would depend on abnormal visuospatial perception and in some dyslexics it would help to account for their poor performance, especially when reading long words.

In addition to the oculomotor sequence impairment, even the delayed and incomplete correction of the visual axes disconjugation occurring immediately after the landing of the saccade[401] could depend on abnormal spatial relationship perception. In fact, the sudden and adequate vergence movement aimed at correcting this temporary gap [Bucci et al., 2008; Kapoula & Vernet, 2009] is believed to pertain to the sensory domain [Jainta and Kapoula, 2011]: therefore the perceptive distortion of the visual space might be implicated in its failure. In summary, the adaptation of the saccadic amplitude to the length of the word and the ability to compensate the physiological desynchronization of the saccadic versions when reading reinforces the alleged link between ocular motility and visuoperception, a link defined *sensory-driven feedback loop* (Jainta & Kapoula, 2011). In our opinion, in a subtype of patients a visuoperceptive distortion would affect such a *sensory-driven feedback loop*. This visuoperceptive distortion would consist in a reinforcement of the physiological vertical anisotropy, so that the lexical string is perceived as contracted, “shrunk” along its horizontal axis. Due to this contraction, in visual dyslexics the first and the last saccade would fall closer to the ends of the words compared to normal readers[402]. In fact in such a visuoperceptual condition their optimal viewing position turns out to be shifted, creating an oculomotor disorientation.

Finally, the perturbation of the saccadic pattern would be responsible for the higher number of fixations, the greater frequency and the lower amplitude of forward saccades and the increased number of backward saccades.

In conclusion, a primitive visuoperceptive anomaly would affect the oculomotor pattern and not vice versa. In addition, the illusory reduced distance between adjacent letters are expected to increase the reciprocal effect of lateral masking: an event that helps to cause visual confusion and reading slowdown.

The subject is further complicated by the unstable ocular dominance responsible for the fixation instability, since fixation instability deteriorates especially visual localization[403] of the letters that make up words. The theory of the fixation instability deserves a special

[400] From this study, however, do not emerge the expected reduction of the saccadic accuracy in patients. This finding seems in contrast with the hypothesis of the perceptual shrinking, that on the contrary implies FEMs to be inaccurate (in agreement with a large body of evidence). However, compared to our dyslexic sample, the age of the patients in the group recruited in the German study was higher (11-16 years). In older kids it is possible that reading experience modulates the saccadic pattern, re-balancing the displacement of the optimal viewing position of the words. This gradual adjustment would allow patients to learn to localize the actual optimal viewing position in order to direct the saccade with sufficient precision.

[401] See chapter 10

[402] And in fact in dyslexics (especially in the case of words longer than 10 letters), the last and first fixation on the word is closer to its farthest ends compared to controls (distance from the end of the string: 51 minarc vs. 125 minarc in normal reders; distance from the beginning of the string: 56 minarc vs. 124 minarc in normal readers).

[403] Also documented in extralexical tasks [Riddell et al., 1990].

consideration not only for its impact on the scientific community but also for the reported rehabilitative results.

Spatial relationships perception alteration characterized by abnormal vertical anisotropy is an interesting aspect of the visuoperceptive impairment in developmental dyslexia, when present. Our studies show that in about half of the normal readers the visual space tends to be shrunk along the horizontal coordinate. The degree of such a distortion in average is double in a subgroup of dyslexics, worsening the effect of lateral masking and leading to saccadic perturbation.

Therefore, vertical anisotropy and saccadic disorders[404] are the two elements we believe to be the pillars of the neurophthalmological argument in developmental dyslexia. It is remarkable in some ways how our hypothesis seems to be able to explain the other visuoperceptive anomalies reported in the literature: in the first part of this treatise it is shown that increased vertical anisotropy could affect motion perception, in a measure could enhance the negative effect the modest contrast sensitivity reduction may have on the visual span and eventually could impair shape recognition.

Fixation instability is an aggravating factor.

Among the reasons why the perceptual shrinking seems to be a solution worthy of further investigations is, last but not least, the concordance with the signs and the symptoms typically reported by patients: for example the frequent confusion between contiguous letters and syllables is better explained by this approach rather than invoking a primitive saccadic imbalance, that, if anything, could lead to the exchange of characters placed at a certain distance between themselves and not side by side; the prevalence of errors for mirror letters, typical of the dyslexic lexical pattern, may be easier to understand considering that the discrimination threshold for specular letters, especially if flanked by other characters, is higher compared to non-mirror characters. In addition it is anisotropic, therefore particularly sensitive to increased asymmetry in spatial relationship perception[405].

Under an ecological perspective, it is outstanding that the environment could be able to influence the isotropic mapping of images on the visual cortex since the representation of a natural image *per se* is endowed with a certain degree of anisotropy: a country landscape shows faster decay along the vertical coordinate, which translates into a preponderant development of is spatial relationship along the horizontal coordinate. On the contrary, the urban landscape is characterized by a mainly vertical development [Baddeley & Hancock, 1991].

Therefore, exposure to the everyday environment may affect the anisotropy of the visual system.

---

[404] Besides unstable dominance.

[405] A complementary explanation involves higher levels of image processing and suggests in addition to lateral masking reinforcement a deficit of the so-called side *discrimination*. The side discrimination is a function that allows to recognize two stimuli that differ because one is rotated or is the mirror image of the other: this is the case of some letters, such as p, q, d, b. On the contrary, due to the symmetry generalization (pertaining to the right parietal cortex) a given object is recognized irrespective of its position or rotation and from any perspective it be examined [Jaśkowski & Rusiak, 2005]. Therefore, it was suggested that dyslexics are less skilled than normal readers to identify mirror letters due to defective side discrimination [Jaśkowski & Rusiak, 2005], in presence of a normal or supernormal symmetry generalization [Corballis et al., 1985a, b]. On this basis, Lachmann postulated that the hyperactivation of the symmetry generalization may inhibit the side discrimination, accounting for the confusion between mirror letters [Lachmann, 2002]. In line with this solution, Pontius observed in 4/5 of his patients difficulties in detecting the rotation of a figure, and related this feature to the frequent confusion of mirror letters along the two cardinal axes [Pontius, 1981].

It is curious that the estimated prevalence of dyslexia in the isle of White was only 5% compared to 10% and more in the central districts of London [Yule et al., 1973].

There is no doubt that the diagnosis of developmental dyslexia is up to the neuropsychiatrist. It is a challenging task because a single standardized test aimed at detecting this clinical condition is not available, to date. Moreover, developmental dyslexia cannot be diagnosed exclusively by means of exams in the phonological-auditory or in the visual field [American Academy of Pediatrics, 2011].

On the contrary, as stated by the American Academy of Pediatrics, the diagnosis and the treatment of a child with dyslexia depends on the constant collaboration of a multidisciplinary team [American Academy of Pediatrics, 2011].

This authoritative source and the other researchers, however, do not deny the possibility for the ophthalmologist to diagnose a visuoperceptive disorder in dyslexics or suspected dyslexics. A serious and focused approach in this direction can be very useful to classify patients and to develop rigorous rehabilitative solutions.

Indeed, this is the goal of our protocol, without pretending to investigate the problem beyond our clinical field. Although the diagnosis of dyslexia is not a neuro-ophthalmological matter, its early detection and management can benefit from the clinical and experimental research in vision science. The use of tests aimed at assessing the magnocellular function along the visual pathway as critical fusion frequency of coherent motion detection[406] could allow to identify children at risk of dyslexia in prelexical age, therefore before the deficient function shows [Talcott et al., 1998].

Also the attentional function and in particular the assessment of the forming resolving field seems to be promising in this respect.

Apart from excluding (or treating) concurrent (and potentially aggravating) ophthalmological conditions and helping in the early diagnosis, the neurophthalmological approach can contribute to the typification of each patient. Since dyslexics are not homogeneous in their clinical features, it is likely they are not homogeneous in the pathogenesis, too: therefore, the classification of dyslexia is a crucial moment for the management of every single patient. Since the model advanced by Boder in the seventies, several other classifications have been suggested. In most of them, the form with a prevailing phonological component is opposed to the type with prevailing orthographic or visuoperceptive factors. Yet, this perspective does not fully explain the semeiological spectrum of dyslexics: indeed, phonological and visual factors rather than being mutually exclusive seem to be complementary. Irrespective of the dyseidetic or dysphonetic class, or better *within* each of these classes, the visuoperceptive impairment can occur to a different extent and with different characteristics which, in turn, need to be categorized. Therefore, the

[406] According to a recent longitudinal study, motion perception is an early marker of dyslexia and would enable the early diagnosis since the last year of kindergarten (age: 5) [Boets et al., 2011]. In the investigation, coherent motion perception was estimated in 31 preschool children (mean age: 5 years and 6 months). Children were classified as suspected dyslexic after assessing their lexical prerequisites, and subsequently confirmed as dyslexics. Their motion perception threshold was compared with the results obtained in an age-matched group expected to develop normal reading function. Coherent motion threshold measured during the last year of kindergarten turned out to be higher in suspected (and subsequently confirmed) dyslexics compared to their peers that would prove normal readers. The next year (first grade), motion perception was improved in both samples and the prior difference was no more detectable. Therefore, motion perception enhancement observed in first grade seems to be consequent to lexical training and not due to improved sensibility to dynamic stimuli per se. Thereby, according to this study motion perception is an early indicator of dyslexia for children in prelexical age, but its causal role is ruled out.

advanced classification addressed to the visuoperceptive impairment is not another classification of developmental dyslexia (it would not be up to us), but a categorization of dyslexic patients solely based on the kind of perceptive defects they are affected from.

As discussed, a main visuoperceptive anomaly in dyslexia deals both with reinforcement of the lateral masking stemming from abnormal spatial relationship anisotropy and with fixation instability depending on unstable ocular dominance. In these cases the difficulty may involve the analysis of words and (on a more local scale) of letters, that is to say the fragmentation of the string into its single features and their subsequent processing. Alternatively or in addition, the impairment is expected to occur at a global level, dealing with the configuration of the word as a whole: It has to do with the *synthesis* of the single features after their *analytical* processing has been completed. The difference between the two forms, therefore, relies on the level of the perceptual impairment: analysis in the first case, synthesis in the second.

Of course, the ultimate goal of this approach lies in the rehabilitation of the visual component, an aspect that has been too often underestimated. Indeed, the American Academy of Pediatrics states that doctors should recommend only evidence-based treatments and the ophthalmologist should inform parents on the actual lack of proven efficacy of the visual therapy [American Academy of Pediatrics, 2011]. In 2003 less than 5% of the studies on dyslexia were addressed to the rehabilitation [Tressoldi et al., 2003]. Presumably (and correctly), the proportion refers to investigations made with scientific criteria. Even if the number of these rigorous investigations has grown, it is still small, whereas reports of questionable validity, poorly designed experiments without solid rationale basis and mainly derived from anecdotal attempts have multiply with impressive rate.

The major academic American bodies agree that there is no scientific evidence, to date, supporting that children with reading problems can improve by means of treatments based on the visual training, including exercises on eye muscles, visual tracking and colored lenses. This does not mean that visual rehabilitation is ruled out, but that proven evidence about its effectiveness is lacking, to date. Indeed, in his review on the role of the modern technology in the diagnosis and treatment of developmental dyslexia, Colbert pinpointed that the visuoperceptive techniques are promising [Colbert et al., 2003]. Really, visual rehabilitation seems promising when given to receptive patients, that is to say if the target of the subjects to be treated has been previously established by using appropriate classification criteria.

In Italy, eight different treatments adopted in clinical practice have been compared [Tressoldi et al., 2003]. Of these techniques, three involve visual perception: the stimulation of the attentional focus by masking the text on the right side of the fixation point[407] (Davis-Piccoli treatment), a paradigm based on the visual interemispheric stimulation according to Bakker, and the so-called *sublexical treatment* with perceptual masking, based on the model of the moving window described by Geiger. Compared to the other (linguistic) protocols available, these treatments turned out to be more effective in improving reading rate and (except the first) in increasing lexical accuracy.

Still, no doubt that treating the visuoperceptive defects is only a part of the strategy aimed at rehabilitating patients affected by developmental dyslexia, since developmental dyslexia is a single aspect of a multifaceted condition: a condition which seems to extend well beyond the reading ability.

[407] With a sheet of paper.

Indeed, it is likely that the chromosomal modifications underlying developmental dyslexia promote a much more generalized condition, whose reading disability is just one aspect. Phylogenetically, dyslexia-related malfunctioning genes would survive since they are responsible also for tasks that only a few centuries ago (that is to say in times of marked illiteracy) were more important compared to the concurrent inability to read. Thereby, dyslexia can be imagined as the price to be paid to better perform skills that in the past, when reading was not crucial, were more important.

It has been argued that the magnocellular defect not only provides lexical disadvantage but it is even dangerous, since reduced motion perception, reduced sensitivity to some auditive frequencies, poor motor coordination and the other reported M-related defective functions would expose patients to a risk in daily life. Yet, a loss of a few log unit fractions for the sensory functions or a slight postural unbalance in motor tasks probably are not so crucial for surviving. Indeed, it is surprising that the allele responsible for defective magnocellular development is so widespread despite its potential "lethality". Yet, when the reading demand in a modern cultural environment requires higher visuoperceptive performances, the phenotypic expression of that allele turns out to be decisive.

Surprisingly, as if to repay patients and their families for the troubles it is responsible of, our condition seems to carry significant advantages to the dyslexic child: for example protective effect from blood hypertension and cardiovascular diseases [Taylor & Stein, 2002] and talents in many speculative and practical fields.

In conclusion, as reminded by Stein & Talcott [1999], dyslexics are not condemned to an eternal incompetence. On the contrary, there are many examples of talents that dyslexic children have developed in other areas of their lives. There are a lot of talented dyslexic people in history who were probably dyslexic: for example, Leonardo, Albert Einstein, Winston Churchill, Thomas Edison, Walt Dysney just to name a few. It has been suggested that the secret talent of dyslexics is their ability to approach a problem from a global perspective so as to find the solution via holistic approach rather than considering separately the single components it is made of.

This advantage would be related to an enhancement of the long-range parvocellular connections, a possible compensatory response to the M-cells deficit. This way, the parvocellular network not only preserves its original function (processing fine details) but in addition is enriched by the ability to integrate its function on a larger, more global, more "magnocellular" scale.

Among the famous dyslexics is Sir. Winston Churchill (1874-1965).

Quoting one of his most picturesque aphorisms is probably the best way to close the narration of a debate that despite the great speculative effort remains fairly unsolved:

Now this is not the end.
It is not even the beginning of the end.
But it is, perhaps, the end of the beginning.

References

Aleci C. *Analisi delle curvature, percezione dei rapporti spaziali e qualità della visione in campo neurofisiologico ed oftalmologico.* Doctoral dissertation, Turin, 2003.

American Academy of Pediatrics. (2011). *Joint Tecnical Report-Learning Disabilities, Dyslexia, and Vision.* Pediatrics, 127: 818-852.

Baddeley RJ & Hancock PJ. (1991). *A statistical analysis of natural images matches psychophysically derived orientation tuning curves.* Proceedings of the Royal Society of London B, 246:219-223.

Biscaldi M, Gezeck S, Stuhr V. (1998). *Poor saccadic control correlates with dyslexia.* Neuropsychologia, 36: 1189-1202.

Boets B, Vandermosten M, Cornelissen P, Wouters J, Ghesquiére P. (2011).*Coherent motion sensitivity and reading development in the transition from prereading to reading stage.* Child Development, 82: 854-869.

Brannan J, Williams M. (1987). *Allocation of visual attention in good and poor readers.* Perception & Psychophysics, 41: 23-28.

Bucci MP, Bremond-Gignac D, Kapoula Z. (2008). *Poor binocular coordination of saccades in dyslexic children.* Graefes Archive for Clinical and Experimental Ophthalmology, 246: 417-428.

Chambers CD, Payne JM, Stokes MG, Mattingley JB. (2004). *Fast and slow parietal pathways mediate spatial attention.* Nature Neuroscience, 7: 217-218.

Colbert JE, McGraw TM, Wenrich JR, Burdette K. (2003). *The role of technology in the diagnosis and treatment of dyslexia: A research synthesis.* Charleston, VW: AEL, Institute for the Advancement of Emerging Technologies in Education. http://www.ael.org/page2.htm?&index=788&pd=1&pv=x.

Corballis MC, Macadie L, Beale IL. (1985a). *Mental rotation and visual laterality in normal and reading disabled children.* Cortex 1985; 21: 225-236.

Corballis MC, Macadie L, Crotty A, Beale IL. (1985b) *The naming of disoriented letters by normal and reading-disabled children.* J Child Psychol Psychiatry 1985; 26: 929-938.

Eden GF, Stein JF, Wood HM, Wood FB. (1995). *Temporal and spatial processing in reading disabled and normal children.* Cortex, 31: 451-468.

Gandhi SP, Heeger DJ, Boynton GM. (1999). *Spatial attention affects brain activity in human primary visual cortex.* Proceedings of the National Academy of the United States of America, 96: 3314-3319.

Hockfield S, Sur M. (1990). *Monoclonal CAT 301 identifies Y cells in cat LGN.* Journal of Clinical Neurology, 300: 320-330.

Jainta S, Kapoula Z. (2011). *Dyslexic children are confronted with unstable binocular fixation while reading.* PLoS ONE, 6: 1-10.

Jaśkowski P, Rusiak P. (2005). *Posterior parietal cortex and developmental dyslexia.* Acta Neurobiologiae Experimentalis, 65: 79-94.

Kowler E, Anton S. (1987). *Reading twisted text: implications for the role of saccades.* Vision Research, 27: 45-60.

Lachmann T. (2002). *Reading disability as a deficit in functional coordination.* In: Basic Functions of Language, Reading, and Reading Disability, Witruk, Friederici & Lachmann Eds,. Kluwer Academic Pub, Dordrecht, Holland.

Laycock R, Crewther SG. (2008). *Towards an understanding of the role of the 'magnocellular advantage' in fluent reading.* Neuroscience and Biobehavioral Reviews, 32: 1494-1506.

MacKeben M, Trauzettel-Klosinski S, Reinhard J, Dürrwächter U, Adler M, Klosinski G. (2004). *Eye movement control during single-word reading in dyslexics.* Journal of Vision, 4 (5): 388-402.

Martinez A, DiRusso F, Anilo-Vento L, Sereno MI, Buxton RB, Hillyard SA. (2001). *Putting spatial attention on the map: timing and localization of stimulus selection processes in striate and extrastriate visual areas.* Vision Research, 41: 1437-1457.

Morandi F, Hipp C, Koch C. (2007). *Activity in the visual cortex in modulated by top-down attention locked to reaction time.* Journal of Cognitive Neuroscience, 19: 331-340.

Neggers SF, Huijbers W, Vrijlandt CM, Vlaskamp BN, Schutter DJ, Kenemans JL. (2007). TMS pulses on the frontal eye fields break coupling between visuospatial attention and eye movements. Journal of Neurophysiology, 98: 2765-2778.

Rayner K. (1998). *Eye movements in reading and information processing: 20 years of research.* Psychological Bulletin, 124: 372-422.

Renvall A, Hari R. (2002). *Auditory cortical responses to speech-like stimuli in dyslexic adults.* Journal of Cognitive Neuroscience, 14: 757-768.

Riddell PM, Fowler MS, Stein JF. (1990). *Spatial discrimination in children with poor vergence control.* Perception & Motor Skills, 70: 707-718.

Stein JF, Talcott J. (1999). *Impaired neuronal timing in developmental dyslexia-the magnocellular hypothesis.* Dyslexia, 5: 59- 77.

Stein JF, Walsh V. (1997). *To see but not to read: the magnocellular theory of dyslexia.* Trends in Neurosciences, 20: 147-152.

Steinman BA, Steinman SB, Lehmkuhle S. (1997). *Transient visual attention is dominated by the magnocellular stream.* Vision Research, 37: 17-23.

Talcott JB, Hansen PC, Willis-Owen C, McKinnell IW, Richardson AJ, Stein J. (1998). *Visual magnocellular impairment in adult developmental dyslexics.* Neuro-Ophthalmology, 20: 187-201.

Taylor KE, Stein JF. (2002). *Dyslexia and familiar high blood pressure: An observational pilot study.* Archives of Disease in Childhood, 86: 30-33.

Tressoldi PE, Vio C, Lorusso ML, Facoetti A, Iozzino R. (2003). *Confronto di efficacia ed efficienza tra trattamenti per il miglioramento della lettura in soggetti dislessici.* Psicologia Clinica dello Sviluppo, 3: 481-493.

Vernet M, Kapoula Z. (2009). *Binocular motor coordination during saccades and fixations while reading: A magnitude and time analysis*. Journal of Vision, 9 (7): 1-13.

Vincent A, Deacon R, Blamire AW, Pendlebury S, Salmond C, Johansen-Berg H, Dalton P, Rajogopalan B, Styles P, Stein JF. (2000). *Behavioural and cerebellar MRS findings in mice exposed in utero to serum from mothers of children with neurodevelopmental disorders.* Proceedings of the International Society of Magnetic Resonance Medicine, 1080.

Yantis S, Jonides J. (1984). *Abrupt visual onsets and selective attention: evidence from visual search.* Journal of Experimental Psychology: Human Perception and Performance, 10: 601-621.

Yantis S, Jonides J. (1996). *Attentional capture by abrupt onsets: new perceptual objects or visual masking?* Journal of Experimental Psychology: Human Perception and Performance, 22: 1505-1513.

Yule M, Rutter M, Berger M, Thompson B. (1973). *Over and under achievement in reading.* British Journal of Educational Psychology, 44: 1-12.

Epilogue

"*To be able to read is not an option - it is a right*".

The definition of disease given by the World Health Organization is *the absence of health*. A state of health is a state of complete physical, mental and social well-being. In alternative, *disease* can be defined as a morphological, functional and /or psychic anomaly that leads the individual to suffer. So, how can it be denied that developmental dyslexia is a disease? And how can it be doubted that the functional anomalies of the magnocellular system have begun to cause the suffering since the individual found himself plunged into a cultural environment that required lexical performance to a greater extent, and not previously, when in a rural society he was busy working in the fields? In spite of those who argue that dyslexia is not a disease but a simple "biodiversity" (as if to exorcise its destructive potential), for its clinical characteristics and from a medical rather than psychological perspective we insist on considering it a real pathological condition.

In February 2010 the World Dyslexia Forum was held in Paris at the UNESCO headquarters and was attended by more than 250 delegates from 90 countries of the world. Patron of the event was Her Royal Highness the Grand Duchess Maria Teresa of Luxembourg.

Some striking points have arisen in that occasion. The 85% of young misfits of Toronto, Canada, suffer from unrecognized learning disabilities, and as such untreated. From 75 to 95% of prisoners in the jails of this country have experienced significant reading problems and all teenagers who committed suicide in Ontario turned out to have the same problem. Beside the bewilderment, there is concern for the lack of recognition of this condition in several countries such as the Arab countries, but to a certain extent even in the western world. As an example, in the United Kingdom its estimated prevalence is up to 10% but only 2.5% of cases are diagnosed and officially recognized[408].

In the battle against developmental dyslexia the scientific progress clashes with the difficulties of an interdisciplinary condition, which requires early diagnosis and rehabilitation strategies based on the modern experimental investigation. People involved in neuro-ophthalmology and vision sciences cannot avoid to participate, since *"[...] reading, first of*

---

[408] Stein J. [2001]. The magnocellular theory of developmental dyslexia.Dyslexia, 7: 12-36.

all, is a visual task and the research about dyslexia should consider this aspect likewise important"[409].

Clinical trials are urgently required so as to compare different training and rehabilitative programs as well as to devise customized treatments. A specific training is necessary for teachers and professionals, too, so far hampered by costs and lack of consensus on the most effective protocols to be adopted.

Finally, an educational approach and a rehabilitative methodology aimed at developing all sensory modalities in the context of a fruitful interdisciplinary collaboration is desirable.

In the interest of hundreds of thousands of children it is a duty to persist in rigorous research and free exchange of ideas and information among everyone involved in this field.

Without prejudice.

"Only after nouns and definitions, visual perceptions and sensations are laboriously rubbed together, only after they have been discussed in kind discussions in which envy does not dictate either the question or the answer, wisdom and intelligence spurt on everything, with all the intensity the human force is capable".

Plato, Lett. VII, 344b

Turin, January, the 20th, 2012.

[409] Laycock R, Crewther SG. [2008]. Towards an understanding of the role of the 'magnocellular advantage' in fluent reading. Neuroscience and Biobehavioral Reviews, 32: 1494-1506.

Appendices

Appendix A: On the Optimal Perceptive Characteristics of a Text

In the first of a series of articles, the effect of some visuoperceptive parameters on the readability of a text has been discussed in detail [Legge et al., 1985]. Although this topic goes beyond the purposes of the book, it is worthwhile providing readers with a list of the ideal characteristics a written page should have to be easily read.

Luminance of the text

When luminance level is raised from 0.3 cd/m^2 to 300 cd/m^2, the lexical speed improves by 86% [Legge et al., 1985]. The concomitant increase of the contrast sensitivity at high luminance values [Blommaert & Timmers, 1987] helps to account for this improvement. It is a good rule, therefore, to make sure that the illumination of the text is satisfying, avoiding any source of reflection (natural or artificial) on the page: for this reason the printed paper should be dull rather than glossy.

Reading Distance

Recently, it has been observed that a reduced reading distance may further deteriorate the lexical function of dyslexics: the closer is the page, the higher is the fusional demand, the less stable is fixation [Jainta & Kapoula, 2011]. Fixation stability[410] improves significantly by moving away the text from the usual reading distance of about 40 cm to 1 meter.

[410] Fixation stability is computed as the standard deviation of the visual axes movements in the time unit.

Font Size

Both in adults [Erdmann & Neal, 1968; Blommaert & Timmers, 1987] and in children [Cornelissen et al., 1991] recognition threshold of letters and words depends on the print size, so that below a given value the reading rate is reduced. A study dating back to the sixties found the optimal size of the character to be at least 0.4 degrees [Howell & Kraft, 1960]. Later on, it was observed that enlarging the print size up to 2.8 degrees the readability of the text tends to improve. In summary, the lexical function is optimal for sizes between 0.3 and 2 degrees while for smaller or larger sizes the performance tends to worsen [Legge et al., 1985][411].

The reduction of the readability for character sizes above 2 degrees could be due to the increased time required by the oculomotor system to process the string; in particular, the effect would depend on the longer time consumed by the saccades: since larger print size implies a longer string, increased saccadic width (thereby longer duration of each saccadic movement) and/or increased saccadic frequency is expected.

At the conventional reading distance of 33 cm, the usual print size (10-14 points) subtends a visual angle of 0.37 -0.46 deg per letter. The typical print size in Italian children's books ranges from 5 to 10 mm (0.72-1.43 deg at reading distance). Large sizes (1.43 deg) may increase the lexical speed in pupils up to 7 years of age while the advantage disappears in older children. [Hughes & Wilkins, 2002]. This gain is probably related to the positive effect that he enlargement of the characters has on fixation stability. Therefore, unstable fixation in dyslexics can be minimized by increasing the print size up to about 2 degrees: by using this strategy, in fact, it is observed that the number of lexical errors decreases in patients who showed this problem [Cornelissen et al., 1991]. As a matter of fact, the widening of the print size leads to larger interletter spacing. In turn, wider separation between adjoining characters increases the tolerance in case their bilateral projection on the foveal region were imprecise for unstable fixation, and at the same time it tends to neutralize the strengthened lateral masking in patients.

Character Contrast

A marked reduction of the contrast of the letters causes lexical performance deterioration. In normal readers, reading rate halves if contrast sensitivity lowers by at least 1 log unit [Legge et al., 1987]. Yet, such a contrast sensitivity impairment cannot account for the reading disability of dyslexic patients, whose deficit does not exceed 0.1-0.2 logarithmic units.

Still, reduced contrast sensitivity tends to expand the lateral masking, making letters more crowded, thereby more difficult to recognize. The contrast amount required by dyslexics to process words correctly is greater by 0.3 log units compared to the contrast needed to identify single letters. In conclusion, reading material for dyslexics should be printed with higher contrast than usual.

[411] Size interval ranging from 0.06 to 24 degrees.

Print Quality as Contrast Amplitude Modulation

By considering in a broad sense contrast as the difference or the ratio between the luminance of a dark bar compared to the luminance of the background, its function in the spatial domain is well represented as a square wave, since luminance level is expected to be constant across the bar and then changes abruptly into the luminance of the background. Bars that make up letters in this case are sharp, so are the resulting characters. If the luminance instead of being constant across the bar is minimal at the center and increases gradually toward its boundary, the square wave turns into sinusoidal or triangular (or trapezoidal).

In this case the contrast across the bar is maximum in the central part and decreases toward the edges. The faster is the decremental gradient, the more blurred is the bar.

Applied to characters, this means reduced readability (figure 1).

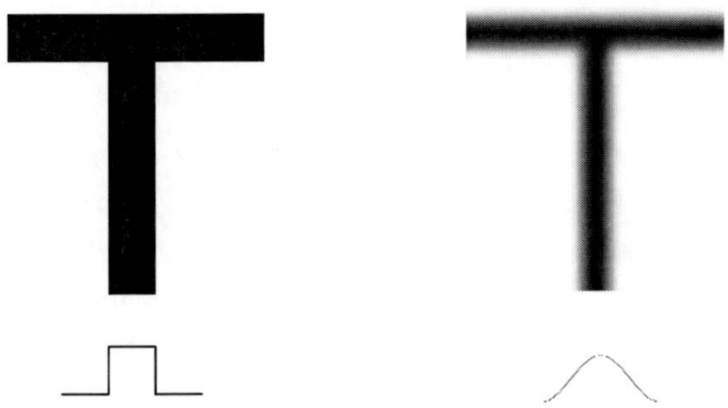

Figure 1. Contrast amplitude modulation. Left: square wave. The luminance value of a dark bar compared to the light background is uniform; right: sinusoidal wave. The luminance of the bar is not constant but it is minimal at its center and increases gradually toward the boundaries.

If contrast turns out to be reduced by 50% at the midpoint between the center of the stroke and its edges, the legibility of the character is made harder. If it were reduced by 75%, readability would be even more demanding. On the contrary, if it were reduced only by 25%, readability would be easier, and further easier if in the same point contrast were reduced just by12.5%.

In substance, the contrast modulation across the stroke can be regarded as the expression of the printing quality, Since, evidently, poor printing quality reduces the readability, it has been estimated that optimal reading condition requires a modulation of 0.6-0.3 cycles /character [Ginsburg, 1978] while reading begins to be hampered for values greater than 0.5 cycles/character [Legge et al., 1985].

Contrast Polarity between Print and Background

Even if some evidence suggests that reading improves when white letters are printed on a black background [Sloan, 1977], other studies failed to support this argumentation [Tinker, 1963; Cavonius & Bauer, 1980; Legge et al., 1985], especially if the character size is small [Tinker, 1963]. Therefore, reading performance does not seem to depend on the contrast polarity between text and background.

Printing Hue

Text printed so as to enhance the activity of the M-system is read better than when letters are in color, since colored print it is argued to stimulate the P-system [Omtzigt et al., 2002][412].

Printing Style

When preparing lexical material suitable for dyslexics, it has to be considered that the recognition of letters is faster for some fonts[413] (for example Minimal compared to Serif: Sanocki, 1987).

Text Presentation

In accordance with the argued reinforcement of the lateral masking in many dyslexics, patients read better when presented with one word at a time. On the contrary, in this condition a normal reader is disadvantaged [Hill & Lovegrove, 1993; Pepper & Lovegrove, 1999]. Therefore, it has been suggested to make use of special cardboard masks to be placed on the sheet and shifted along the line in order to help the attentional focus and hinder the disturbing effect of the context.

By increasing interletter distance, reading rate is found to improve in patients putatively affected by abnormal crowding [Aleci et al., 2012]. The exact amount of the spacing widening, however, depends on the subject, therefore should be assessed previously. To this purpose, the REPORT computes the optimal spacing for the patient under examination, as well as the expected reading rate increase in syl/sec and per cent compared to the conventional interletter distance.

References

Aleci C,Piana G, Piccoli M, Bertolini M. (2012). *Developmental dyslexia and spatial relationship perception.* Cortex, 48: 466-476.

Bauer D, Cavonius CR. (1980). *Improving the legibility of video display units through contrast reversal.* In: Ergonomic Aspects of Video Displays Terminals, Grandjean & Vigliani Eds., Taylor & Francis, London, UK.

Blommaert FJ, Timmers H. (1987). *Letter recognition at low contrast levels: effects of letter size.* Perception, 16: 421-432.

[412] In addition, the processing rate and reading comprehension in dyslexics seem to improve if the page is illuminated by a blue light instead of a white or a red one [Williams et al., 1990].

[413] See also part II, chapter 4.

Cornelissen P, Bradley L, Fowler S, Stein JF. (1991). *What* **children** *see affects how they read.* Developmental Medicine & Child Neurology, *33*: 755-762.

Erdmann RL, Neal AS. (1968). *Word legibility as a function of letter legibility, with word size, word familiarity, and resolution as parameters.* Journal of Applied Psychology, 52: 403-409.

Ginsburg AP. (1978). *Visual Information Processing Based on Spatial Filters Constrained by Biological Data.* Vols I and II, Dissertazione di Dottorato, Cambridge University, in Aerospace Medical Research Laboratory Report; AMLR-TR, Wright-Patterson AFB, Ohio.

Hill R, Lovergrove W. (1993). *One word at a time: A solution to visual deficit in SRD's?* In: Facets of dyslexia and its remediation, Wright SF & Groner R Eds., Amsterdam.

Howell W, Kraft C. (1960). *Size, blur, and contrast as variables affecting the legibility of alphanumeric symbols on radar-type displays.* WADC Technical Report 1960; Wright-Patterson AFB, Ohio.

Hughes LE, Wilkins A. (2002). *Reading at a distance: implications for the design of text in children's big books.* British Journal of Educational Psychology, 72: 213-226.

Jainta S, Kapoula Z. (2011). *Dyslexic children are confronted with unstable binocular fixation while reading.* PLoS ONE, 6: 1-10.

Legge GE, Pelli DG, Rubin GS, Schleske MM. (1985). *Psychophysics of reading-I. Normal vision.* Vision Research, 25: 239-252.

Legge GE, Rubin GS, Luebker A. (1987). *Psychophysics of reading-V. The role of contrast in normal vision.* Vision Research, 27: 1165-1175.

Omtzigt D, Hendriks AW, Kolk HH. (2002). *Evidence for magnocellular involvement in the identification of flanked letters.* Neuropsychologia, 40: 1881-1890.

Pepper K, Lovergrove W. (1999). *The effects of different types of text presentation on children with a specific reading disability.* In: Reading and dyslexia: Visual and attentional processes, Everatt Ed., Routledge, London, UK.

Sanocki T. (1987). *Visual knowledge underlying letter perception: Font-specific, schematic tuning.* Journal of Experimental Psychology, 13: 267-278.

Sloan LL. (1977). *Reading Aids for the partially sighted: A systematic classification and procedure for prescribing.* Williams and Wilkins Eds., Baltimore, MD.

Tinker MA (1963). *Legibility of Print.* Iowa State University Press, Ames.

Williams MC, LeCluyse K, Bologna N. (1990). *Masking by light as a measure of visual integration time in normal and disabled readers.* Clinical Vision Sciences, 5: 335-343.

Appendix B: Development Stages of Some of the Visual Functions Potentially Involved in Developmental Dyslexia

Reading Rate

From the second grade of school (7-8 years) to the college, the average reading rate increases of about 14 words of standard length[414] per minute per year [Carver, 1990].

Contrast Sensitivity

Contrast sensitivity reaches adult values around the 7th year of life [Ellemberg et al., 1999].

Coherent Motion Perception

Coherent motion perception has been observed since the 8th month of age with electrophysiological techniques [Hirai & Hiraki, 2005]. It is fully developed around the 10th - 11th year of age [Gunn et al., 2002]. The latency of the visual potentials evoked by dynamic stimuli in 10 years old children, in fact, matches the latency recorded in kids aged 14 [Kubová et al., 1996; Kuba et al., 2001].

Given the supposed relationship between motion perception and relative positional encoding among the characters [Cornelissen et al., 1998], it is worthwhile reporting that positional encoding improves with age up to the fifth grade (10-11 years) [Farkas & Smothergill, 1979].

Ocular Dominance

Ocular dominance consolidation starts at the age of 4 and is complete at the age of 15 [Ygge et al., 2005].

Saccadic Binocular Discrepancy

The amount of the temporary slight *dysconjunction* between the two visual axes at the end of the saccadic movements during reading[415] decreases progressively up to the age of 11-12 years [Yang & Kapoula, 2003, 2004].

[414] A standard length word is made up of six characters of text, including punctuation and spaces [Carver, 1990].
[415] See chapter 13.

Crowding

Crowding is subject to a developmental process consisting in a gradual reduction of the critical spacing, that proceeds at least up to the fifth year of life [Atkinson & Braddick, 1983; Atkinson et al., 1988; Kwon & Law, 2006]. The age-related variation of crowding in the normal population has been evaluated as *crowding ratio* [Atkinson et al., 1988]. The crowding ratio is the ratio between the visual acuity measured with single letters and in presence of other neighboring characters: according to this paradigm, a crowding ratio greater than 1 is suggestive of lateral masking.

The authors observed that lateral masking is greater in preschool children (age 3-4 years: crowding ratio = 1.8) and decreases until the 5th -7th year of age (crowding ratio = 1.2), matching the crowding ratio of the adulthood [Atkinson et al., 1988]. The reduction of crowding with age has been confirmed in a more recent study [Bondarko & Semenov, 2005]. Concomitant with the reduction of crowding, a progressive widening of the visual span, which continues up to the 12th -13th year of age[416], takes place [Kwon & Legge, 2006; Kwon et al., 2007].

Local /global Processing

It is argued that in tender age the visual processing of a configuration at the global level precedes the visual processing at the local level [Lux et al., 2008], so that the visual system moves from a first global evaluation to a more accurate (local) analysis of the configuration [Koch & Ullman, 1985]. The precedence of the global function on the local one, however, declines more and more with age and in 65 years old subjects this relationship is reversed [Oken et al., 1999; Slavin et al., 2002, Lux et al., 2008]. Given the parallelism on the one hand between global processing and distributed attention, on the other hand between local processing and focused attention, it is arguable that in normal readers the form resolving field tends to narrow with age, causing the attentional focus to strengthen to the detriment of the distributed mode [Oken et al., 1999].

The reduced steepness of the right slope of the form resolving field in dyslexics compared to normal readers suggest that this global/local switch is difficult in the former and supports the hypothesis of delayed development of visual attention.

Critical Print Size (CPS)

Both in normal readers and in dyslexics, the CPS tends to decrease with age.

In normal readers the CPS is 0.23 logMAR at the age of 6, it drops to 0.17 logMAR at the age of 7-8 and turns 0.09 logMAR from the 8th to the 9th year of age [Hughes & Wilkins, 2002; Kwon et al., 2007].

In dyslexic the CPS is 0.30 logMAR from the 7th to the 8th year of age, 0.20 logMAR from the 8th to the 9th year, and decreases to 0.18 logMAR at the age of 10 [O'Brien et al., 2005].

---

[416] See Manny et al. [1987] for a counter evidence.

Shape Perception

The perception of shapes generated by textures reaches its full development around 11-12 years of age (around 7 years for the shapes generated by the coherent motion of a random dot configuration: Parrish et al., 2005). If estimated with parallel and concentric Glass pattern[417], the development of shape perception is complete at the age of 9 [Lewis et al., 2004].

References

Atkinson J, Anker S, Evans C, Hall R, Pimm-Smith E. (1988). *Visual acuity testing of young children with the Cambridge Crowding Cards at 3 and 6 m.* Acta Ophthalmologica, 66: 505–508.

Atkinson J, Braddick O. (1983). *Assessment of visual acuity in infancy and early childhood.* Acta Ophthalmologica, 61: 18-26.

Bondarko V, Semenov L. (2005). *Visual acuity and the crowding effect in 8- to 17-year-old schoolchildren.* Human Physiology, 31: 532-538.

Carver RP. (1990). *Reading rate: A review of research and theory.* Academic Press Ed., San Diego, CA.

Cornelissen P, Hansen PC, Gilchrist I, Cormack F, Essex E, Frankish C. (1998). *Coherent motion detection and letter position encoding.* Vision Research, 38: 2181-2191.

Ellemberg D, Lewis TL, Liu CH, Maurer D. (1999). *Development of spatial and temporal vision during childhood.* Vision Research, 39: 2589-2602.

Farkas MS, Smothergill DW. (1979). *Configuration and position encoding in children.* Child Development, 50: 519-523.

Glass L. (1969). *Moirè effect from random dots.* Nature, 223: 578-580.

Gunn A, Cory E, Atkinson J, Braddick O, Wattam-Bell J, Guzzetta A, Cioni G. (2002). *Dorsal and ventral stream sensitivity in normal developmental hemiplegia.* Cognitive Neuroscience and Neuropsychology, 13: 843-847.

Hirai M, Hiraki K. (2005). *An event-related potentials study of biological motion perception in human infants.* Cognitive Brain Research, 22: 301-304.

Hughes LE, Wilkins A. (2002). *Reading at a distance: implications for the design of text in children's big books.* British Journal of Educational Psychology, 72: 213-226.

Koch C, Ullman S. (1985). *Shifts in selective visual attention: Towards the underlying neural circuitry.* Human Neurobiology, 4: 219-227.

Kuba M, Szanyi J, Gayer D, Kremlacek J, Kubová Z. (2001). *Electrophysiological testing of dyslexia.* Acta Medica (Hradec Kralove), 44: 131-134.

Kubová Z, Kuva M, Peregrin J, Nonakova V. (1996). *Visual evoked potential evidence for magnocellular system deficit in dyslexia.* Physiological Research, 45: 87-89.

Kwon MY, Legge GE. (2006). *Developmental changes in the size of the visual span for reading: Effects of crowding* [Abstract]. Journal of Vision, 6 (6): 997.

Kwon MY, Legge GE, Dubbels BR. (2007). *Developmental changes in the visual span for reading.* Vision Research, 47: 2889-2900.

[417] The pattern of Glass [Glass, 1969] is a figure formed by the overlapping of two random dots fields, the second of which is generated via linear or non linear transformation of the first. In this way, different configurations are obtained, such as circles or spirals.

Lewis TL, Ellemberg D, Maurer D, Dirks M, Wilkinson F, Wilson HR. (2004). *A window on the normal development of sensitivity to global form in Glass patterns*. Perception, 33: 409-418.

Lux S, Marshall JC, Thimm M, Fink GR. (2008). *Differential processing of hierarchical visual stimuli in young and older healty adults: Implications for pathology*. Cortex, 44: 21-28.

Manny RE, Fern KD, Loshin DS. (1987). *Contour interaction function in the preschool child.* American Journal of Optometry and Physiological Optics, 64: 686-692.

O'Brien BA, Mansfield JS, Legge GE. (2005). *The effect of print size on reading speed in dyslexia*. Journal of Research in Reading, 28: 332-349.

Oken BS, Kishiyama SS, Kaye JA, Jones DE. (1999). *Age-related differences in global-local processing: Stability of laterality differences but disproportionate impairment in global processing.* Journal of Geriatric Psychiatry and Neurology, 12: 76-81.

Parrish EE, Giaschi DE, Boden C, Dougherty R. (2005). *The maturation of form and motion perception in school aged children.* Vision Research, 45: 827-837.

Slavin MJ, Mattingley JB, Bradshaw JL, Storey E. (2002). *Local-global processing in Alzheimer's disease: an examination of interference, inhibition and priming.* Neuropsychologia, 40: 1173-1186.

Yang Q, Kapoula Z. (2003). *Binocular coordination of saccades at far and at near in children and adults.* Journal of Vision, 3: 554-561

Yang Q, Kapoula Z. (2004). *Saccade-vergence dynamics and interaction in children and in adults.* Experimental Brain Research, 156: 212-223.

Ygge J Aring E, Han Y, Bolzai R, Hellstrom A. (2005). *Fixation stability in normal children.* Annals of the New York Academy of Sciences, 1039: 480-483.

Appendix C: The Reading Performance Test (Report)

A way to determine whether the impairment of a visuoperceptive function affects the ability to read, is to create an experimental situation that makes the visual processing of the text based on that function more difficult. If dyslexics read worse in this anomalous situation while the normal readers are not (or not much) affected, then the integrity of the function referred to that visual situation can be considered an important condition for the normal lexical process.

For example, a solution suitable to evaluate the lexical ability in condition of experimental visual stress makes use of the reduction of the print size. Although it has long been known that below a certain print size the accuracy of all readers drops[418] [Erdmann & Neal, 1968; Blommaert & Timmers, 1987], children with unstable dominance tend to make a greater number of errors compared to stable dominants and tend to turn words into nonsense words (or non-words) [Cornelissen et al., 1991].

---

[418] It is assumed that the print sizes we are referring to are above the recognition threshold, so that in these cases the decreased lexical performance cannot be attributed to reduced visibility of the letters.

The effect is claimed to depend on fixation instability caused by unstable dominance. Therefore, the reduction of the print size as a stressful lexical condition enhances the effect of unstable ocular dominance (thereby unstable fixation) when reading, favoring the positional exchange between neighboring characters.

Now, decreased font size does not imply solely the reduction of the character size: it involves the reduction of the visual space occupied by the string as well, which in turn leads to the narrowing of the space between the letters: it follows that the deleterious effect of the fixation instability is associated to a strengthening of the lateral masking. Crowding (and in particular the critical spacing that is its characterizing parameter) has been evaluated in several clinical investigations by means of a psychometric function, the *frequency-of-seeing curve*. The frequency-of-seeing curve is plotted by means of two different paradigms: by measuring the percentage of correct answers (i.e. the frequency of recognition) as a function of the distance between target and distractors or by estimating the contrast threshold that enables to recognize the target as a function of the distance between target and distractors.

The curve shows a steep gradient at the beginning and then stabilizes (*ceiling effect*). In both paradigms, however, the evaluation of the crowding effect occurs out of the normal reading process. As pointed out almost 40 years ago by McConkie & Rayner [1975], the level of crowding depends on the characteristics of the stimulus and on the task the subject is required to perform. For this reason, even if the evaluation of crowding in the extra lexical context (e.g. by presenting tachistoscopically triplets of letters or numbers) can reveal some peculiarities in dyslexics, it does not help to understand how these peculiarities affect the reading performance.

Therefore, we decided to develop a psychophysical technique aimed at estimating the effect of lateral masking directly on the lexical function, without changing the print size. In particular, given the relationship that links vertical anisotropy and crowding, we have devised a test aimed at providing for each patient:

- Information about the lexical performance in conditions of reinforcement (visuoperceptive stress) and release (ameliorative effect) of the lateral masking obtained through the *anisotropization* (i.e. dilation or contraction) of the visual space occupied by the string.
- Information on the presence of a compensatory effect on the vertical anisotropy (thereby on the lateral masking) provided by the dilation of the visual space filled by the string (*horizontal anisotropization*); in case, information on the lexical gain achievable by this compensatory manipulation of the visual space.
- Information on the extent of the critical spacing.

The Reading Performance Test (REPORT) measures reading rate as a function of the level of "shrink" and "stretch" applied to strings made of words and non-words[419].

On a high-resolution LCD screen, 11 presentations are displayed in randomized succession.

Each presentation (or trial), is made of 4 words[420] placed side by side and composed of, 3, 4, 3 and 2 syllables[421] or 5 non-words placed side by side and composed of, 2, 2, 2, 3 and 3

[419] For the rationale of this approach refer to part II, chapter 3 [Aleci et al., 2012].

[420] The difference between the lexical performance measured with words arranged into a sentence or presented in random order can be defined as *context gain*. It has been estimated that in a sentence the probability to

syllables. Trials are displayed unmodified (i.e. in their normal spatial relationship) or stretched /contracted to a predetermined extent along the horizontal axis (*anisotropization*)[422].

The adopted anisotropization levels are such as to test interletter distances ranging from 0.2 up to 0.51 degrees[423].

In each trial, the lexical sample is different from each other. Letters are displayed on a light background[424] and subtend a mean visual angle of 0.4 degrees (i.e. well above the recognition threshold) at the examination distance of 70 cm. The subject is required, without being urged to the best performance, to read aloud[425] each presentation in binocular conditions. Each presentation remains visible on the screen the time necessary to complete the operation. The instrument measures the reading rate as syllables per second and computes the number of errors for each value of anisotropization[426] via a wireless tablet activated by the technician.

After the first set of presentations a new sequence is given (made of lexical material different from the previous one) in order to obtain two estimates for each value of anisotropization. The best estimate of each couple of trials is automatically selected by the instrument during the data processing.

The full examination includes a test with words and a test with non-words. In the former it is presented lexical material suitable to the age of the child (from the 3rd to the 5th grade). The normative data for each class have been previously obtained in the normal scholar population (see Appendix E).

In order to have comparable results in subsequent examinations when the test is performed by different operators, the software measures in advance the reaction time of the technician to auditory stimuli. When processing the data, the software computes the reading

understand the next word based on the context (that is, relying on the reading of the previous words) is 20-35% [Stanovich & Stanovich, 1995]. Since the REPORT is a tool designed to assess the visuoperceptive function and intends, therefore, to rule out as much as possible the linguistic-cognitive element, words are presented in extra lexical context, that is to say not arranged into a sentence. The scope is to avoid the effect of the contextual gain.

421 Font Free Monospace.

422 In the REPORT, the anisotropization of the string implies an inversely proportional change of the visual space occupied by the string itself along the two cardinal coordinates: as a result, after the horizontal spatial manipulation the area filled by the words remains constant.

423 Interletter spacings are calculated center-to-center, in agreement with the current literature. Single values: 0.2, 0.23, 0.25, 0.27, 0.28, 0.31, 0.36, 0.4, 0.44, 0.47, 0.51 degrees.

424 Letter luminance: 0.3 cd/m^2, backg round luminance: 85 cd/m^2.

425 Even if reading aloud is not the physiological way to read, it can be regarded as the simpler way to measure reading rate and accuracy. Therefore, subjects who undergo the REPORT are required to reading aloud, in line with many experiments performed on dyslexics.

426 In literature, reading ability is estimated in terms of speed and accuracy, and the latter depends on the number of reading errors. However, the most common measure of the reading performance is the former [MacKeben et al., 2004], which in fact is considered the most sensitive marker of dyslexia in adults [Lefly & Pennington, 1991]. In transparent languages, reading slowly is a tract so characteristic that it has been suggested to rename developmental dyslexia in transparent languages as *speed dyslexia* [Wimmer, 1993]. Therefore, at the beginning we preferred to ignore the accuracy (which does not take into account reading rate) replacing it with a new index, the reading efficiency. The reading efficiency complements the reading rate with the number of errors, in order to provide a parameter that reflects the ability to read fluently (i.e. properly and quickly).

When testing the prototype, however, it became clear that the high number of graphs and indices generated by reading rate and efficiency would make the interpretation of the exam too difficult, potentially misleading and counter intuitive. For this reason, in the final version reading efficiency has been removed and replaced with simple histograms showing the amount of errors made per each anisotropization value. Errors are considered omissions, wrong pronounce and exchange of letters or syllables [Martelli et al., 2009].

rate after having subtracted the obtained reaction time of the operator from the reading time measured trial after trial in the patient.

In figure 1 is shown an example of printout.

Before starting to analyze the collected data, the system performs Grubb's test for detecting outliers and, in case, removes the unreliable values[427]. Depending on the responses, the test provides an indication about the overall performance of the subject in comparison to a normal reader of the same age.

For each of the two experimental conditions (words and non-words) two graphs and some lexical indices are reported in the printout.

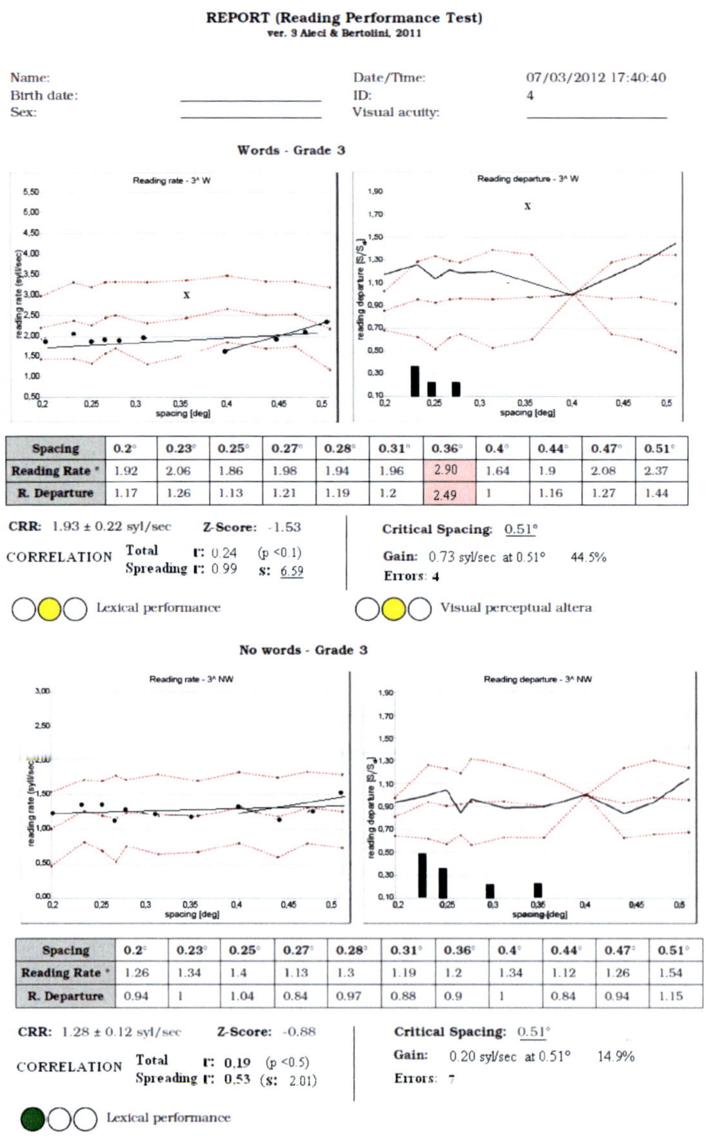

REPORT (Reading Performance Test)
ver. 3 Aleci & Bertolini, 2011

Name:
Birth date: ______
Sex: ______
Date/Time: 07/03/2012 17:40:40
ID: 4
Visual acuity: ______

Words - Grade 3

Spacing	0.2°	0.23°	0.25°	0.27°	0.28°	0.31°	0.36°	0.4°	0.44°	0.47°	0.51°
Reading Rate *	1.92	2.06	1.86	1.98	1.94	1.96	2.90	1.64	1.9	2.08	2.37
R. Departure	1.17	1.26	1.13	1.21	1.19	1.2	2.49	1	1.16	1.27	1.44

CRR: 1.93 ± 0.22 syl/sec Z-Score: -1.53
CORRELATION Total r: 0.24 (p <0.1)
Spreading r: 0.99 s: 6.59

Critical Spacing: 0.51°
Gain: 0.73 syl/sec at 0.51° 44.5%
Errors: 4

Lexical performance
Visual perceptual altera

No words - Grade 3

Spacing	0.2°	0.23°	0.25°	0.27°	0.28°	0.31°	0.36°	0.4°	0.44°	0.47°	0.51°
Reading Rate *	1.26	1.34	1.4	1.13	1.3	1.19	1.2	1.34	1.12	1.26	1.54
R. Departure	0.94	1	1.04	0.84	0.97	0.88	0.9	1	0.84	0.94	1.15

CRR: 1.28 ± 0.12 syl/sec Z-Score: -0.88
CORRELATION Total r: 0,19 (p <0.5)
Spreading r: 0,53 (s: 2.01)

Critical Spacing: 0.51°
Gain: 0.20 syl/sec at 0.51° 14.9%
Errors: 7

Lexical performance

Figure 1. The printout of the Reading Performance Test (REPORT).

[427] Outliers are marked with a red square in the graphs and are not considered in the statistical analysis.

The scattergram on the left (Reading Rate) plots reading rate as a function of the anisotropization level, from the maximum contraction (0.2°, left) to the maximum dilation value (0.51°, right), taking 0.4° as the reference interletter spacing. This interval has been chosen after considering two earlier studies [Huckauf et al., 1999; Huckauf & Heller, 2002], and it matches the interletter distance commonly adopted in the Italian lexical material. The upper broken line refers to the normative average trend according to the age of the patient, the two lower ones correspond to the first and the second SD below the normative values. On these graphs, the result of a double linear regression analysis (*total regression* and *spreading regression*) is reported. The two regression lines together with the respective correlation coefficient *r* aim at detecting a reading rate trend[428] starting from the value of maximum contraction (*total r*) and from the reference spacing (*spreading r*). The graphs on the left side, therefore, provide an overview of the actual lexical performance compared to the normative one across the spectrum of anisotropization, in order to assess whether increased interletter spacing has a compensatory effect on the lexical speed of words (upper part) and non-words (lower part). The graphs on the right side (*Reading Departure*) amplify the trend, showing the deviation of the performance compared to normal readers as a function of the string anisotropization, regardless of the absolute result. Therefore, in the right panel it is shown whether and (in case) at what level of anisotropization the reading rate of the subject departs from the rate expected in age-matched normal readers. To help the judgment, two dotted lines delimit the range of +2 / -2 SD referred to the variation measured in the normal age-matched population. The graphs on the right, therefore, enable a detailed study of the variation of the performance compared to the trend measured in the normal age-matched population across the spectrum of anisotropization. Below the two pairs of graphs, is a table reporting the results measured for each interletter spacing, and expressed both as syllables per second (*reading rate*) and as deviation from the reference spacing (*reading departure*).

Below the table are some lexical indexes:

- *Cumulative Reading Rate (CRR ±SD):* is the sum of the reading rate measured at each value of spacing divided by the number of intervals. The CRR is reported as syl/sec and as Z-score[429]. Evidently, the CRR is a global index of the reading performance.

Total r: is the linear correlation coefficient over the entire interval of anisotropization. Whether the total r is *clinically indicative*[430] is deduced from the associated value of statistical significance (*p*). If r is clinically indicative, p is underlined.

---

[428] The correlation is expected to be positive (ameliorative), but in certain circumstances (for example saccadic hypometry), a reverse trend could be observed.

[429] In our case, the Z-score specifies how many standard deviations the actual reading rate is below the mean normal value. Z-score is defined as: (CRRdyslexic-CRRnormal)/SD_{CRR}normal.

[430] Due to the low probability of detecting a statistically significant correlation with only two measures of lexical performance for each level of anisotropization, a trend that would be significant with a greater number of trials can be rejected (because masked by artifacts, especially in case of children). Therefore, to avoid false negative estimates, in these cases a different criterion of judgment has been applied. A statistical level of significance p in the patient lower than the level referred to the highest correlation coefficient found in the reference values (normal readers) denotes that the correlation in the patient is presumably higher compared to the higher correlation level recorded in the normal population, irrespective of the achievement of the statistical significance (i.e. $p < 0.05$). In this case, the coefficient of correlation, even if it is not statistically significant, is considered clinically indicative and reported underlined. Otherwise, *p* is in brackets. For example, in a child (3rd grade), a level of significance p referred to the total r when reading words ≥ 0.22 is not clinically indicative; on the contrary, if p is <0.22, the total r is considered as clinically indicative, even if p is far from being statistically significant (≤ 0.05). Note that to be clinically indicative, p is expected to be lower than 0.12 in the same child one year later (4th grade).

- *Spreading r*: is the correlation coefficient over the interval of anisotropization ranging from the reference value to the value of maximum dilation of the string (0.4°-0.51°). On the right is reported the correspondent slope of the linear model (*s*).

If in the patient *s* localizes beyond +1 SD calculated on the normative data, it is considered *clinically indicative* and underlined. A *clinically indicative* slope therefore indicates that the increase of the interletter spacing leads to reading rate improvement greater than that expected in the normal population.

- *Critical Spacing (CS)* is the angular value that corresponds to the maximum performance at the end of an incremental trend. The calculation of the CS assumes that starting from the maximum stretch condition, reading rate increases with the widening of the interletter spacing and then stabilizes (ceiling effect). A specific logic algorithm enables the software to perform the computation minimizing the artifactual components. The algorithm considers some parameters and criteria to filter the noise and to identify along the trend the peak or *plateau* corresponding to the interval of interest. If the critical spacing is greater than the normative one, it is reported underlined. Below are given some examples (Figure 2).

The last two panels show that the ameliorative trend can culminates beyond the reference value of spacing. Indeed, this is the most interesting case, which suggests the critical spacing of the subject to be so widened that the interletter distance commonly found in most of the texts (0.4 °) results to be within the zone of influence of the lateral masking.

-*Gain:* this index quantifies the expected reading rate improvement if the interletter distance is increased by a given amount. When present, the gain is reported as syl/sec and percentage.

In figure 1 (upper part), for example, by increasing the interletter spacing from 0.4 ° to 0.51 °, the expected gain is 0.73 syl/sec. This means that by widening the distance between the characters by 0.11°, the subject is expected to read words by 44.5% faster than at the ordinary interletter distance.

In this case, the spreading r is clinically indicative with the best performance (which in this case corresponds to the CS) to 0.51°.

-*Reading errors:* when present, reading errors are reported in the right side of the printout, under the gain. Their distribution across the anisotropization spectrum is represented in the right graph as histograms whose height is proportional to their number.

In addition to graphs and indexed, the printout provides two performance indicators for both the words and non-words experimental condition. The left indicator is based on the cumulative reading rate and informs whether CRR localizes within -1 SD compared to the normative values (green), between -1 and -2 SD (yellow) or beyond -2 SD (red). The right indicator informs about the presence of an impairment of the visuoperceptive component and "lights up" in case the left indicator is yellow or red. The indicator on the right can turn green, yellow or red depending on the occurrence of one or more of the following alternatives:

1) total r positive and clinically indicative. 2) spreading r with positive slope and clinically indicative. 3) critical spacing wider compared to the normative values.

If none of the three criteria is satisfied, the indicator would be green; if the first or second criterion is satisfied it would be yellow; if the third criterion or the first two criteria are satisfied, the indicator would be red.

Au automatic report is printed at the end of the examination (Immediate Automatic Description, IAD).

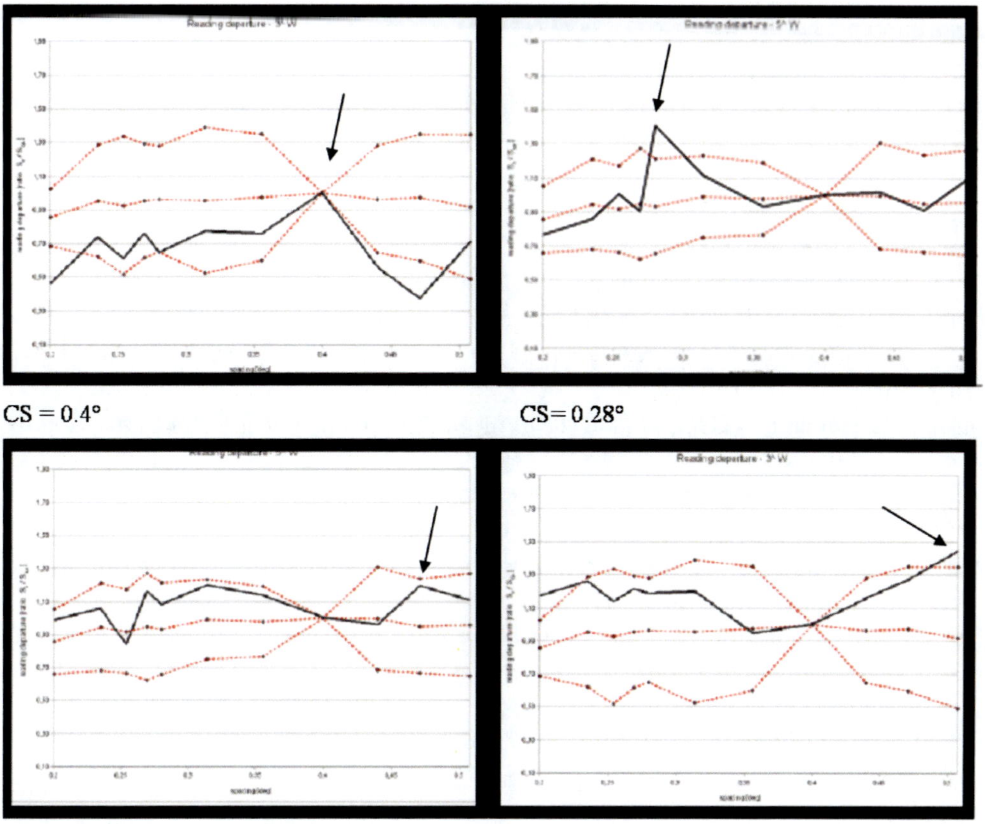

CS = 0.4° CS= 0.28°

CS= 0.47° CS= 0.51°

Figure 2. REPORT. Critical spacing.

In summary, the Reading Performance Test has been devised to provide information about the effects of the visuospatial distortion on the lexical function and in no way it can be considered suitable to diagnose developmental dyslexia. Really, the diagnosis of dyslexia is up to neuropsychiatrists or logopedists.

Even if the REPORT is an experimental *avant-garde*, it can show to be an useful aid to assess the kind and degree of visuoperceptive involvement in every single patient. Probably its main drawback is test-retest reliability. High reliability is expected to be difficult to achieve when testing children with a psychophysical technique demanding a stressful task like the REPORT. The examination requires the maximum number of collected answers being arranged with the shortest examination time, in order to prevent an attentional drop in the patient and excessive time commitment for the operator.

Data interpretation (apart from the occurrence of artifactual measurements) is another problematic aspect. The automatic detection of outliers attempts to minimize this drawback.

To make more difficult for the REPORT to outline a common pattern in the dyslexic population, is the fact that despite what it was believed, the coefficient of Bouma is not constant. As a matter of fact, the coefficient of Bouma shows large individual variations among normal readers [Pelli et al., 2007] and is found to be doubled in the dyslexic population (SD: 0.3 in normal readers vs. 0.59 in dyslexics) [Martelli et al., 2009].

References

Aleci C,Piana G, Piccoli M, Bertolini M. (2012). *Developmental dyslexia and spatial relationship perception.* Cortex, 48: 466-476.

Blommaert F J, Timmers H. (1987). *Letter recognition at low contrast levels: effects of letter size. Perception,* 16: 421 – 432.

Cornelissen P, Bradley L, Fowler S, Stein JF. (1991). *What* children *see affects how they read.* Developmental Medicine & Child Neurology, 33: 755-762.

Erdmann RL, Neal AS. (1968). *Word legibility as a function of letter legibility, with word size, word familiarity, and resolution as parameters.* Journal of Applied Psychology, 52: 403-409.

Huckauf A, Heller D. (2002). *What various kinds of errors tell us about lateral masking effects.* Visual Cognition, 9: 889-910.

Huckauf A, Heller D, Nazir TA. (1999). Lateral masking: *Limitations of the feature interaction account.* Perception & Psychophysics, 61: 177-189.

Lefly DL, Pennington BF. (1991). *Spelling errors and reading fluency in compensated adult dyslexics.* Annals of Dyslexia, 41: 143-162.

MacKeben M, Trauzettel-Klosinski S, Reinhard J, Dürrwächter U, Adler M, Klosinski G. (2004). *Eye movement control during single-word reading in dyslexics*. Journal of Vision, 4: 388-402.

Martelli M, Di Filippo G, Spinelli D, Zoccolotti P. (2009). *Crowding, reading, and developmental dyslexia*. Journal of Vision, 9 (4), 14: 1-18.

McConkie GW, Rayner K. (1975). *The span of the effective stimulus during a fixation in reading,* Perception & Psychophysics, 17: 578–586.

Stanovich KE, Stanovich PJ. (1995). *How research might inform the debate about early reading acquisition.* Journal of Research in Reading, 18: 87-105.

Wimmer H. (1993). *Characteristics of developmental dyslexia in a regular writing system.* Applied Psycholinguistics, 14: 1-33.

Appendix D: Examples of Clinical Cases

Example 1 -Lexical Disability without Visuoperceptive Alteration

S MP., female, age 10 5th grade.

Slow reading with many errors, frequent confusion b/d, a/e, b/s. Dystocia. At birth intensive care for 4 days + incubated for 15 days. At the moment good health, no allergies.

Visual acuity: 60/60 bilaterally. Orthophoria, normal fusional amplitude for close vision, normal stereopsis.

Normal saccadic movements.

Ocular dominance: right in right-hander.

Eidomorphometry (IR%): HT 5; VT: 5; SRA: 0.

REPORT:

Words: the Z-score, well beyond -2SD, indicates that the cumulative reading rate across the spectrum of anisotropization is definitely reduced. An outlier (red square) is detected at 0.28 deg and ruled out from the analysis.

The critical spacing cannot be determined.

The correlation coefficient *Total r* is 0.59, not significant (p=0.08) neither clinically indicative, meaning that the progressive widening of the interletter spacing from 0.2 to 0.51 degrees does not improve the lexical performance to a greater extent compared to normal readers. The same absence of trend can be deduced from the correlation coefficient *Spreading r*, computed on the range of spacing from 0.4 to 0.51 degrees (*spreading r* =0.42), the improvement of the reading rate in the subject is not greater than the trend estimated in the age-matched normal population: the slope of the linear function is negligible (s: 1.7). Thereby, *s* is not underlined but put in brackets. It follows that the widening of the interletter interval would be of little avail for this patient, since the reading rate gain would be no more than 0.27 syl/sec, that is to say just 12.7% at 0.51 deg of spacing compared to the reference value.

The trial resulted to be free from reading errors.

In summary, when asked to read words, the child showed reduced reading rate without evident visuoperceptive alterations: the left indicator (reading performance) is red, whereas the right one (visuoperceptive impairment) is green.

Non-words: Z-score localizes at -2 SD, meaning that the cumulative reading rate across the spectrum of anisotropization is reduced.

The critical spacing is 0.25 deg, not wider compared to the normal age-matched population.

The correlation coefficient *Total r* is negative (-0.23) and not significant (p=0.46), showing that the progressive widening of the interletter spacing from 0.2 to 0.51 degrees does not improve (if anything worsens) the lexical performance. Even if the *spreading r* is high and statistically significant (0.98), the reading rate improvement (quantified by the slope of the linear function) is negligible, (s: 1.1), and as such not higher compared to the trend estimated in the age-matched normal population: in fact, *s* is not underlined but put in brackets.

It follows that the widening of the interletter interval would be of little avail for this patient, since the reading rate gain would be no more than 0.12 syl/sec, that is to say just 10.4% at 0.51 deg of spacing compared to the reference value.

The trial resulted to be free from reading errors.

Therefore, also for non-words the reading rate is reduced without evident visuoperceptive alterations: the left indicator (reading performance) is red, whereas the right one (visuoperceptive impairment) is green.

Conclusion: normal visual acuity, ocular motility and stereopsis. Normal saccadic pattern, right ocular dominance. The spatial relationship perception is spared.

The cumulative reading rate for words and non-words, as assessed by the Reading Performance Test, localizes beyond and around the -2 SD, respectively. From the minimum interletter distance as well as from the reference one (0.4 deg), the reading rate shows a negligible (i.e. not clinically indicative) improvement when the spacing is enlarged up to 0.51 deg.

In summary, the visuoperceptive involvement is absent with normal saccadic pattern and stable (albeit incongruent) ocular dominance.

TETRA - Patient's Report for Reading Performance Test
Ver. 1.0.98 . Aleci, dicembre 2012

Name: ID: Date/Time:

Words - Grade 5

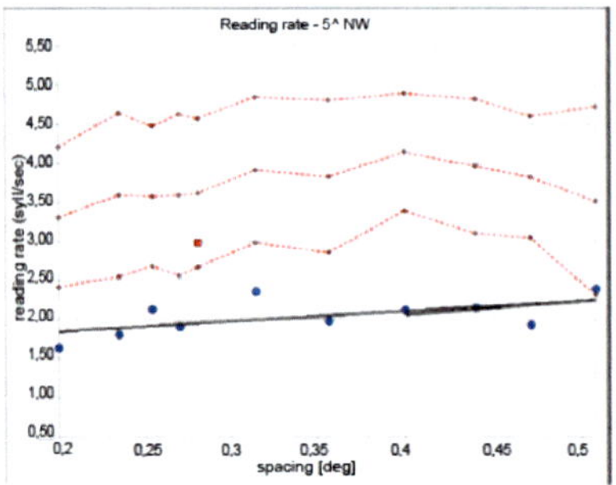

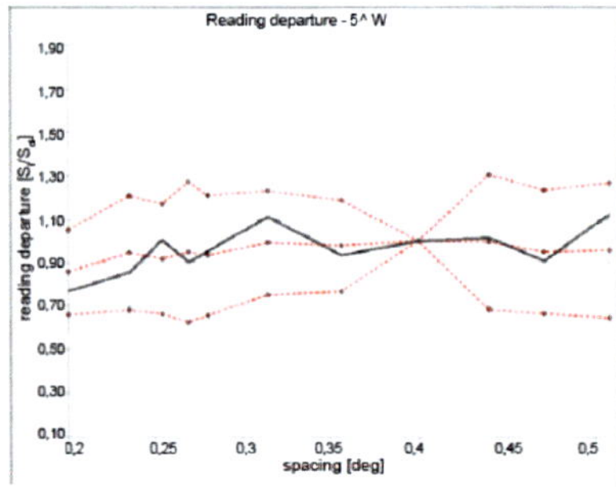

Spacing	0.2°	0.23°	0.25°	0.27°	0.28°	0.31°	0.36°	0.4°	0.44°	0.47°	0.51°
Reading Rate	1.63	1.81	2.13	1.91	2.98	2.36	1.98	2.12	2.15	1.93	2.39
R. Departure	0.77	0.85	1	0.9	1.41	1.11	0.93	1	1.01	0.91	1.13

CRR: 2.04 ± 0.24 syl/sec **Z-Score:** -2.78

CORRELATION **Total** r: 0.59 (p =0.08) **Spreading** r: 0.42 (s: 1.72)

Lexical performance

Critical Spacing: nd

Gain: 0.27 syl/sec at 0.51° (12.7%)

Errors: 0

Visual perceptual alterations

No words - Grade 5

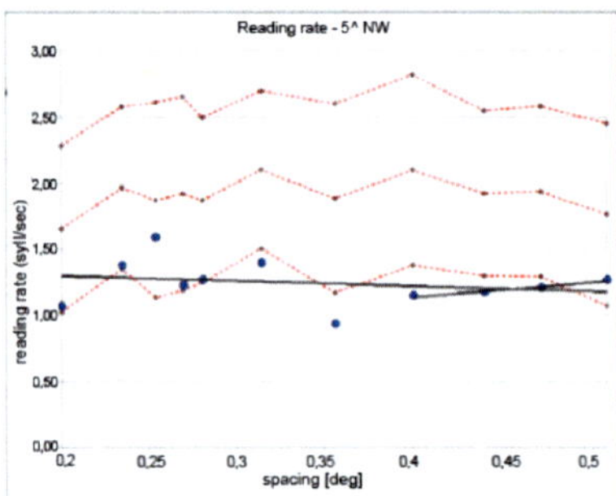

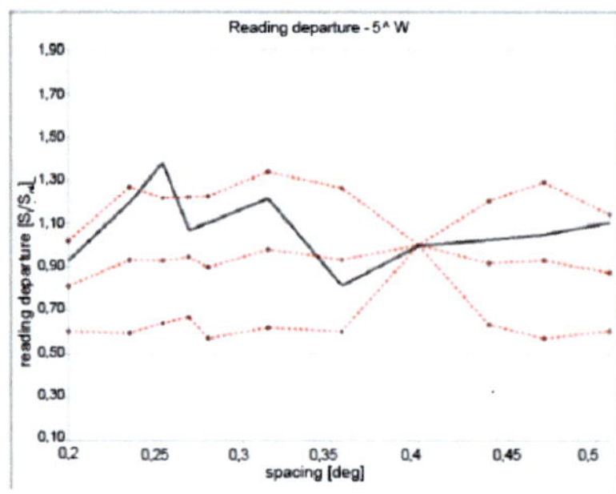

Spacing	0.2°	0.23°	0.25°	0.27°	0.28°	0.31°	0.36°	0.4°	0.44°	0.47°	0.51°
Reading Rate	1.07	1.38	1.59	1.23	1.27	1.4	0.94	1.15	1.18	1.21	1.27
R. Departure	0.93	1.2	1.38	1.07	1.1	1.22	0.82	1	1.03	1.05	1.1

CRR: 1.24 ± 0.17 syl/sec **Z-Score:** -2

CORRELATION **Total** r: -0.23 (p =0.46) **Spreading** r: 0.98 (s: 1.1)

Lexical performance

Critical Spacing: 0.25°

Gain: 0.12 syl/sec at 0.51° (10.4%)

Errors: 0

Visual perceptual alterations

Example 2 - Widening of the Critical Spacing with Saccades Alteration

O.F., female, age 8, 4th grade.

Reading difficulty.

Good health, no allergies.

Visual acuity: 60/60 bilaterally. Orthophoria, normal fusional amplitude for close vision, normal stereopsis.

Saccadic movements: hypermetric.

Ocular dominance: left in left hander.
Eidomorphometry (IR%): HT 5; VT: 4; SRA: 1.
REPORT:

Words: the Z-score, well below -2SD, means that the cumulative reading rate across the spectrum of anisotropization is definitely reduced. The correlation coefficient *Total r* is not significant (0.08, p = 0.8), showing that the progressive enlargement of the interletter spacing from 0.2 to 0.51 degrees does not improve the reading rate. The same is shown by the correlation coefficient *Spreading r* (r = 0). Therefore, in this patient the widening of the interletter interval would be of no avail: in fact, the gain is 0.

The critical spacing is 0.28-0.36 deg, i.e. wider compared to the normal age-matched population, so, it is underlined. To be noted in the graph on the right that the correspondent peak of the reading rate at 0.36 degrees goes beyond the superior red line marking the second standard deviation referred to the normative data.

The trial resulted to be free from reading errors.

The overall outcome reveals reduced reading rate with increased critical spacing, even if the widening of the interletter distance does not provide any ameliorative effect: in fact, the spatial relationship perception is not reduced. Thereby, the left indicator (reading performance) is red as well as the right one (visuoperceptive impairment), informing that a visupoperceptual abnormality (as suggested by the widening of the critical spacing) is affecting the visual system of the patient.

Since the increase of the critical spacing is below the reference spacing (0.4°), in this case the widening of the interletter interval beyond this value does not improve the reading rate. On the contrary, compared to the reference value, a slight narrowing of the interletter spacing (from 0.4° to 0.36°) seems to speed up the lexical function.

Non-words: the Z-score, between -1 and -2SD, means that the cumulative reading rate across the spectrum of anisotropization is reduced. The presence of four peaks is suggestive of low reliability.

The critical spacing (0.27°) is at the limit of the normative range. The correlation coefficient *Total r* is not significant (0.17, p=0.59), showing that the progressive enlargement of the interletter spacing from 0.2 to 0.51 degrees does not improve the reading rate. From the reference value the correlation is far stronger (spreading r= 0.88) and the reading rate tends to improve even if the finding is not clinically significant.

In fact *s* (2.4) is not underlined but put in brackets. The gain is 0,3 syl/sec at 0.51° of spacing, that is 30.6% compared to the reference spacing.

The trial is free from reading errors.

In summary, when asked to read non-words, the child showed reduced reading rate without visuoperceptive alterations: the left indicator (reading performance) is yellow, whereas the right one (visuoperceptive impairment) is green.

Conclusion: normal visual acuity, ocular motility and stereopsis. Left ocular dominance. The spatial relationship perception is spared whereas FEMs are hypermetric.

The cumulative reading rate for words and non-words, as assessed by the Reading Performance Test, localizes beyond and below the -2 SD, respectively. The worsening of the lexical performance at the ordinary interletter spacing compared to the narrower intervals would depend on the defective saccadic pattern, more and more inefficient as the distance to be covered between the sequential letters enlarges.

It could be advisable, therefore, the reduction of the spacing from 0.4 to 0.36-0.31 degrees.

Author's note: in this child after the reduction of the interletter distance by about one tenth of degree the reading rate turned out to improve. The patient is actually adopting in her school textbook the font Arial narrow.

TETRA - Patient's Report for Reading Performance Test

Ver. 1.0.98 . Aleci. dicembre 2012

Name: ID: Date/Time:

Words - Grade 4

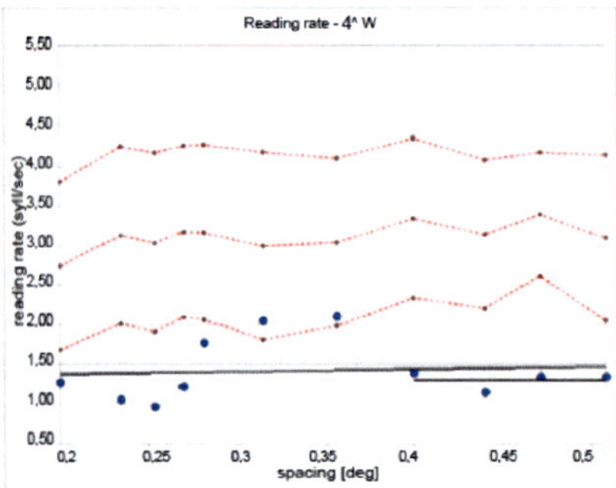

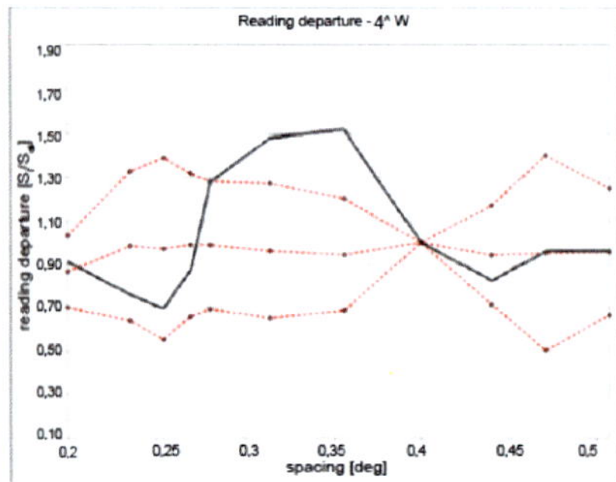

Spacing	0.2°	0.23°	0.25°	0.27°	0.28°	0.31°	0.36°	0.4°	0.44°	0.47°	0.51°
Reading Rate	1.27	1.06	0.97	1.22	1.78	2.06	2.11	1.39	1.15	1.34	1.34
R. Departure	0.91	0.76	0.7	0.88	1.28	1.48	1.52	1	0.83	0.96	0.96

CRR: 1.43 ± 0.39 syl/sec **Z-Score:** -2.61

CORRELATION **Total** r: 0.08 (p =0.8) **Spreading** r: 0 (s: 0.01)

Critical Spacing: 0.28°

Gain: 0

Errors: 0

Lexical performance

Visual perceptual alterations

No words - Grade 4

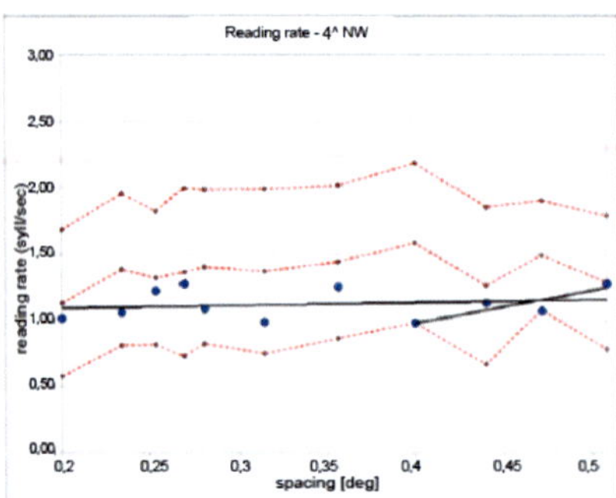

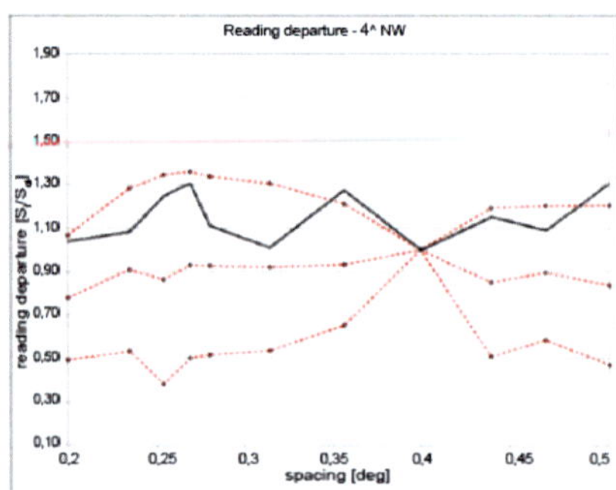

Spacing	0.2°	0.23°	0.25°	0.27°	0.28°	0.31°	0.36°	0.4°	0.44°	0.47°	0.51°
Reading Rate	1.02	1.06	1.22	1.28	1.09	0.99	1.25	0.98	1.13	1.07	1.28
R. Departure	1.04	1.08	1.24	1.31	1.11	1.01	1.28	1	1.15	1.09	1.31

CRR: 1.12 ± 0.11 syl/sec **Z-Score:** -1.44

CORRELATION **Total** r: 0.17 (p =0.59) **Spreading** r: 0.88 (s: 2.41)

Critical Spacing: 0.27°

Gain: 0.3 syl/sec at 0.51° (30.6%)

Errors: 0

Lexical performance

Visual perceptual alterations

Example 3 - Widening of the Critical Spacing Subsequent to Vertical Anisotropy

C.G., female, age 8.5, 3th grade.

Developmental dyslexia and dysgraphia/dysortographia.

Good health, no allergies.

Visual acuity: 56/60 bilaterally. Slight exophoria for close vision, normal fusional amplitude for close vision, normal stereopsis.

Saccadic movements: hypermetric.

Ocular dominance: right in right-hander.

Eidomorphometry: HT 11; VT: 2; SRA: 9.

REPORT:

Words: the Z-score, between -1 and -2SD, means that the cumulative reading rate across the spectrum of anisotropization is reduced.
The critical spacing is 0.47 deg, i.e. wider compared to the normal age-matched population, so, it is underlined.
The trial shows some reading errors localized in the left (narrower) side of the spectrum of anisotropization.
The correlation coefficient *Total r* (0.40) is clinically indicative, so that *p* it is reported underlined (0.23). Therefore, the progressive widening of the lexical string increases the reading rate to a level not observed in the normal age-matched population. A similar trend, even if not clinically indicative, is quantified by the *spreading r* (0.66). The interletter widening seems to improve the lexical performance so that the gain at 0.47° is 0.70 syl/sec, that is to say 39% compared to the reference interval.
The left indicator (reading performance) is yellow, whereas the right one (visuoperceptive impairment) is red, since the increased critical spacing and the positive correlation between string anisotropization and reading rate is suggestive of a visuoperceptive involvement

Non-words: Z-score localizes between the -1 and -2 SD, meaning that cumulative reading rate across the spectrum of anisotropization is reduced.
The critical spacing cannot be determined.
The correlation coefficient *total r* is higher compared to the corresponding one measured with words (0.43), but in this experimental context is not clinically indicative.
Likewise, the *spreading r*, even if higher than the *total r* (0.8), is not significant so that s is put in brackets (However also with non-words the widening of the interletter interval from 0.4 to 0.47 degrees tends to increase the reading rate by 0.32 syl/sec, i.e. 42% compared to the reference interval).
The trial shows some reading errors localized on the left (narrower) side of the spectrum of anisotropization.
Therefore, the left indicator is yellow, the right one is green.

Conclusion: normal visual acuity, ocular motility and stereopsis. right stable ocular dominance. FEMs are hypermetric, and the spatial relationship perception is abnormal and characterized by vertical anisotropy.

The cumulative reading rate for words, as assessed by the Reading Performance Test, localizes between the -1 and the -2 SD and improves in the presence of words when the spacing is enlarged to 0.47 deg. This value, considered as the critical spacing, is wider than normal as a result of the anisotropic shrinking of the visual space along the horizontal axis.

TETRA - Patient's Report for Reading Performance Test

Ver. 1.0.98 , Aleci, dicembre 2012

Name: ID: Date/Time:

Words - Grade 3

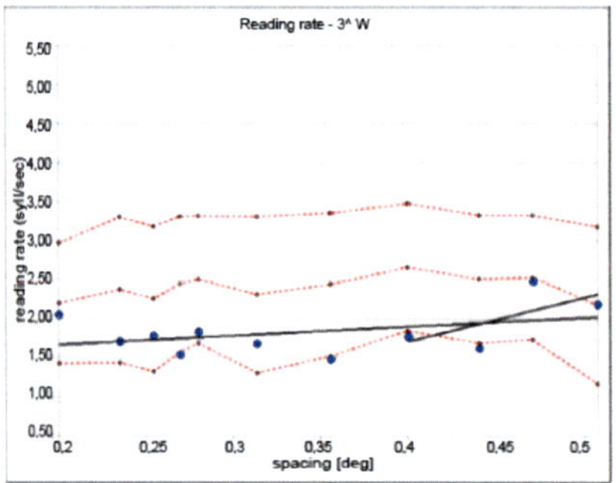

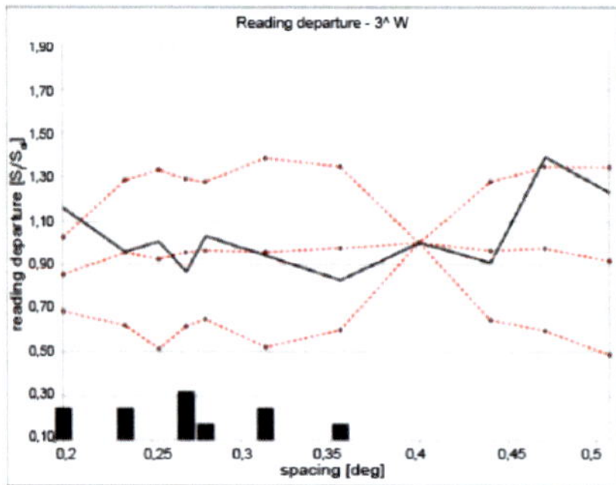

Spacing	**0.2°**	**0.23°**	**0.25°**	**0.27°**	**0.28°**	**0.31°**	**0.36°**	**0.4°**	**0.44°**	**0.47°**	**0.51°**
Reading Rate	2.06	1.71	1.79	1.54	1.84	1.68	1.48	1.78	1.62	2.48	2.19
R. Departure	1.16	0.96	1.01	0.87	1.03	0.94	0.83	1	0.91	1.39	1.23

CRR: 1.83 ± 0.3 syl/sec **Z-Score:** -1.65

CORRELATION **Total** **r:** 0.4 p =0.22

Spreading **r:** 0.66 (**s:** 5.63)

Lexical performance

Critical Spacing: 0.47°

Gain: 0.7 syl/sec at 0.47° 39.3%

Errors: 11

Visual perceptual alterations

No words - Grade 3

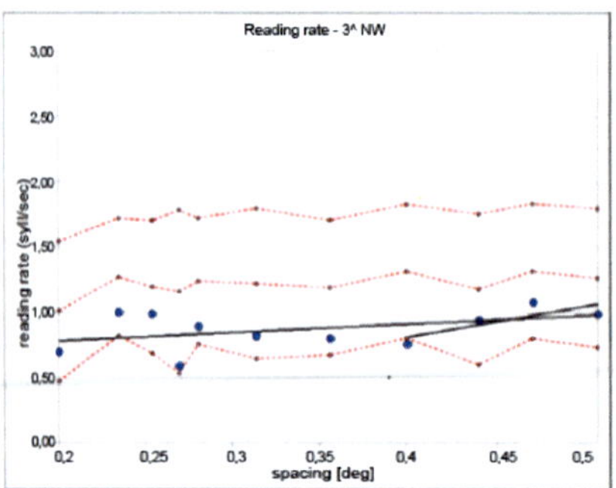

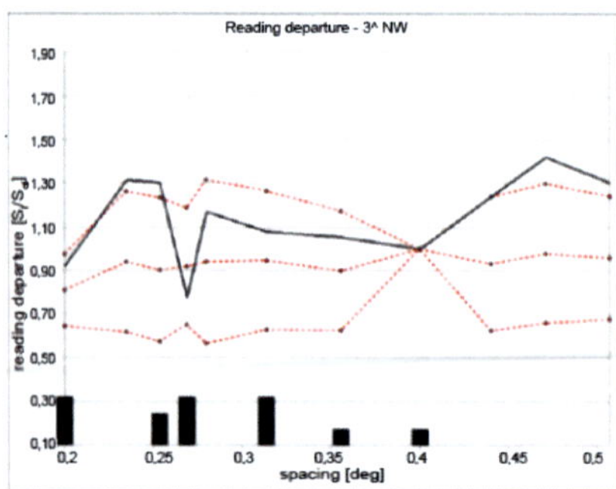

Spacing	**0.2°**	**0.23°**	**0.25°**	**0.27°**	**0.28°**	**0.31°**	**0.36°**	**0.4°**	**0.44°**	**0.47°**	**0.51°**
Reading Rate	0.7	1	0.99	0.59	0.89	0.82	0.8	0.76	0.94	1.08	0.99
R. Departure	0.92	1.32	1.3	0.78	1.17	1.08	1.05	1	1.24	1.42	1.3

CRR: 0.87 ± 0.15 syl/sec **Z-Score:** -1.65

CORRELATION **Total** **r:** 0.43 (p =0.2)

Spreading **r:** 0.8 (**s:** 2.34)

Lexical performance

Critical Spacing: nd

Gain: 0.32 syl/sec at 0.47° (42.1%)

Errors: 13

Visual perceptual alterations

Example 4- Vertical Anisotropy and Dominance Instability without Impairment of the Visuoperceptive Parameters as Assessed at the REPORT

Z.M.., female, age 11, 5th grade.

Developmental dyslexia and dysgraphia.

Good health, no allergies.

Visual acuity: 60/60 bilaterally. Orthophoria for close vision, normal fusional amplitude for close vision, normal stereopsis.

Normal saccadic movements.

Ocular dominance: unstable in right-hander.

Eidomorphometry: HT 9; VT: 5; SRA: 4.

REPORT:

Words: the Z-score, around -0.5 SD, means that the cumulative reading rate across the spectrum of anisotropization is within the normal range.

The critical spacing cannot be determined.

The correlation coefficient *Total r* is not significant (0.4, p=0.22), showing that the progressive widening of the interletter spacing from 0.2 to 0.51 degrees does not improve reading to a higher rate compared to normal readers. The *spreading r*, even if higher than the *total r* (0.65), is not clinically indicative so that *s*, even if considerable, is put in brackets (s= 5.52).

Nevertheless, as a result of the noticeable *s*-value, the widening of the interletter interval from 0.4 to 0.47 degrees tends to improve the reading rate by 0.75 syl/sec, i.e. 19% compared to the reference value.

The trial shows some reading errors.

In summary, when asked to read words, the child showed normal reading rate without visuoperceptive alterations: in fact the left indicator (reading performance) is green. When the left indicator is green, the right one is not visualized.

Non-words: the Z-score localizes between the -1 and -2 SD, meaning that cumulative reading rate across the spectrum of anisotropization is reduced. An outlier (red square) is detected at 0.23 deg and ruled out from the analysis.

The critical spacing is 0.31 deg, not wider compared to the normal age-matched population.

The correlation coefficient *Total r* (-0.63) *is negative and not statistically significant*, meaning that the progressive widening of the interletter spacing from 0.2 to 0.51 degrees does not improve (if anything worsens) the lexical performance when the child reads non-words.

Considering the range of spacing from 0.4 to 0.51 degrees, the correlation coefficient *Spreading r* is not significant, showing that the improvement of the reading rate in the subject is not greater than the improvement estimated in the age-matched normal population: the slope of the linear function (s= 1.15) is therefore put in brackets. It follows that the widening of the interletter interval would be of little avail for this patient: actually, the reading rate gain is expected to be no more than 0.11 syl/sec, that is to say less than 8% at 0.51 deg of spacing compared to the reference value.

The trial shows some reading errors.

In summary, when asked to read non-words, the child showed reduced reading rate without evident effect of her visuoperceptive alteration (revealed by the eidomorphometry) on the lexical function: in fact, the critical spacing is normal and the widening of the interletter distance is not influent on the reading rate. Thereby, the left indicator (reading performance) is yellow, whereas the right one (visuoperceptive impairment) is green.

Conclusion: normal visual acuity, ocular motility and stereopsis. Regular saccadic pattern with unstable ocular dominance and spatial relationship perception affected by vertical anisotropy.

The cumulative reading rate for words, as assessed by the Reading Performance Test, localizes within the normative range with words, whereas it looks to be fairly compromised with non-words. Although unstable dominance and imbalanced spatial relationship perception have been observed, this results do not seems to affect the visual lexical processing.

TETRA - Patient's Report for Reading Performance Test

Ver. 1.0.98 , Aleci, dicembre 2012

Name: ID: Date/Time:

Words - Grade 5

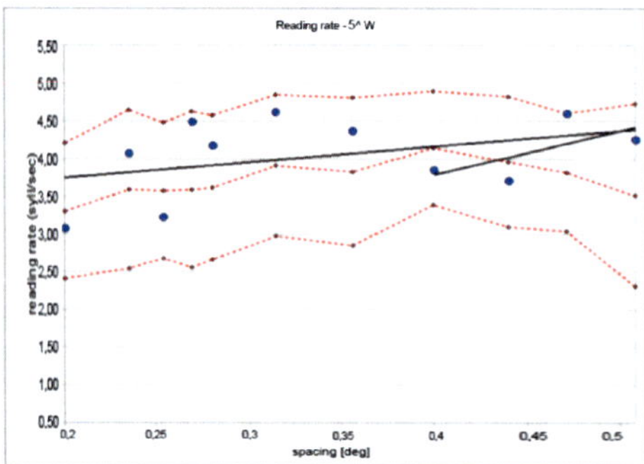

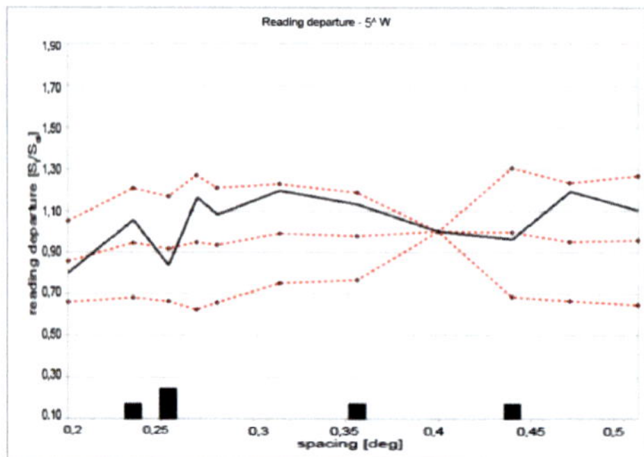

Spacing	0.2°	0.23°	0.25°	0.27°	0.28°	0.31°	0.36°	0.4°	0.44°	0.47°	0.51°
Reading Rate	3.08	4.07	3.23	4.49	4.17	4.62	4.37	3.85	3.71	4.6	4.26
R. Departure	0.8	1.06	0.84	1.17	1.08	1.2	1.14	1	0.96	1.19	1.11

CRR: 4.04 ± 0.52 syl/sec **Z-Score:** -0.65

CORRELATION **Total** **r:** 0.4 (p =0.22)
Spreading **r:** 0.65 **(s:** 5.71)

Lexical performance

Critical Spacing: nd

Gain: 0.75 syl/sec at 0.47° (19.5%)

Errors: 5

No words - Grade 5

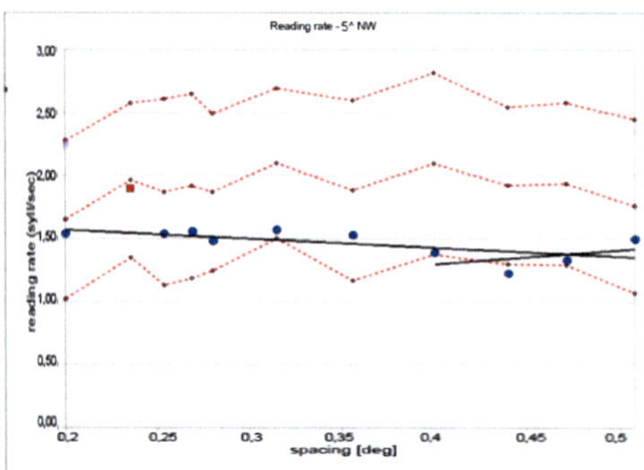

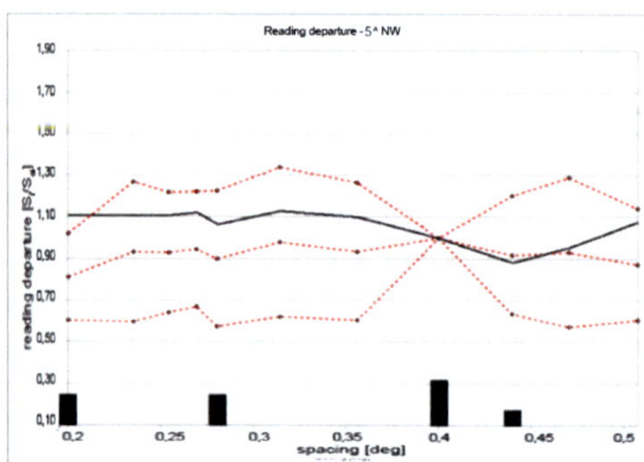

Spacing	0.2°	0.23°	0.25°	0.27°	0.28°	0.31°	0.36°	0.4°	0.44°	0.47°	0.51°
Reading Rate	1.54	1.9	1.54	1.56	1.48	1.57	1.53	1.39	1.23	1.33	1.5
R. Departure	1.11	1.37	1.11	1.12	1.06	1.13	1.1	1	0.88	0.96	1.08

CRR: 1.47 ± 0.11 syl/sec **Z-Score:** -1.66

CORRELATION **Total** **r:** -0.63 (p =0.05)
Spreading **r:** 0.47 **(s:** 1.15)

Lexical performance

Critical Spacing: 0.31°

Gain: 0.11 syl/sec at 0.51° (7.9%)

Errors: 8

Visual perceptual alterations

Example 5- Vertical Anisotropy, Unstable Dominance and Saccadic Hypermetria Affecting the Reading Performance

A.M, male, age 8, 3rd grade.

suspected dyslexia.

Good health, no allergies.

Visual acuity: 60/60 bilaterally. Slight esophoria for close vision, normal fusional amplitude for close vision, normal stereopsis.

Saccadic movements: hypermetric.

Ocular dominance: unstable in right-hander.

Eidomorphometry: HT 9; VT: 5; SRA: 4.

REPORT:

Words: the Z-score, approaching the -1SD, means that the cumulative reading rate across the spectrum of anisotropization is within the normative range, albeit mildly reduced compared to the average performance of age matched normal readers.

The critical spacing (0.4°) is at the limit of the normative range.

The correlation coefficient *Total r* is negligible (r= 0.01), meaning that the progressive widening of the interletter spacing from 0.1 to 0.51 degrees does not improve the lexical performance. An appreciable negative trend is quantified by the *spreading r* (-0.52) and the related slope (*s*= -11), suggesting an evident slow down of the reading rate as the interletter distance is increased starting from the reference value.

Although the critical spacing is not wider compared to the normative value, from 0.1 deg to the critical spacing a pronounced reading improvement can be observed. The correlation coefficient, computed a posterior by the technician, turned out to be highly significant (r= 0.84, p<0.008).

The trial shows some reading errors.

This is a case that requires particular consideration, in the light of the vertical anisotropy and of the saccadic hypermetria found in the child. Vertical anisotropy and fixation instability (this latter being the main consequence of unstable dominance), indeed, may be responsible for the significant increase of the reading rate up to 0.4 deg of spacing, while the evident worsening starting from this interval is expected to depend on the abnormal saccadic pattern.

The left indicator is green. Even if the right indicator is not visualized, this particular example suggests that even in cases of slight reading disabilities a visuoperceptive impairment cannot be ruled out.

Non-words: the Z-score localizes between the -1 and -2 SD, meaning that cumulative reading rate across the spectrum of anisotropization is reduced. Due to the artifactual component, as suggested by the high variability of the trend, it is not advisable to make further considerations.

Conclusion: normal visual acuity, ocular motility and stereopsis. The saccadic pattern is abnormal with unstable ocular dominance and spatial relationship perception affected by vertical anisotropy.

The cumulative reading rate for words, as assessed by the Reading Performance Test, even if slightly reduced compared to the average level of the age-matched normal readers, localizes within the normative range. However, a noticeable ameliorative trend is observed from the maximum shrinking level up to the reference value as a possible consequence of vertical anisotropy. A further worsening till to the maximum interletter spacing can depend on saccadic disarticulation.

TETRA - Patient's Report for Reading Performance Test
Ver. 1.0.98 . Aleci. dicembre 2012

Name: ID: Date/Time:

Words - Grade 3

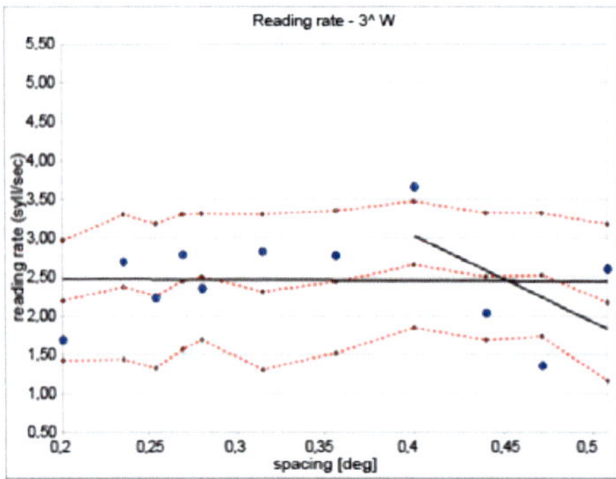

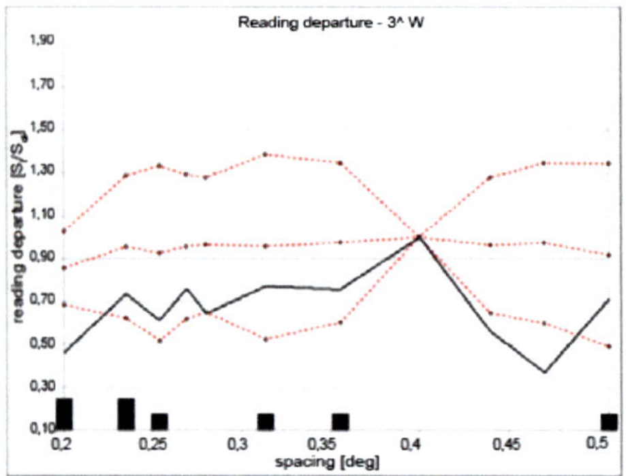

Spacing	0.2°	0.23°	0.25°	0.27°	0.28°	0.31°	0.36°	0.4°	0.44°	0.47°	0.51°
Reading Rate	1.69	2.7	2.24	2.79	2.36	2.83	2.78	3.66	2.05	1.36	2.61
R. Departure	0.46	0.74	0.61	0.76	0.64	0.77	0.76	1	0.56	0.37	0.71

CRR: 2.46 ± 0.62 syl/sec **Z-Score:** -0.93

CORRELATION **Total** **r:** -0.01 (p =0.97)
Spreading **r:** -0.52 (**s:** -11.01)

Lexical performance

Critical Spacing: 0.4°
Gain: 0
Errors: 8

No words - Grade 3

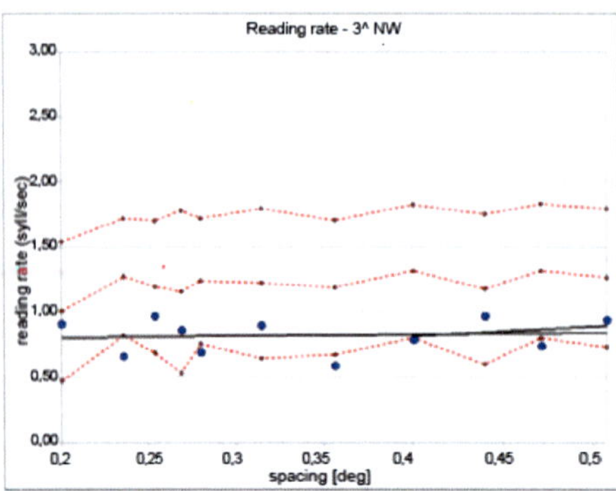

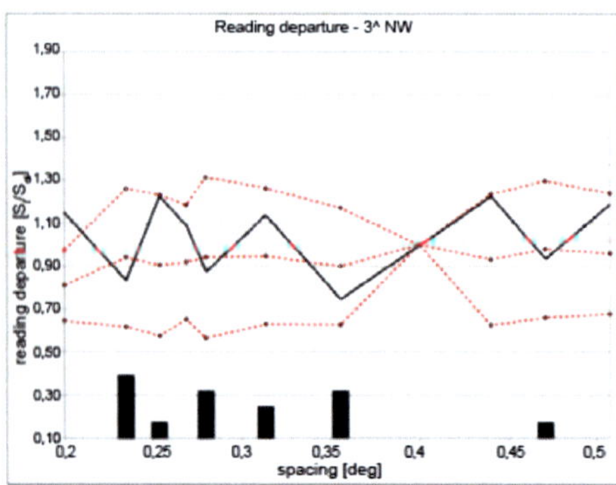

Spacing	0.2°	0.23°	0.25°	0.27°	0.28°	0.31°	0.36°	0.4°	0.44°	0.47°	0.51°
Reading Rate	0.91	0.66	0.97	0.86	0.69	0.9	0.59	0.79	0.97	0.74	0.94
R. Departure	1.15	0.84	1.23	1.09	0.87	1.14	0.75	1	1.23	0.94	1.19

CRR: 0.82 ± 0.13 syl/sec **Z-Score:** -1.74

CORRELATION **Total** **r:** 0.1 (p =0.79)
Spreading **r:** 0.29 (**s:** 0.72)

Lexical performance

Critical Spacing: 0.44°
Gain: 0.18 syl/sec at 0.44° 22.8%
Errors: 14

Visual perceptual alterations

Example 6- Hemianopic Dyslexia

LSM, male, age 36.

Neuro-ophthalmological assessment required after two surgical treatments for left temporal astrocytoma.

Absence of ophthalmological alterations

Visual acuity: 60/60 bilaterally.

The visual field within 30 and 12 degrees from the fixation point shows as follows:

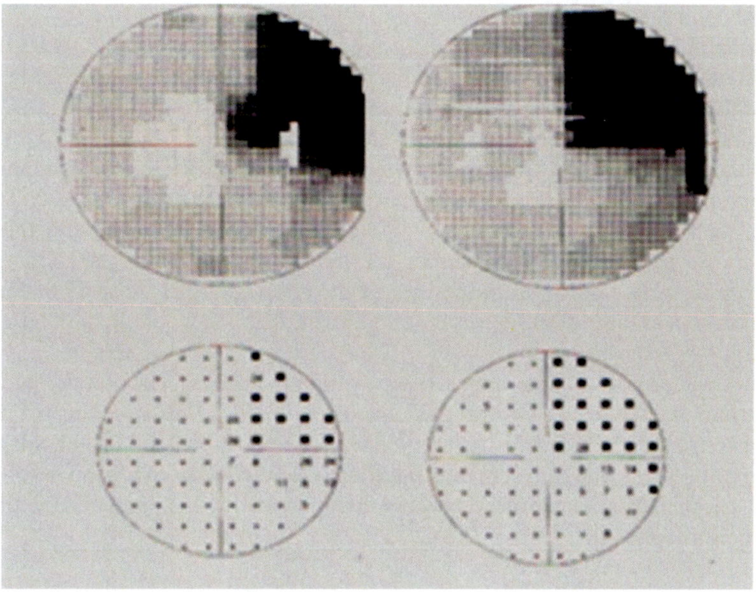

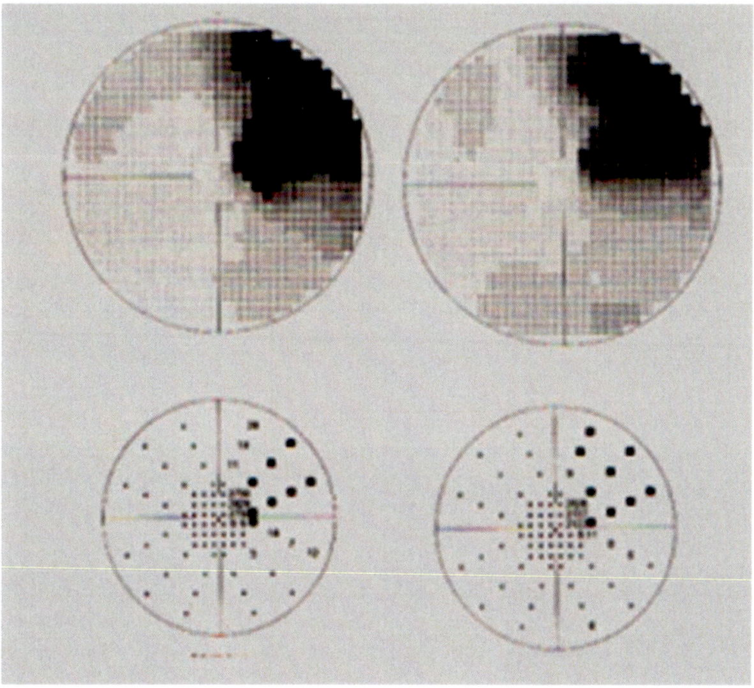

Saccadic movements: hypermetric.
Ocular dominance: unstable in right-hander.
Eidomorphometry: HT 6; VT: 3; SRA: 3.
REPORT:

The reading rate of 2.82 syl/sec for words, corresponds to a Z-score close to the -2 SD[431]; the reading rate of 2.41 syl/sec for non-words corresponds to a Z-score not higher (contrary to what expected) than the mean performance in 5th grade schoolchildren. This estimates mean that the cumulative reading rate across the spectrum of anisotropization is reduced in both experimental conditions, but mainly for words.

A considerable worsening trend, quantified by the *Total r* (words: -0.69, p=0.02; non-words: r= -0.66, p=0.03) is common to both experimental conditions, suggesting a remarkable reduction of the lexical performance as the interletter distance is increased.

This is the crucial finding, irrespective of the other indexes.

The explanation of this peculiar trend relies on the visual field loss, involving the right side of the fixation point. As can be seen in the previous figure, the sensitivity of a consistent portion of the right parafoveal region is lost and just a little portion adjoining the fixation point is available for the parafoveal processing of the syllables. Therefore, the defect prevents the patient from a suitable parafoveal processing of the letters, so that more FEMs are required to read the word. In addition, in this case the impairment is made worse by the defective saccadic pattern.

The final outcome is overall longer reading time with the horizontal anisotropization that hampers further the lexical task. On the one hand, in fact, the widening of the interletter distance shifts farther the adjoining letters liable to be pre-processed by the spared portion of parafovea; on the other hand, it demands additional (and defective) saccades for the letter-by-letter analysis, since this is the only way to compensate for the loss of effectiveness of the parafoveal pre-processing[432].

Conclusion: normal visual acuity ocular motility and stereopsis in right superior quadrantanopia. The saccadic pattern is abnormal with unstable ocular dominance. Spatial relationship perception is spared.

A consistent worsening of the lexical performance is observed from the maximum shrinking level up to the maximum interletter spacing. The effect may depend on the joint effect of impaired parafoveal pre-processing and saccadic perturbation.

In this case the narrowing of the interletter distance in the reading material could improve the lexical function.

---

[431] Z-score computed from 5th grade normative data.

[432] To be noted that the right indicator is green. Actually, the Reading Performance Test has been conceived for developmental dyslexics and not for hemianopes. In dislexics, indeed, the detection of the visuoperceptive impairment relies mainly on the improvement of the reading rate with the widening of the interletter distance as well as on the enlargement of the critical spacing. As a matter of fact, these are not the traits proper to hemianopes.

TETRA - Patient's Report for Reading Performance Test
Ver. 1.0.98 , Aleci, dicembre 2012

Name: ID: Date/Time:

Words - Grade 5

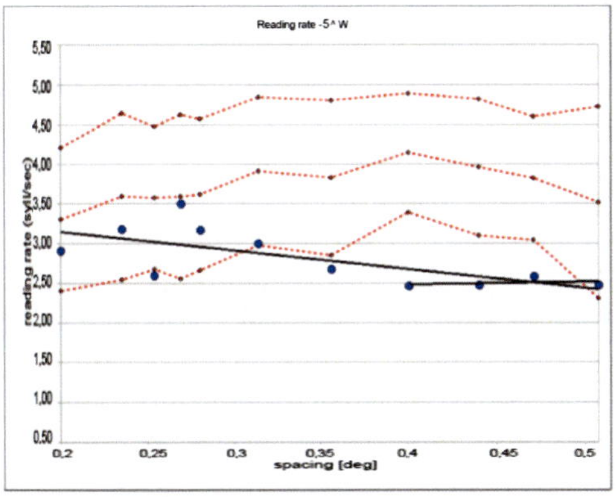

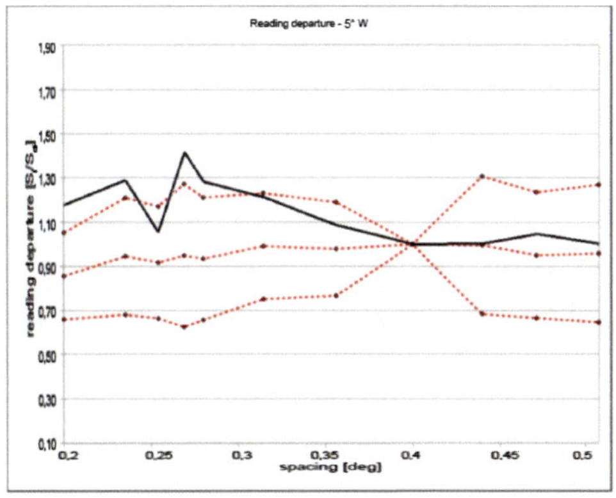

Spacing	0.2°	0.23°	0.25°	0.27°	0.28°	0.31°	0.36°	0.4°	0.44°	0.47°	0.51°
Reading Rate	2.91	3.18	2.6	3.5	3.17	3	2.68	2.47	2.48	2.59	2.48
R. Departure	1.18	1.29	1.05	1.42	1.28	1.21	1.09	1	1	1.05	1

CRR: 2.82 ± 0.35 syl/sec **Z-Score:** -1.95

CORRELATION **Total** **r:** -0.69 (p =0.02)
Spreading **r:** 0.3 (**s:** 0.37)

Lexical performance

Critical Spacing: nd

Gain: 0.12 syl/sec at 0.47° (4.9%)

Errors: 0

Visual perceptual alterations

No words - Grade 5

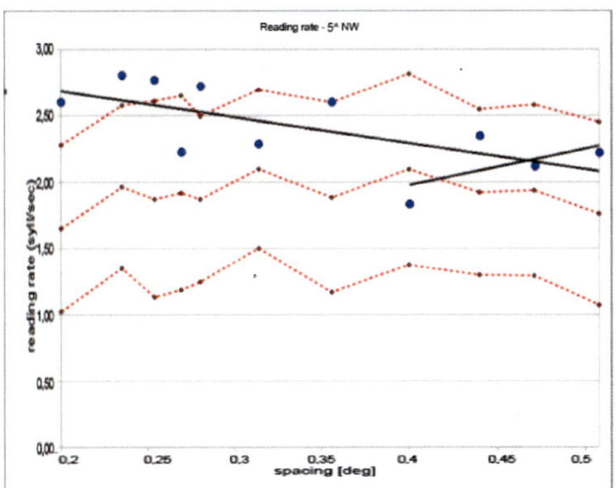

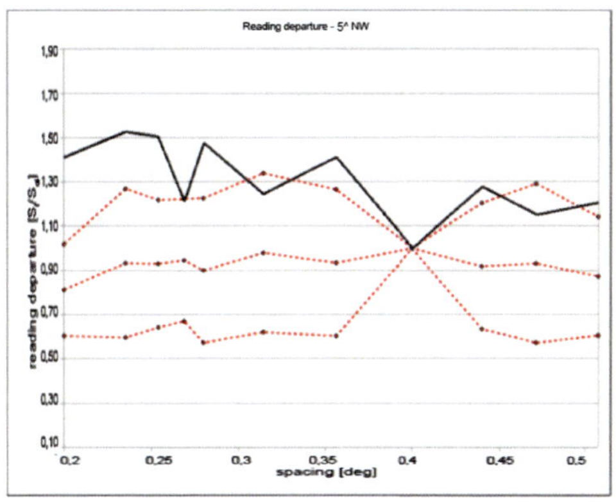

Spacing	0.2°	0.23°	0.25°	0.27°	0.28°	0.31°	0.36°	0.4°	0.44°	0.47°	0.51°
Reading Rate	2.6	2.81	2.77	2.23	2.72	2.29	2.6	1.84	2.35	2.12	2.22
R. Departure	1.41	1.53	1.51	1.21	1.48	1.24	1.41	1	1.28	1.15	1.21

CRR: 2.41 ± 0.31 syl/sec **Z-Score:** -0.25

CORRELATION **Total** **r:** -0.66 (p =0.03)
Spreading **r:** 0.58 (**s:** 2.73)

Lexical performance

Critical Spacing: 0.23°

Gain: 0.51 syl/sec at 0.44° (27.7%)

Errors: 0

Example 7- Unreliable Examination (Artifactual)

M.G, male, age 9, 4th grade.

Dyslexia and dyscalculia.

Visual acuity: 60/60 bilaterally. Exophoria for close vision, normal fusional amplitude for close vision, normal stereopsis.

Saccadic movements: hypometric with compensatory movements of the head.

Ocular dominance: unstable, right in right-hander.

Eidomorphometry: HT 1; VT: 4; SRA: -3.

REPORT:

> Both for words and non-words, the Z-score localizes between the -1 and -2 SD, meaning that cumulative reading rate across the spectrum of anisotropization is reduced. Due to the artifactual component (especially for words) as suggested by the high variability of the trend, it is not advisable to make further considerations.

TETRA - Patient's Report for Reading Performance Test
Ver. 1.0.98 . Aleci, dicembre 2012

Name: ID: Date/Time:

Words - Grade 4

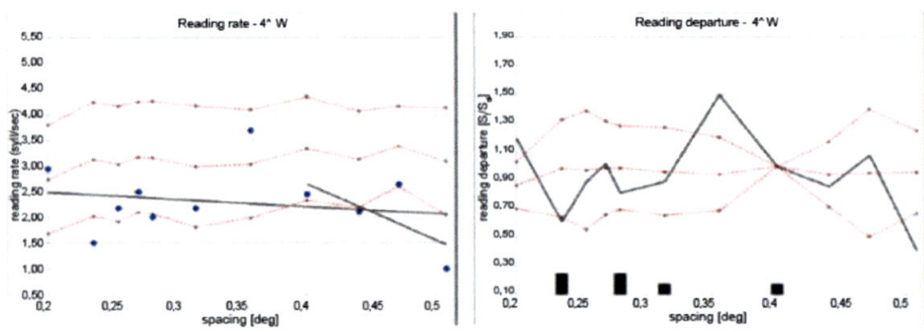

Spacing	0.2°	0.23°	0.25°	0.27°	0.28°	0.31°	0.36°	0.4°	0.44°	0.47°	0.51°
Reading Rate	2.95	1.5	2.19	2.51	2.01	2.19	3.7	2.46	2.11	2.66	1
R. Departure	1.2	0.61	0.89	1.02	0.82	0.89	1.5	1	0.86	1.08	0.41

CRR: 2.3 ± 0.71 syl/sec **Z-Score:** -1.78

CORRELATION **Total** r: -0.2 (p =0.57) **Spreading** r: -0.68 (s: -10.98)

Critical Spacing: 0.36°
Gain: 0.2 syl/sec at 0.47° (8.1%)
Errors: 6

Lexical performance

Visual perceptual alterations

No words - Grade 4

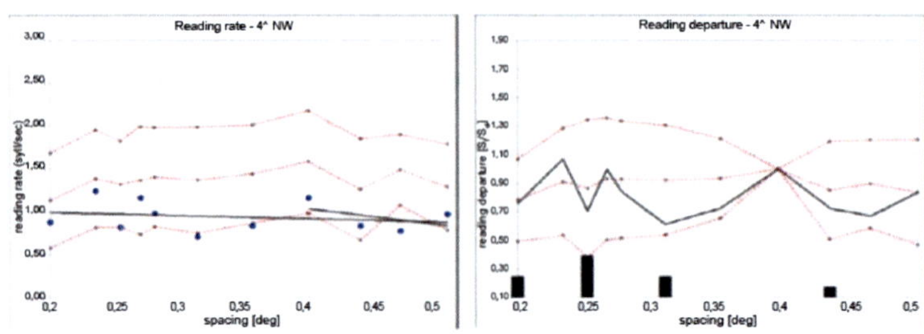

Spacing	0.2°	0.23°	0.25°	0.27°	0.28°	0.31°	0.36°	0.4°	0.44°	0.47°	0.51°
Reading Rate	0.88	1.24	0.82	1.16	0.98	0.71	0.84	1.16	0.84	0.78	0.97
R. Departure	0.76	1.07	0.71	1	0.84	0.61	0.72	1	0.72	0.67	0.84

CRR: 0.94 ± 0.17 syl/sec **Z-Score:** -1.77

CORRELATION **Total** r: -0.22 (p =0.53) **Spreading** r: -0.5 (s: -1.83)

Critical Spacing: nd
Gain: 0
Errors: 9

Lexical performance

Visual perceptual alterations

Appendix E: REPORT - Normative Data and Trend Analysis

A representative sample of the scholar population of 3rd, 4th and 5th grade living in urban and rural areas has been selected. Exclusion criteria were dyslexia, neuropsychiatric or phonological problems, amblyopia, strabismus, visual acuity <50/60 and ophthalmological pathologies. Even if not diagnosed as dyslexics, children whose reading rate was below the second standard deviation, as reported in the operational definition of developmental dyslexia, were excluded.

The standard deviation of the average cumulative reading rate (CRR) has been estimated in each of the three populations. Children whose CRR standard deviation was beyond the second SD calculated on the respective population were considered unreliable and excluded.

In order to allows the comparison of trends irrespective of the absolute lexical level, the values obtained were transformed according to the function:

$$S_{normalized} = S_x / S_{rif\,(0.4)}$$

For each interval of spacing Sx, $S_{normalized}$ deviates from the unit as a function of the discrepancy between the reading rate at Sx and the reading rate at the reference interletter spacing (0.4 deg); in this way a value <1 indicates a worse performance at Sx than at the reference spacing, while a ratio > 1 refers to a better result.

The error bars in the figures refer to the confidence interval (95%).

1a - Reading Rate for Words in the 3rd Grade Population

The graph below depicts the reading rate of words as a function of the anisotropization of the string in the sample of 3rd grade.

The analysis of variance shows significant differences in reading speed as a function of the spacing (ANOVA for repeated measures: $F = 2.01$, $p = 0.03$). In particular, the reading rate is higher at 0.4 degrees compared to 0.2 (Tukey-Kramer [$q = 4.61$]: $q = 5.55$, $p < 0.01$). In addition, a decremental gradient from the reference value toward wider spacing intervals can be observed.

The graph below shows the trend of the reading rate deviation (*departure*) compared to the reference interval (0.4°).

The statistical analysis on the deviation of the reading performance compared to the reference value (*departure*) confirms the effect of the spacing widening on the reading rate (ANOVA for repeated measures: $F = 1.91$, $p = 0.04$). In particular, compared to 0.2 deg, CRR is higher at the reference value of 0.4 deg (Tukey-Kramer [$q = 4.61$]: $q = 5.23$, $p < 0.05$) and at the limit of the statistical significance at 0.36 degrees and at 0.47 degrees (Tukey-Kramer $q = 4.32$ and 4.47 respectively).

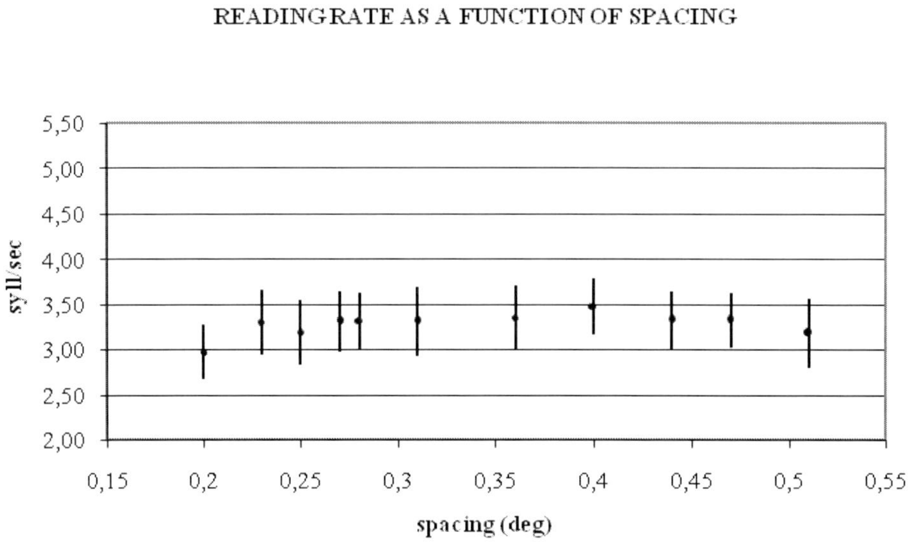

Figure 1.

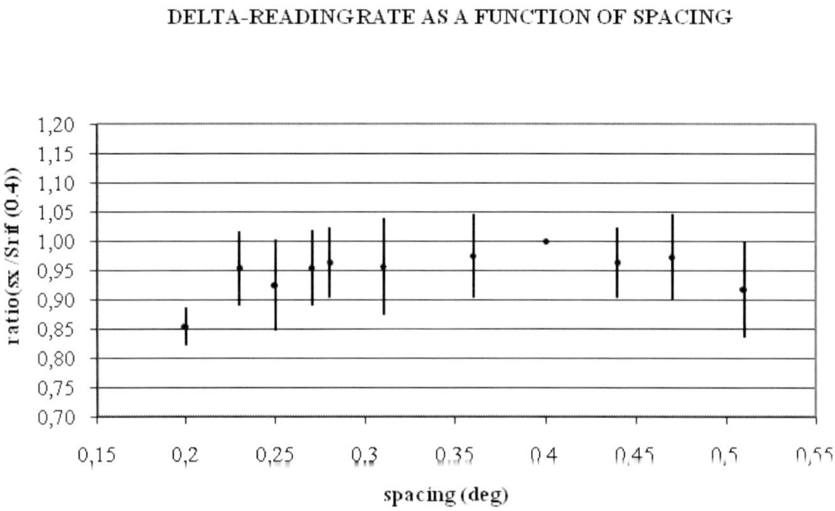

Figure 2.

From the reference value, the reduction of the reading rate with the increase of the spacing remains evident.

As a consequence of this non-monotonic behavior, the linear regression analysis performed on the previous data[433] does not show a statistically significant trend referred to the reading rate across the whole spectrum of anisotropization (i.e. of interletter spacing) considered.

Instead, from the reference interval, the reading rate as a function of the interletter spacing shows a significant worsening ($r = -0.94$, $p = 0.03$) (table I).

[433] Departure.

Table I.

	Linear regression (0.2-0.51°)	*Linear regression (0.4-0.51°)*
r	0.37	-0.94
r^2	0.13	0.93
slope	0.45	-2.5
p	0.25	0.03

Therefore, it can be concluded that reading rate tends to increase with the widening of the inter letter spacing from 0.2 to 0.4 degrees. An expansion of the spacing from 0.4 to 0.51 degrees causes a statistically significant reversal of the trend, with a reduction of the reading rate.

If the critical spacing when reading were assumed to corresponds to the inter letter distance at which the lexical performance ends up raising and stabilizes, from the data reported in this sample, it can be deduced that in the 3rd grade schoolchildren for words it extends up to 0.4 degrees.

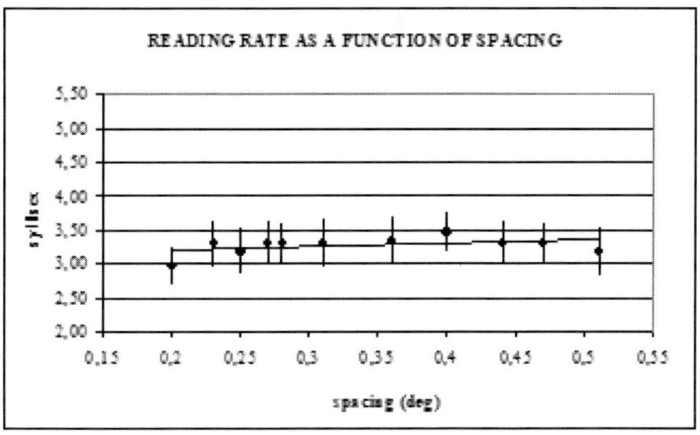

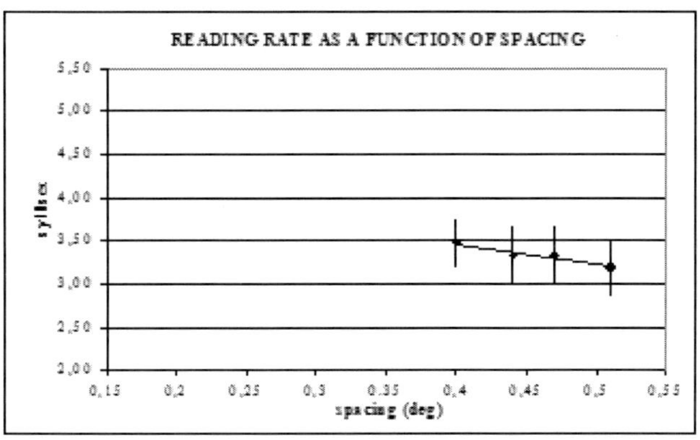

Figure 3.

2a- Reading Rate for Words in the 4rt Grade Population

The graph below represents the reading rate of words as a function of the anisotropization of the string in the sample of 4th grade.

READINGRATE AS A FUNCTION OF SPACING

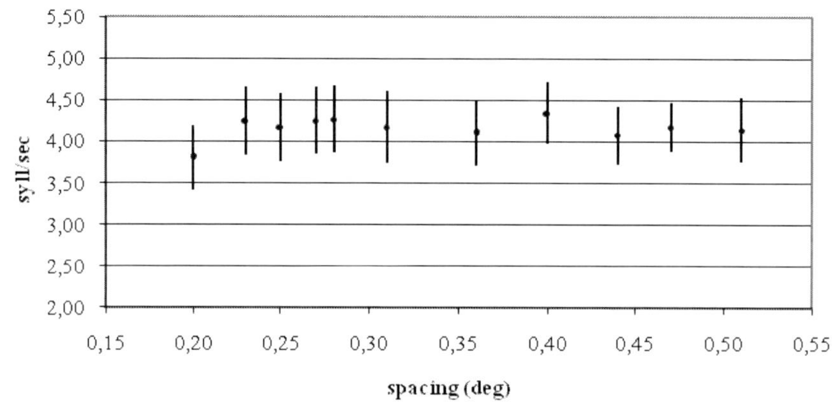

Figure 4.

Although the analysis of variance does not show significant differences in reading rate as a function of the spacing (ANOVA: $F = 0.50$, $p = 0.88$), the performance tends to improve from 0.2 to 0.23 degrees, then remains unchanged up to the reference spacing.

The graph below shows the trend of deviation (*departure*) of the reading rate as a function of the interval of reference for each interletter spacing.

DELTA-READINGRATE AS A FUNCTION OF SPACING

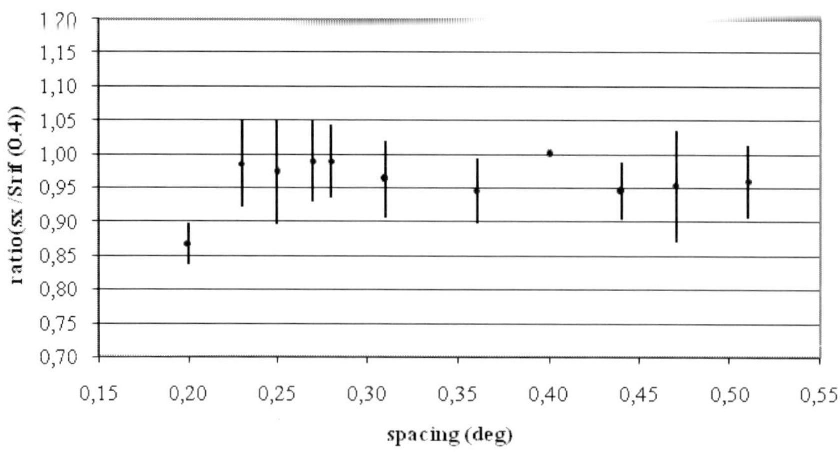

Figure 5.

The statistical analysis on the deviation of the reading performance compared to the reference value (*departure*), shows a ameliorative effect of the spacing widening on the reading rate (ANOVA for repeated measures: $F = 1.91$, $p = 0.04$): in particular, the improvement is significant when the spacing is widened from 0.2 to 0.27, 0.28 and 0.4 degrees (Tukey-Kramer [$q = 4.60$]: $q = 4.67$, $p < 0.05$, $q = 4.65$, $p < 0.05$, $q = 5.05$, $p < 0.05$ respectively).

As depicted from the table and the graphs below, the change of the reading rate as a function of the spacing across the spectrum of anisotropization does not follow a significant linear model.

Similarly to what is found in the sample of the third grade, starting from the reference spacing the increased anisotropization along the horizontal axis tends to worsen the reading performance, even if the trend is not statistically significant ($r = -0.60$, $p = 0.39$) (Table II).

Table II.

	Linear regression (0.2-0.51°)	*Linear regression (0.4-0.51°)*
r	0.17	-0.60
r^2	0.03	0.36
slope	0.23	-1.5
p	0.60	0.39

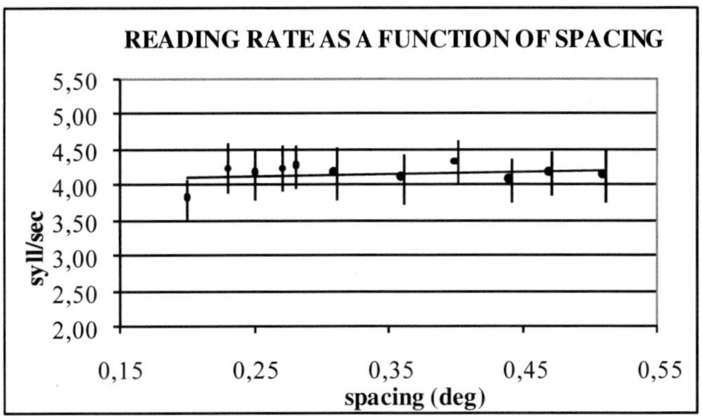

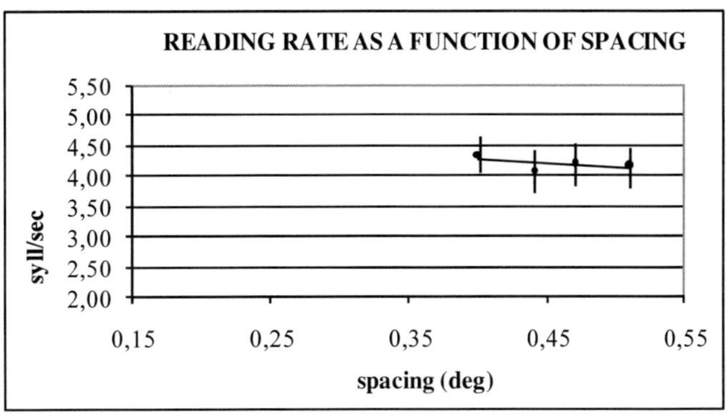

Figure 6.

Since the reading rate tends to improve with the widening of the inter letter distance from 0.2 to 0.23 deg, becoming significant at 0.27 deg, and then a plateau up to 0.4 degrees takes place, it can be deduced that for words in the fourth grade schoolchildren the critical spacing is narrower compared to the corresponding population of third grade and extends up to 0.27 degrees.

A further widening of the interletter distance from 0.4 to 0.51 degrees determines a reversed trend (even if not statistically significant) with reduced reading rate.

3a- Reading Rate for Words in the 5th Grade Population

The graph below represents the reading rate of words as a function of the anisotropization of the string in the sample of the 5th grade.

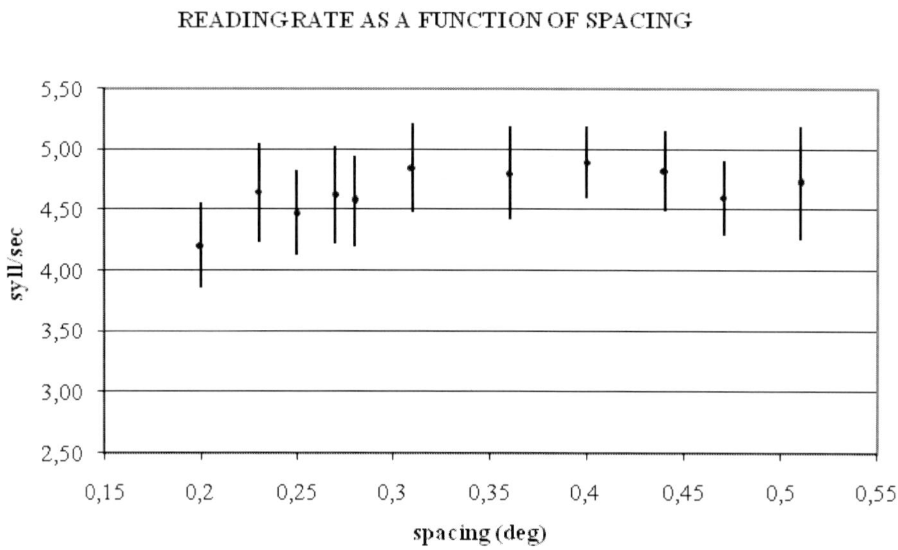

Figure 7.

In this case the analysis of variance shows a significant reading rate variation as a function of spacing (ANOVA for repeated measures: F = 3.29, p = 0.0005): in particular reading rate increase is significant from 0.2 to 0.31, 0.36, 0.4, 0.44 and 0.51 degrees (Tukey-Kramer [q = 4.61]: q = 5.86, p <0.01, q = 5.49, p <0.01, q = 6.30, p <0.001, q = 5.64, p <0.01, q = 4.72, p <0.05 respectively).

The graph below shows the trend of the reading rate deviation (departure) in reading rate compared to the reference interval (0.4°).

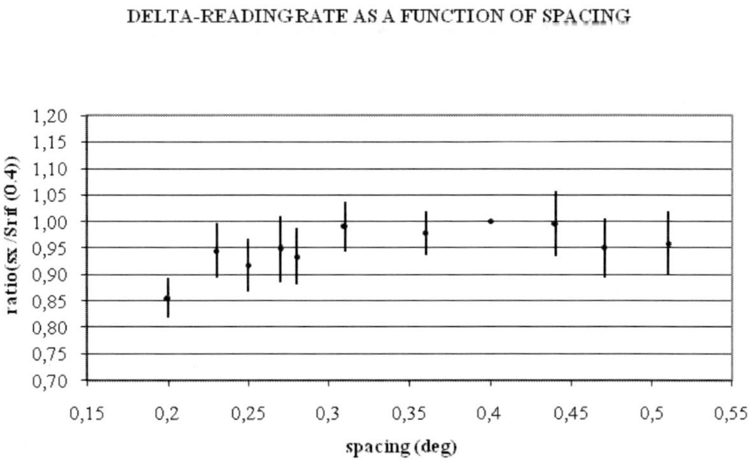

Figure 8.

The statistical analysis on the variation of the reading performance compared to the reference value shows that the effect of the interletter spacing on the reading rate is extremely significant (ANOVA for repeated measures: $F = 3.17$, $p = 0.0008$): in particular, compared to 0.2 deg, the improvement at 0.31, 0.36, 0.4 and 0.44 deg is confirmed (Tukey-Kramer [$q = 4.61$]: $q = 5.79$, $p < 0.01$, $q = 5.21$, $p < 0.05$, $q = 6.16$, $p < 0.01$, $q = 5.98$, p <0:01 respectively).

As shown from the table and graphs below, the linear regression analysis shows a ameliorative, quasi-significant trend of the reading rate across the spectrum of anisotropization. Similarly to what is found in the sample of the 3rd and the 4th grade, starting from the reference value the interletter widening leads to a worsening in the reading rate, even if not statistically significant ($r = -0.71$, $p = 0.28$).

In conclusion, the widening of the inter letter spacing increases the reading rate, which becomes statistically significant at 0.31 degrees. A further anisotropization does not produce any additional ameliorative effect.

Therefore, in the 5th grade schoolchildren the critical spacing for words is 0.31 degrees and is thereby lower than the critical spacing estimated in the population of the third grade, and similar to that of the population of the fourth grade.

As in the previous two cases, a widening the spacing from 0.4 to 0.51 degrees reverses the trend.

Table III.

	Linear regression (0.2-0.51°)	*Linear regression (0.4-0.51°)*
r	0.58	-0.71
r^2	0.34	0.51
slope	1.1	-1.9
p	0.06	0.28

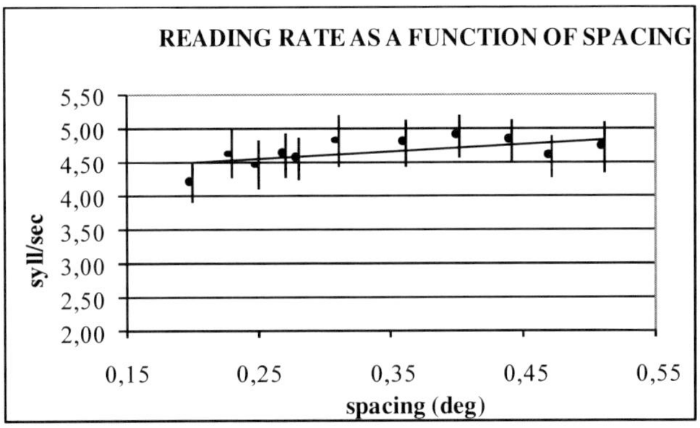

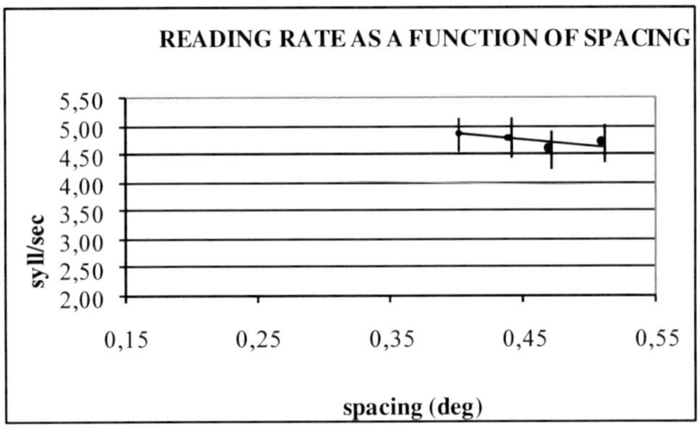

Figure 9.

1b- Reading Rate for Non-words in the 3rd Grade Population

The graph below represents the reading speed of non-words as a function of the anisotropization of the string in the sample of 3rd grade.

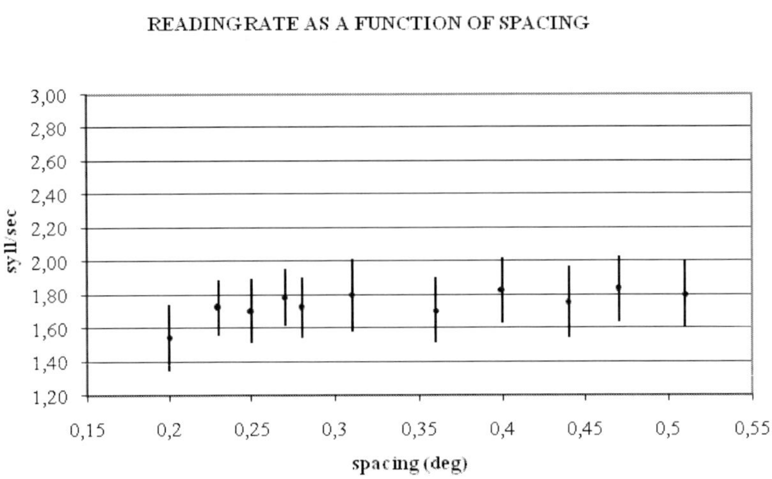

Figure 10.

The analysis of variance does not show significant differences in reading rate as a function of the spacing (ANOVA: F = 0.62, p = 0.78). Examining the scattergram, however, it can be noted that the improvement of the performance with the increase of the spacing reaches a plateau around 0.23 degrees.

The graph below shows the trend of the reading rate deviation (*departure*) compared to the reference interval (0.4°).

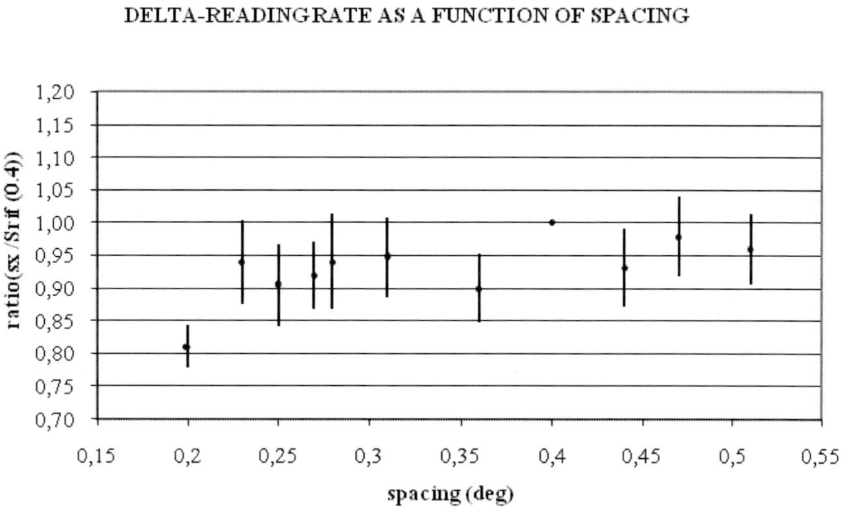

Figure 11.

Yet, the statistical analysis on the variation of the reading performance compared to the reference value reveals a significant effect of spacing (ANOVA: F = 3.04, p = 0.001): in particular, compared to 0.2 degrees, reading rate increases at 0.31, 0.4, 0.47 and 0.51 degrees (Tukey-Kramer [q = 4.60]: q [0.2-0.31] = 4.80, p <0.05, q [0.2-0.4] = 6.67, p <0.001, q [0.2-0.47] = 5.93, p <0.01, q [0.2-0.51] = 5.26, p <0.05 respectively).

As shown in the table and graphs below, the change of the reading rate as a function of the spacing across the spectrum of anisotropization does not follow a significant linear model.

Similarly to words, even for non-words increasing the interletter spacing from the reference value does not show any ameliorative effect (r = -0.12, p = 0.87).

Table IV.

	Linear regresson (0.2-0.51°)	*Linear regression (0.4-0.51°)*
r	0.68	-0.12
r^2	0.46	0.01
slope	0.54	-0.1
p	0.06	0.87

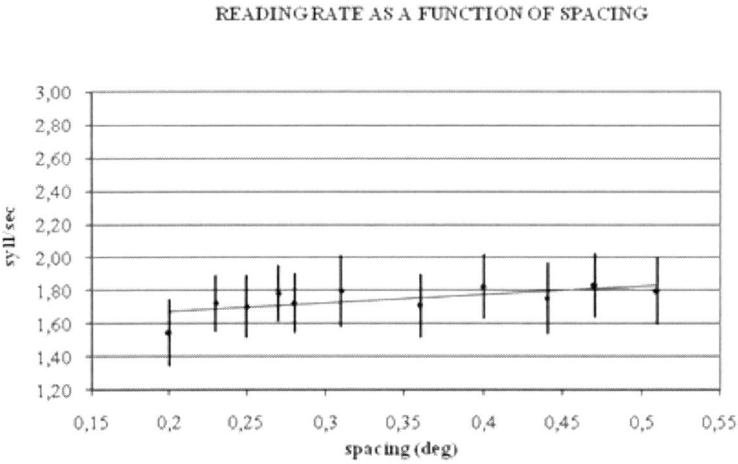

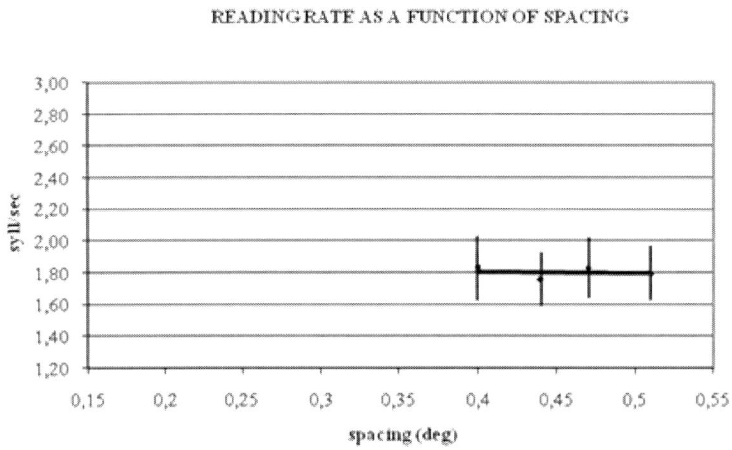

Figure 12.

In conclusion, the widening of the inter letter spacing from 0.2 to 0.31 degrees leads to a statistically significant increase of the reading rate, then the trend stabilizes. Since a further anisotropization does not produce any additional ameliorative effect, in the case of non-words the critical spacing in the 3rd grade schoolchildren seems to localize around 0.31 degrees. This is an interval unexpectedly lower compared to that found with words (0.4°).

However, examining the scattergram, a further improvement of the reading rate from 0.31 to 0.4 degrees is conjecturable. This improvement, even if not significant, looks to be consistent as its amount is up to 36% of the improvement observed in the transition from 0.2 to 0.31 degrees.

Therefore, waiting for a larger normative sample, the cutoff of 0.31° as critical spacing has been considered as a bias and even for non-words the critical spacing is supposed to be 0.4°. In fact, enlarging the interletter distance beyond 0.4 degrees does not allow any further reading rate improvement.

2b- Reading Rate for Non-words in the 4th Grade Population

The graph below represents the reading rate of non-words as a function of the anisotropization of the string in the sample of 4th grade.

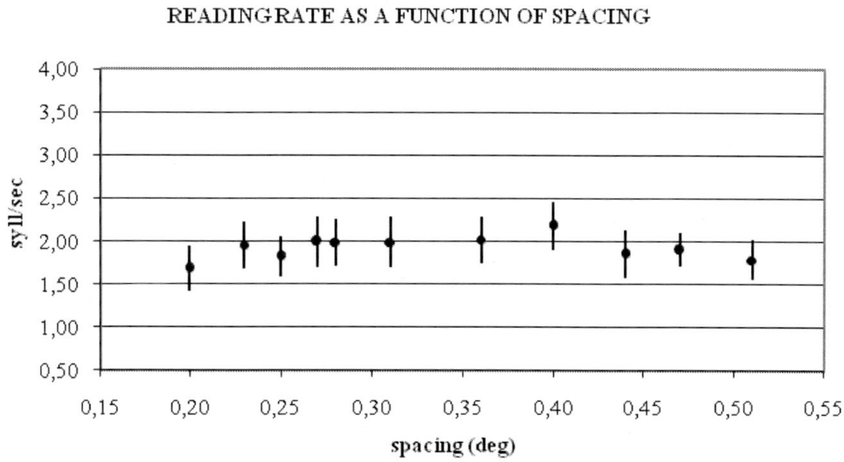

Figure 13.

Significant differences are found in the reading rate as a function of the spacing of the alphabetic symbols (ANOVA for repeated measures: $F = 2.93$, $p = 0.002$): in particular the reference spacing performance (0.4 degrees) is greater compared to both that of maximum shrinking (Tukey-Kramer [$q = 4.63$]: q [0.2-0.4] = 6.36, $p < 0.001$) and, at the opposite side of the spectrum, that of maximum dilation (q [0.4-0.51] = 5.01, $p < 0.05$). Differences at the limit of significance are found at 0.2 vs. 0.36 ($q = 4.26$), 0.25 vs. 0.4 ($q = 4.56$) and between 0.4 vs. 0.44 ($q = 4.19$).

The graph below shows the trend of the reading rate deviation (*departure*) compared to the reference interval (0.4°).

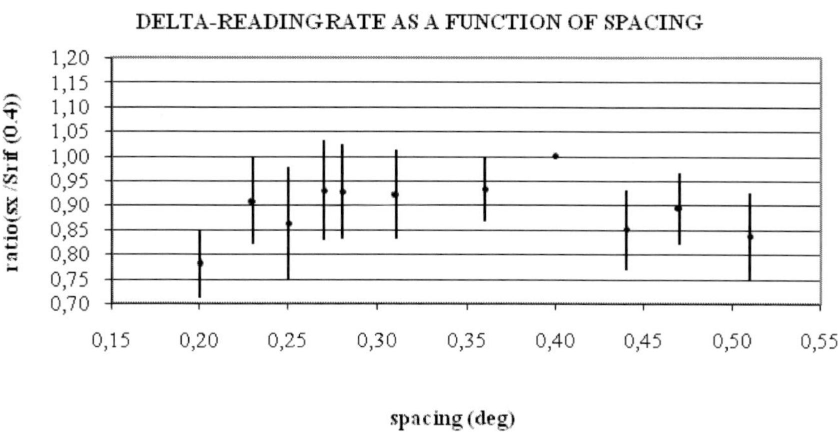

Figure 14.

The statistical analysis on the variation of the reading performance compared to the reference value reveals a significant effect of spacing (ANOVA for repeated measures: $F = 2.72$, $p = 0.004$): in particular, the increase of the reading rate from 0.2 to 0.4 degrees turns out to be significant (Tukey-Kramer [$q = 4.63$]: $q = 6.13$, $p < 0.01$).

The reduction of the reading rate from 0.4° to the value of maximum dilation is at the limit of the significance ($q = 4.49$).

As shown from the table and graphs below, the change of the reading rate as a function of the spacing across the spectrum of anisotropization does not follow a significant linear model.

Similarly to what was found in the previous cases, the increase of the spatial relationships along the horizontal axis from the reference value shows a worsening trend, even if not statistically significant ($r = -0.85$, $p = 0.14$).

Table V.

	Linear Regression (0.2-0.51°)	*Linear Regression (0.4-0.51°)*
r	0.1	-0.85
r^2	0.01	0.73
slope	0.13	-3.2
p	0.76	0.14

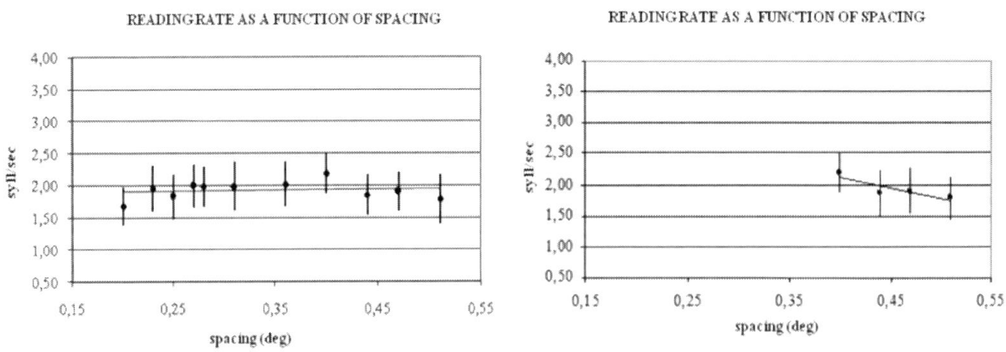

Figure 15.

In summary, by widening the interletter spacing from 0.2 to 0.4 degrees, an increase of the reading rate takes place. In the 4th grade schoolchildren population, the critical spacing for non-words is larger than for words and extends up to 0.4 degrees.

The enlargement of the interletter distance beyond 0.4 degrees tends to reverse the trend.

3b- Reading Rate for Non-Words in the 5th Grade Population

The graph below represents the reading rate of non-words as a function of the anisotropization of the string in the sample of 5th grade.

The analysis of variance shows significant differences in reading rate as a function of the spacing (ANOVA for repeated measures: $F = 4.24$, $p = 0.0001$); in particular, the reading rate increase is significant from 0.2 to 0.25, 0.27, 0.31, 0.36 and 0.4 degrees (Tukey-Kramer [q =

4.60]: q = 4.92, p <0.05, q = 5.53, p <0.01, q = 6.19, p <0.001, q = 4.75, p <0.05, q = 8.22, p <0.01, q = 4.72, p <0.05, respectively). In addition, reading rate increases when the interletter spacing is widened from 0.28 to 0.4 degrees (q = 4.81, p <0.05) and decreases from 0.4 to 0.51 degrees (q = 5.47, p <0.01).

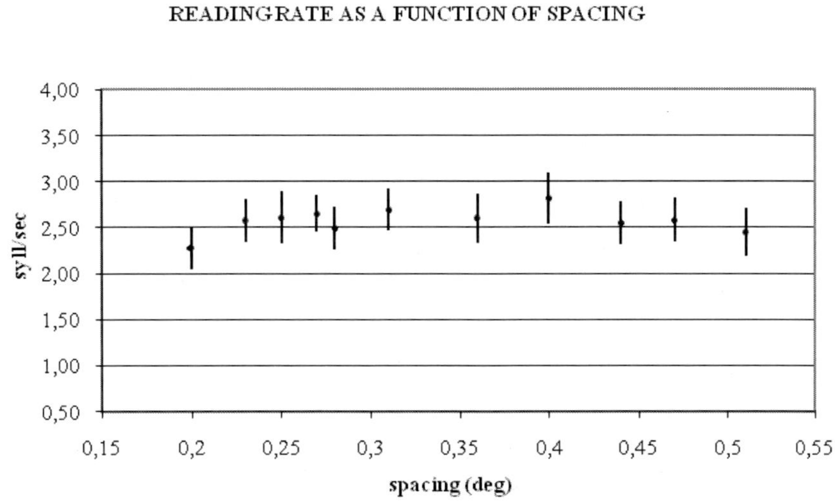

Figure 16.

The graph below shows the trend of the reading rate deviation (*departure*) compared to the reference interval (0.4°).

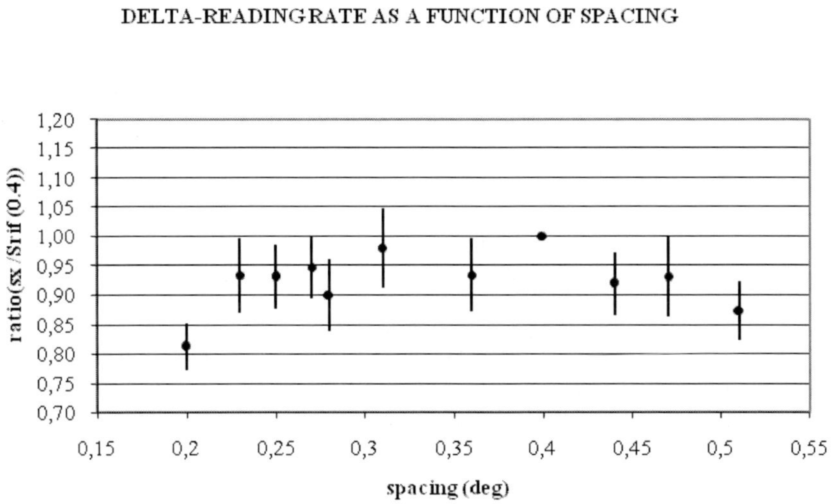

Figure 17.

The statistical analysis on the deviation of the reading performance from the reference value confirms a significant effect of the spacing on the reading rate (ANOVA for repeated measures: F = 4.18 p = 0.0001): in particular the increase of the reading rate is significant from 0.2 to 0.23, 0.25, 0.27, 0.31, 0.36, 0.4 and 0.47 degrees (Tukey-Kramer [q = 4.60]: q =

4.92, $p < 0.05$, $q = 4.82$, $p < 0.05$, $q = 5.46$, $p < 0.01$, $q = 6.81$, $p < 0.001$, $q = 4.95$, $p < 0.05$ $q = 7.63$, $p < 0.001$, $q = 4.91$, $p < 0.05$ respectively). The significant reading rate increases from 0.28 to 0.4 degrees found in the non-normalized data, in this case localizes at the limits of the statistical significance ($q = 4.04$).

Moreover, the reading rate reduction from 0.4 to 0.51 degrees is confirmed ($q = 5.13$, $p < 0.05$).

As shown from the table and graphs below, the change of the reading rate as a function of the spacing across the spectrum of anisotropization does not follow a significant linear model.

In agreement with the analysis of variance, the increase of the spatial relationships along the horizontal axis from the reference value shows a worsening trend, even if not statistically significant ($r = -0.90$, $p = 0.09$).

Table VI.

	Linear Regression (0.2-0.51°)	*Linear Regression (0.4-0.51°)*
r	0.17	-0.90
r^2	0.03	0.82
slope	0.23	-3.1
p	0.6	0.09

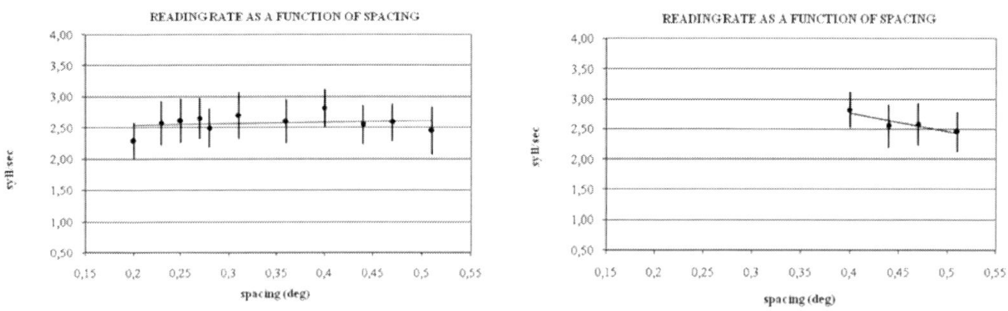

Figure 18.

In conclusion, with the increase of the inter letter distance starting from the minimum value of spacing considered an increase of the reading rate can be observed from 0.2 to 0.28°, followed by a further significant increase till to the reference value (0.4°).

It can be deduced that in the 5th grade schoolchildren population the critical spacing for non-words is larger than for words and extends up to 0.4 degrees.

A further expansion from 0.4 to 0.51 degrees reverses the reading rate trend.

The summary of the critical spacing and the slope of the reading rate-related linear model referred to the two regression analyses in the three classes of age, for both words and non-words, is reported in the table below[434].

The lexical function considered in terms of reading rate is therefore affected by the inter letter distance in school-age children, both in the presence of words and in the case of the experimental administration of non-words.

[434] Computed on the non-normalized data.

Based on the findings reported in literature, it can be assumed that the reading improvement with the increase of the interval between characters is related to the crowding effect, therefore, to the critical spacing.

We can therefore draw the following considerations:

Table VII.

Class	Critical Spacing (deg)	Gradient 0.2→0.51 (slope)	Gradient 0.4→0.51 (r) (slope)
III grade- words	0.4	0.45	-2.5
IV grade-words	0.27	0.23	-1.5
V grade- words	0.31	1.1	-1.9
III grade- non-words	(0.4)	0.54	-0.1
IV grade- non-words	0.4	0.13	-3.2
V grade- non-words	0.4	0.23	-3.1

1. in the presence of words, the critical spacing in younger children (third grade) extends up to 0.4 degrees. In more developed children (fifth and fourth grade) it decreases at 0.31 to 0.27 degrees. The narrower lateral masking in the more developed individuals is in line with the age-related crowding reduction reported in literature (see Appendix B).
2. in the experimental condition of non-words, in which the lexical material is free from linguistic content, the critical spacing is wider compared to words, that is to say 0.4 degrees irrespective of the age of the sample. The equivalence of the result for words and non-words in the 3rd grade children should mean that during the early lexical acquisition the linguistic content does not have a substantial ameliorative effect on the lexical task, in accordance with the adoption of the sublexical strategy. On the contrary in older children, who start to use the lexical route and can rely also on the linguistic content, the critical spacing tends to be narrower for words.

In an Italian study, the lexical performance (expressed as vocal reaction time) has been measured in a group of normal readers (average age: 12.4 years) for words made up of letters with spacing from 0.24 to 0.59 degrees[435]. No significant differences were found up to 0.41 degrees, while a further enlargement to 0.59 degrees led to the decrease of the lexical performance. It is interesting to consider how the absence of an ameliorative trend with the widening of the interletter spacing in normal readers found in this investigation is in agreement with the linear regression analysis reported in normal readers (average age: 9.1 ± 2 years) in a personal study[436] and is confirmed by the reported normative data obtained by means of the Reading Performance Test in the pupils of 3rd, 4th, and 5th grade.

Our findings suggest that in normal subjects the increase of the inter letter distance beyond 0.4 degrees tends to degrade the lexical function.

---

[435] Spinelli D, De Luca M, Judica A, Zoccolotti P. (2002). Crowding effects on word identification in developmental dyslexia. Cortex, 38: 179-200.

[436] Aleci C, Piana G, Piccoli M, Bertolini M. (2012). Developmental dyslexia and spatial relationship perception. Cortex, 48: 466-476. See chapter 3 in this section.

Index

C

E

F

G

H

I

J

K

L

M

N

O

P

Q

R

S

T

U

V

W